BLEACHING TECHNIQUES IN RESTORATIVE DENTISTRY

This book is dedicated to the memory of Dr Edward Greenwall (1901–1990) and Dr Joe Greenwall (1896–1990). These brothers pioneered dentistry as a profession in our family under great hardship and sacrifice.

It is dedicated to my father Dr Ryno Greenwall, in dental practice since 1956, for his constant support and guidance through my life and my professional career.

It is also dedicated to my husband, Henry, and our sons, Andrew, Joseph and Edward, for their encouragement, love and friendship.

Who is wise? He who learns from every man; as it is said, from all my teachers I grew wise.

(Psalms 119:99)

BLEACHING TECHNIQUES IN RESTORATIVE DENTISTRY

An Illustrated Guide

Edited by

Linda Greenwall, BDS, MGDSRCS, MRDRCS, MSc, FGDP
Private practice, London, UK

With contributions from

George A Freedman, DDS, FFACD
Associate Director, Esthetic Dentistry Education Center
SUNY at Buffalo, USA, and private practice, Toronto, Canada

Valeria V Gordan, DDS, MS
Operative Dentistry, University of Florida, Gainesville, USA

Van B Haywood DDS
Oral Rehabilitation, University of Georgia, Augusta, USA

Martin Kelleher BDS, MSc, FDS
Consultant Dentist, King's College School of Dentistry
and private practice, London, UK

Gerald McLaughlin DDS
SUNY at Stony Brook, USA

Ilan Rotstein DDS
Endodontics, Hadassah Faculty of Dental Medicine
Hebrew University, Jerusalem, Israel

MARTIN DUNITZ

© 2001 Martin Dunitz Ltd, a member of the Taylor & Francis group

Although every effort has been made to ensure that all owners of copyright material
have been acknowledged in this publication, we would be glad to acknowledge in
subsequent reprints or editions any omissions brought to our attention.

First published in the United Kingdom in 2001
by Martin Dunitz Ltd, The Livery House, 7–9 Pratt Street, London NW1 0AE

Although every effort has been made to ensure that drug doses and other information
are presented accurately in this publication, the ultimate responsibility rests with the
prescribing physician. Neither the publishers nor the authors can be held responsible
for errors or for any consequences arising from the use of information contained
herein. For detailed prescribing information or instructions on the use of any product
or procedure discussed herein, please consult the prescribing information or
instructional material issued by the manufacturer.

A CIP record for this book is available from the British Library.

ISBN 1-85317-772-5

Distributed in the United States and Canada by:
Thieme New York
333 7th Avenue
New York, NY 10001
USA
Tel. 212 760 0888

Composition by Scribe Design, Gillingham, Kent, UK
Printed and bound in Singapore by Kyodo

CONTENTS

FOREWORD *Van B Haywood*   vi

PREFACE   vii

ACKNOWLEDGEMENTS   viii

1 Discoloration of teeth   1

2 A brief history of tooth bleaching   24

3 The bleaching materials   31

4 Treatment planning for successful bleaching   61

5 The home bleaching technique   88

6 Home bleaching trays: how to make them   116

7 Power bleaching and in-office techniques   132
George A Freedman, Gerald McLaughlin and Linda Greenwall

8 Intracoronal bleaching of non-vital teeth   159
Ilan Rotstein

9 Combining bleaching techniques   173

10 Bleaching and the microabrasion technique   193

11 Integrating bleaching with restorative dentistry   205

12 Combining bleaching with direct composite resin restorations   224
Valeria V Gordan

13 Safety issues   244
Martin Kelleher

14 Marketing   250

Appendix I Legal considerations relating to dental bleaching in Europe and the UK   255
Martin Kelleher

Appendix II Home bleaching instruction and consent form   259

Index   263

FOREWORD

Should we bleach people's teeth or not? That still seems to be a question in the minds of some dentists. While the profession has been bleaching teeth for over 100 years, there has never been such an interest in bleaching as now. That interest is partially related to the interconnection of the world through television, the aesthetic appearance of television announcers, actors and models, the impact of movies (in which even the bad guys have good-looking teeth), and the relatively affluent and fashion-conscious times in which we live. However, that interest is also due to the introduction about 10 years ago of the most simple, safe, efficient method for changing the colour of teeth, Nightguard Vital Bleaching or at-home bleaching with 10% carbamide peroxide in a custom-fitted tray. Because this technique can be offered by any dentist with minimal cost to the patient, all other types of bleaching are also enjoying a revival of interest.

Dentist-prescribed, home-applied bleaching has been cited by Dr Gordon Christensen as 'the most important behavior changing procedure available to dentists'. While there were early concerns for safety and efficacy, the evidence in double-blinded clinical and laboratory research as well as millions of patient treatments has addressed those concerns. Recently, the American Dental Association published its conclusion that 'the preponderance of scientific evidence currently available in the literature supports the safety of the ADA-accepted home-use and dentist-prescribed tooth-bleaching products when properly applied and monitored'.

Then should we bleach teeth? Absolutely YES! Not only is there an aesthetic gain for the patient at minimal risk and cost, but this procedure preserves tooth structure and simplifies restorative procedures for the dentist as well. Research has shown that the color of dentine is being changed which offers conservative treatment options for tetracycline-stained teeth as well as other intrinsic stains. I applaud Dr Linda Greenwall for striving to publicize further the current knowledge about bleaching. I pray that patients will not continue to be subjected to needless crowns or veneers, or be embarrassed with discolored teeth when bleaching could resolve their problem and improve their quality of life.

Van B Haywood
Professor, Department of Oral Rehabilitation
University of Georgia, USA

PREFACE

Everyone wants to have whiter teeth. Does that mean that we can provide bleaching treatments for every patient? Yes, well almost! There are a vast number of patients in dental practices who will be asking for these services. Dentists need to know the indications and contraindications and how to do these bleaching procedures.

Bleaching treatments are not new, and attempts to bleach teeth were even performed in the previous century. They involved the patient sitting for many hours in front of a heated bleaching lamp and the treatments were very costly and unpredictable. We now have bleaching techniques that are simple and more predictable.

The idea that teeth can be lightened and whitened in a simple way, by using a night-guard, was a pioneering discovery, which led to the publication of the first article by Haywood and Heymann in 1989. Since then the scope of bleaching treatment we have available to offer our patients has increased exponentially.

The amount of information that is now available on bleaching is vast and there has been a tremendous surge of clinical and in-vitro research on bleaching. There is still much research to be undertaken and there are many areas in bleaching where our clinical and academic knowledge is not evidence-based and what we use on an everyday basis is purely empirical. The dental companies have become involved in the bleaching market very quickly as they stand to gain financially from the patient demand for whiter teeth. There are many products on the market and this can be confusing to many dentists, especially in selecting materials to use for their patients and in selecting whitening toothpastes and other adjunctive products.

Bleaching treatments can be incorporated into all kinds of restorative dentistry and it is the purpose of this book to help dentists to success-fully incorporate the wide variety of bleaching treatments into their practices through the many sequences of illustrations: how to start the bleaching treatments, 'how-to-do-it', how to select the patients as well how as to inform dentists about the bleaching techniques. Although the book is meant for clinicians, both undergraduate and postgraduate, it can also be used to demonstrate to patients what is involved in the bleaching techniques and the type of results that can be achieved.

There are not many laboratory techniques used in the bleaching treatments; however, the making of the appropriate bleaching trays is essential and there is a special chapter on how to make and design these trays. This section can be used by laboratory technicians or for those dentists who wish to make trays at the chairside or teach their dental assistants to make them.

As dentists are very busy people, they may not have time to read the entire text in one go. The book is meant to be user-friendly so that it can be paged through or the relevant sections quickly scanned where necessary. There are sample forms of the kind that can be used in dental practice for patients. However, since the legal considerations are specific for each country, dentists wishing to provide bleaching services for their patients should be acquainted with their country's legal standing before undertaking any bleaching treatments.

There are many different names used for the bleaching treatments that are available. The terminology used in the book will be kept simple: different names will be mentioned in each chapter as appropriate and then the simplest, most descriptive term will be used.

I have included a list of references and further reading at the end of each chapter. I have tried to include as much of the research as possible, but where the research is lacking I have included other clinical references. I would value readers' comments and feedback, so please write to me, care of the publishers.

Linda Greenwall

ACKNOWLEDGEMENTS

It would not have been possible to write this book without the assistance of a considerable number of people. I would firstly like to acknowledge my patients who went through the bleaching procedures and treatments. Their comments and incidental findings have been helpful and honest and helped me collate the information in the book.

Unless otherwise stated, most of the illustrations, tables, photos and slides are my own. However, as we in the UK have been legally only allowed to bleach teeth comparatively recently, there may be a shortage of clinical cases presented. I am immensely grateful to Dr Ted Croll, Dr Dan Fischer, Dr Valeria Gordan, Dr Van B Haywood and Dr Martin Kelleher for the slides they have lent me to be included in the book.

I should like to thank Dr Colin Hall Dexter who allowed me to adapt his patient questionnaire and charting form for my practice and Dr Eddie Levin for giving me further insights into the golden proportion and his special golden proportion gauge.

Thanks go to my dental technicians, Mick Kedge and Cliff Quince from Kedge and Quince Laboratory, for the help and assistance they have given me over the years. The photos of the making of the bleaching trays are taken in their laboratory. Most of the laboratory work shown is theirs. I should also like to thank Keith Moore of Photocraft for taking the interior photographs in the dental surgery and treatment rooms.

I feel most indebted to the contributing authors, Dr George Freedman, Dr Valeria Gordan, Dr Martin Kelleher, Dr Gerald McLaughlin and Professor Ilan Rotstein–all experts in their fields–who have shared their unique expertise in the book. I should also like to acknowledge Professor Bernard G N Smith, who encouraged me to undertake original research into bleaching during my master's degree (1990–2), and Robert Peden of Martin Dunitz Publishers, who encouraged me to write this book and saw it through from an idea to final publication.

Finally, I wish to thank my dental staff in the practice for their continual support, encouragement and dedication to improving, building and striving for excellence in the dental practice. I would also like to thank my mother for encouraging me to open my own practice so that I could fulfil an ideal dream and for taking care of the babies while I was balancing building a busy practice with a young family.

Linda Greenwall

The publishers would like to acknowledge permission to use figures or text reprinted or adapted from other publications:

P. Abbott, Aesthetic considerations in endodontics: internal bleaching. *Pract Periodont Aesthetic Dent* (1997) **9**(7):833–40.

K. Eaton, K. Nathan, The MGDS examination: a systemic approach. 3. Part 2 of the examination: diagnosis, treatment planning, execution of treatment, maintenance and appraisal, writing-up log diaries, *Primary Dental Care* (1998) **5**:113–18.

T.S. Fasanaro, Bleaching teeth: history, chemicals and methods used for common tooth discolorations. *J Esth Dent* (1992) **4**:71–8.

P.A. Hayes, C. Full and J. Pinkham, The etiology and treatment of intrinsic discoloration, *J Canad Dent Assoc* (1986) **3**:217–20.

V.B. Haywood, History, safety and effectiveness of current bleaching techniques and application of the Nightguard Vital Bleaching technique, *Quintessence Int* (1992) **23**(7):471–88.

V.B. Haywood, Nightguard Vital Bleaching: current concepts and research. *J Am Dent Assoc* (1997) **128**(suppl):19–25.

M.G.D. Kelleher and F.J.C. Roe, The safety-in-use of 10% carbamide peroxide (Opalescence) for bleaching teeth under the supervision of a dentist. *Br Dent J* (1999) **187**(4):190–3.

R.H. Leonard, Efficacy, longevity, side effects and patient perceptions of Nightguard Vital Bleaching, *Compend Contin Educ Dent* (1998) **9**(8):766–81.

T.P. Van der Bengt, C. Eronat and A.J.M. Plasschaert, Staining patterns in teeth discolored by endodontic sealers, *J Endodont* (1986) **12**:187–91.

DISCOLORATION OF TEETH

INTRODUCTION

Tooth discoloration is a common problem. People of various ages may be affected, and it can occur in both primary and secondary teeth. The aetiology of dental discoloration is multifactorial, while different parts of the tooth can take up different stains. Extrinsic discoloration increases with increasing age and is more common in men (Eriksen and Nordbo 1978); it may affect 31% of men and 21% of women (Ness et al 1977). The result is a complex of physical and chemical interactions with the tooth surface. The aim of this chapter is to assess the aetiology of tooth discoloration and the mechanisms by which teeth stain.

COLOUR OF NATURAL HEALTHY TEETH

Teeth are polychromatic (Louka 1989). The colour varies among the gingival, incisal and cervical areas according to the thickness, reflectance of different colours and translucency in enamel and dentine (see Figure 1.2). The colour of healthy teeth is primarily determined by the dentine and is modified by:

- the colour of the enamel covering the crown
- the translucency of the enamel which varies with different degrees of calcification
- the thickness of the enamel which is greater at the occlusal/incisal edge of the tooth and thinner at the cervical third (Dayan et al 1983).

CLASSIFICATION OF DISCOLORATION

Many researchers classify staining as either **extrinsic** or **intrinsic** (Dayan et al 1983, Hayes et al 1986, Teo 1989). There is confusion

Table 1.1 Aetiology of tooth discoloration

Extrinsic stains
Plaque, chromogenenic bacteria, surface protein denaturation
Mouthwashes, e.g. chlorhexidine,
Beverages (tea, coffee, red wine, cola)
Foods (curry, cooking oils and fried foods, foods with colorings, berries, beetroot)
Dietary precipitate
Illness
Antibiotics (erythromycin, amoxicillins)
Iron supplements

Intrinsic stains
Pre-eruptive
Disease:
– Haematological diseases
– Liver diseases
– Diseases of enamel and dentine

Medication:
– Tetracycline stains
– Other antibiotics use
– Fluorosis stains

Post-eruptive
Trauma
Primary and secondary caries
Dental restorative materials
Ageing
Smoking
Chemicals
Some food stuffs (long-term use causes deeper intrinsic staining)
Minocycline
Functional and parafunctional changes

concerning the exact definitions of these terms. Feinman et al (1987) describes extrinsic discoloration as that occurring when an agent stains or damages the enamel surface of the teeth, and intrinsic staining as occurring when internal tooth structure is penetrated by a discolouring agent. According to his definitions, the terms staining and discoloration are used synonymously. However, extrinsic staining will be defined here as staining that can be easily removed by a normal prophylactic cleaning (Dayan et al 1983). Intrinsic staining is defined here as endogenous staining that has been incorporated into the tooth matrix and thus cannot be removed by prophylaxis.

Some discoloration is a combination of both types of staining and may be multifactorial. For example, nicotine staining on teeth is extrinsic staining which becomes intrinsic staining. The modified classification of Dzierkak (1991) and Hayes et al (1986) and Nathoo (1997) will be used as a guide.

STAINS DURING ODONTOGENESIS (PRE-ERUPTIVE)

These alter the development and appearance of the enamel and dentine on permanent teeth.

DEVELOPMENTALLY DEFECTIVE ENAMEL AND DENTINE

Defects of enamel development can be caused by, for example, amelogenesis imperfecta (Figure 1.3), dentinogenesis imperfecta (Figure 1.4) and enamel hypoplasia. The defects in enamel are either hypocalcific or hypoplastic (Rotstein 1998). Enamel hypocalcification is a distinct brownish or whitish area found on the buccal aspects of teeth (see Figure 1.5). The enamel is well formed and the surface is intact. Many of these white and brown discolorations can be removed with bleaching in combination with microabrasion (see Chapter 10). Enamel hypoplasia is developmentally defective

enamel. The surface of the tooth is defective and porous and may be readily discoloured by materials in the oral cavity. Depending on the severity and extent of the dysplasia, the enamel surface may be bleached with varying degrees of success.

FLUOROSIS

This staining is due to excessive fluoride uptake with the developing enamel layers. The fluoride source can be from the ingestion of excessive fluoride in the drinking water or from overuse of fluoride tablets or fluoride toothpastes (Shannon 1978). It occurs within the superficial enamel, and appears as white or brown patches of irregular shape and form (Figure 1.7). The acquisition of stain, however, is post-eruptive. The teeth are not discoloured on eruption, but as the surface is porous they gradually absorb the coloured chemicals present in the oral cavity (Rotstein 1998). Staining due to fluorosis manifests in three different ways: as simple fluorosis, opaque fluorosis, or fluorosis with pitting (Nathoo and Gaffar 1995). Simple fluorosis appears as brown pigmentation on a smooth enamel surface, while opaque fluorosis appears as grey or white flecks on the tooth surface. Fluorosis with pitting occurs as defects in the enamel surface and the colour appears to be darker (Figure 1.7B).

Stannous fluoride treatment causes discoloration by reactions of the tooth with the tin ion (Shannon 1978). No intraoral discolorations occur from topical use of fluoride at low concentrations. The severity and degree of staining are directly related to the amount of fluoride ingested during odontogenesis.

TETRACYCLINE

Tetracycline is a broad-spectrum bacteriostatic antibiotic (van der Bijl and Ptitgoi-Aron 1995) which is used to treat a variety of infections. The tetracycline antibiotics are a group of related compounds that are effective against Gram negative and Gram positive bacteria. It is well known that the administration of tetracycline during odontogenesis causes unsightly discoloration of both primary and secondary dentitions. The discoloration varies according to the type of tetracycline used (see Table 1.2). The staining effects are a result of chelation of the tetracycline molecule with calcium ions in hydroxyapatite crystals, primarily in the dentine (Swift 1988). The tetracycline is incorporated into the enamel and dentine. The chelated molecule arrives at the mineralizing predentine–dentine junction via the terminal capillaries of the dental pulp (Patel et al 1998). The brown discoloration is due to photooxidation, which occurs on exposure of the tooth to light.

The staining can be classified according to the developmental stage, banding and colour (Jordan and Boksman 1984):

- **First degree** (mild tetracycline staining) is yellow to grey, which is uniformly spread through the tooth. There is no banding (see Figure 1.8).
- **Second degree** (moderate staining) is yellow-brown to dark grey (see Figure 1.9).
- **Third degree** (severe staining) is blue-grey or black and is accompanied by significant banding across the tooth (see Figures 1.10 and 1.11).
- **Fourth degree** (intractable staining) has been suggested by Feinman et al (1987), designated for those stains that are so dark that bleaching is ineffective (see Figure 1.12).

All degrees of stain become more intense on chronic exposure to artificial light and sunlight. The severity of pigmentation depends on three factors: time and duration of administration, the type of tetracycline administered, and the dosage (Shearer 1991, Dayan et al 1983).

First and second degree staining are normally amenable to bleaching treatments (Haywood 1997). Prolonged home bleaching has been reported in the literature to be successful for tetracycline cases. This may take between three and six months or longer (see Figure 1.13). The bleaching material penetrates into the dentine structure of the

Table 1.2 Tetracycline stains (adapted from Hayes et al 1986)

Drug	Colour stain on teeth
Chlortetracycline (Aureomycin)	Grey-brown
Demethylchlortetracycline (Ledermycin)	Yellow
Oxytetracycline (Terramycin)	Yellow – least amount
Tetracycline (Achromycin)	Yellow
Doxycycline (Vibramycin)	No reported changes
Minocycline	Black

tooth and causes a permanent colour change in the dentine colour (McCaslin et al 1999).

ILLNESS AND TRAUMA DURING TOOTH FORMATION

The effects of illness, trauma and medication (e.g. porphyria, infant jaundice, vitamin deficiency, phenylketonuria, haematological anaemia) cumulative effect creating stains and defects, which cannot be altered by bleaching. Staining may result from haematological disorders such as erythroblastosis foetalis (Atasu et al 1998), porphyria, phenylketonuria, haemolytic anaemic, sickle cell anaemia and thalassaemia. As the coagulation system is affected, discoloration occurs due to the presence of blood within the dentinal tubules (Nathoo 1997). Bilirubinaemia in patients with liver dysfunction can cause bilirubin pigmentation in deciduous teeth (Watanabe et al 1999).

STAINS AFTER ODONTOGENESIS (POSTERUPTIVE)

MINOCYCLINE

Minocycline is a semisynthetic second-generation tetracycline derivative (Goldstein 1998). It is a broad-spectrum antibiotic that is highly plasma bound and lipophilic (McKenna et al 1999). It is bacteriostatic and produces greater

Table 1.3 Tooth discoloration: causes and colours (from Abbott 1997, with permission)

Cause	Colour
Extrinsic discoloration	
Cigarettes, pipes, cigars, chewing tobacco	Yellow-brown to black
Marijuana	Dark brown to black rings
Coffee, tea, foods	Brown to black
Poor oral hygiene	Yellow or brown shades
Extrinsic and intrinsic discoloration	
Fluorosis	White, yellow, brown, grey, or black
Ageing	Yellow
Intrinsic discoloration	
Genetic conditions,	
e.g. amelogenesis imperfecta	Brown, black
Systemic conditions,	
e.g. jaundice	Blue-green or brown
porphyria	Purple-brown
Medications during tooth development,	
e.g. tetracycline, fluoride	Brown, grey or black
Body by-products,	
e.g. bilirubin	Blue-green, brown
haemoglobin	Grey, black
Pulp changes,	
e.g. pulp canal obliteration	Yellow
pulp necrosis	
– with haemorrhage	Grey, black
– without haemorrhage	Yellow, grey-brown
Iatrogenic causes,	
e.g. trauma during pulp extirpation	Grey, black
tissue remnants in pulp chamber	Brown, grey, black
restorative dental materials	Brown, grey, black
endodontic materials	Grey, black

antimicrobial activity than tetracycline or its analogues (Salman et al 1985). The drug is used to treat acne and various infections. Its lipophilicity facilitates penetration into body fluids, and after oral administration the minocycline concentration in saliva is 30 to 60% of the serum concentration (McKenna et al 1999). Minocycline is absorbed from the gastrointestinal tract and combines poorly with calcium.

Those adolescents and adults who take the drug are at risk from developing intrinsic staining on their teeth, gingivae, oral mucosa and bones (Bowles and Bokmeyer 1997). It causes tooth discoloration by chelating with iron to form insoluble complexes. It is also thought that the discoloration may be due to its forming a complex with secondary dentine (Salman et al 1985). The discoloration does not resolve after discontinuation of therapy.

The resultant staining is normally milder than that from tetracycline and may be amenable to bleaching and lightening, although it is case specific.

PULPAL CHANGES

Pulp necrosis

This can be the result of bacterial, mechanical or chemical irritation to the pulp. Substances can enter the dentinal tubules and cause the teeth to discolour. These teeth will require endodontic treatment prior to bleaching, the latter using the intracoronal method (see Chapter 8) or the outside/inside technique (see Chapter 9).

Intrapulpal haemorrhage due to trauma

Accidental injury to the tooth can cause pulpal and dentinal degenerative changes that alter the colour of the teeth (see Figure 1.14). Pulpal haemorrhage may occur giving the tooth a grey, non-vital appearance (Nathanson and Parra 1987). The discoloration is due to the haemorrhage, which causes lysis of red blood cells. Blood disintegration products such as iron sulphides enter the dentine tubules and discolour the surrounding dentine, which causes discoloration of the tooth (Baratieri et al 1995). Sometimes the tooth can recover from such an episode (Marin et al 1997) and the discoloration can reverse naturally without bleaching. These discoloured teeth should be vitality tested, because those that are still vital (see Chapter 4) can be successfully bleached using the home bleaching technique (see Chapter 5).

Dentine hypercalcification

This results when there is excessive irregular dentine in the pulp chamber and canal walls. There may be a temporary disruption in blood supply followed by the disruption of

odontoblasts (Rotstein 1998). Irregular dentine is laid down in the walls of the pulp chamber. There is a gradual decrease in the translucency of these teeth which results in a yellowish or yellow-brown discoloration. These teeth can be bleached with good results (see Chapter 9).

DENTAL CARIES

Dental caries (both primary and secondary) may confer a discoloured appearance) (Kleter 1998) occurring around areas of bacterial stagnation (see Figure 1.16), or leaking restorations. Arrested caries has a brown discoloration because the breakdown products react with decalcified dentine (Eriksen and Nordbo 1978) similar to the discoloration of the pellicle.

RESTORATIVE MATERIALS AND DENTAL PROCEDURES

Eugenol causes an orange-yellow stain. Endodontic materials (such as silver points) and pulpal remnants may cause a grey or pink appearance. Darkening of tooth crowns following root canal treatment has been attributed to the use of discoloring endodontic materials (see Figure 1.17) such as those containing silver as a constituent part of the endodontic sealer. A study by van der Burgt et al (1986a) showed that all endodontic sealers tested caused discoloration in the dentine while there was no penetration into the enamel. This discoloration is visible three weeks after application of the endodontic sealer (van der Burgt 1986b).

Silver amalgam may cause the tooth to take on a grey appearance due to the silver salts that get incorporated into the dentinal tubules. Discoloration in the tooth may be due to the physical presence of the amalgam, corrosion products or secondary caries (Kidd et al 1995) (see Figures 1.18–1.20). Colour change alone next to the margin of a restoration should not justify replacement (Kidd et al 1995). Leaking composite restoration can

---

Table 1.4 What are the mechanisms that cause non-vital teeth to discolor?

- Tissue degradation during the necrotic process (Baratieri 1995).
- Trauma causing rupture of blood vessels. This results in haemolysis of red blood cells, which release haemoglobin and haematin derivatives. Iron in red blood cells may be aspirated into dentinal tubules. This may also occur if there is uncontrolled haemorrhage during endodontic treatment.
- Intracanal medications such as phenolics and iodoform-based medications can cause gradual discoloration. The dentine is penetrated causing oxidation.
- Silver points may corrode inside the root canal.
- Coronally placed leaking restorative materials.
- Endodontic cement.
- Inadequate coronal access leaves pulp remnants and necrotic tissue in the pulp chamber.
- Contamination of the pulp cavity during endodontics.
- Insufficient irrigation and debridement.

Table 1.5 Discoloration caused by endodontic sealer (adapted from van der Burgt et al 1986a)

Endodontic sealer	Colour
Grossman's cement, zinc oxide eugenol, endomethasone and N2	Orange/red stain
Diaket, tubuli seal	Mild pink
AH26	Grey
Riebler's paste	Dark red stain

cause the tooth to appear more yellow (Kidd 1991). Several types of stain adjacent to tooth-coloured restorations are recognized by clinicians. Open margins may allow chemicals to enter and discolour the underlying dentine (Rotstein 1998). There may also be white or brown spots of secondary caries (see Figure 1.21). Metal pins and prefabricated posts when placed in the anterior teeth can become visible underneath composite restorations. This causes discoloration of these teeth. Removal of these pins and replacement of leaking restorations is indicated.

AGEING

Colour changes in the teeth result from surface and subsurface changes (Solheim 1988) (Figure 1.22). The degree of manifestation is related to tooth anatomy, structural hardness, and the amount of use and abuse. The following factors are encountered with increasing age.

*   *Enamel changes.* There may be both thinning and texture changes (Morley 1997).
*   *Dentine deposition.* Secondary and tertiary dentine deposition, pulp stones and dentine ageing all cause the tooth to appear darker.
*   *Salivary changes.* Salivary content and composition may change with advancing age (Solheim 1988). Bleaching treatment is normally successful in this age group provided there is sufficient enamel available to bleach (see Chapter 5).

FUNCTIONAL AND PARAFUNCTIONAL CHANGES

Tooth wear may give a darker appearance to the teeth, because of the loss of tooth surface (Smith and Knight 1984).

*   *Erosion* is the progressive loss of hard dental tissues by a chemical process not involving bacterial action (Watson and Tulloch, 1985, Bishop et al 1997). This dissolution of enamel by acid causes the tooth to appear discoloured (Shaw and Smith 1999) as the dentine is more yellow in colour (see Figure 1.23).
*   *Attrition* is defined as wear of the occlusal surfaces or approximal surfaces of the tooth caused by mastication or contact between occluding surfaces (Watson and Tulloch, 1985) (see Figure 1.24). It affects the occlusal and incisal surfaces (Bishop et al 1997).
*   *Abrasion* is defined as the loss by wear of tooth substance or a restoration by factors other than tooth contact (Watson and Tulloch 1985). It is usually caused by abnormal rubbing of a non-dental object such as a pipe, hairclip and musical instrument. It is often caused by over vigorous tooth brushing (Bishop et al 1997). This loss of enamel, causes exposure of dentine which makes the tooth appear more yellow.

Function and parafunction may cause loss of the incisal edges and exposure of underlying dentine, which is susceptible to colour change from absorption and deposition of reparative dentine (see Figure 1.25). Fracture lines develop as white cracks but darken upon exposure to absorptive surface stains (see Figures 1.25 and 1.22). Changes in colour and texture affect the colour and light reflectiveness.

DAILY ACQUIRED STAINS

Daily acquired stains are typical of the extrinsic stains. They cause superficial colour changes, which are removed by prophylaxis.

- *Plaque*. Pellicle and calculus on the surface of the tooth can give it a yellow appearance (see Figure 1.26).
- *Tobacco use*. The products of tobacco dissolve in the saliva and lower its pH, facilitating penetration of pits and fissures (Dayan et al 1983). This gives the tooth a brown/black appearance.
- *Food and beverages*. Consumption of food and drink such as coffee (see Figure 1.27), tea (see Figure 1.28), red wine and berries (Faunce 1983), curry, and colas results in surface and absorptive staining.
- *Poor oral hygiene*. Poor oral hygiene (Dayan et al 1983) may result in green (see Figure 1.29), black-brown and orange staining (see Figure 1.30) which is produced by chromogenic bacteria. These deposits are normally seen in children and are found on the buccal surfaces of maxillary teeth (Eriksen and Nordbo 1978).
- *Good oral hygiene*. A black type of staining can often occur in children. It is normally found in patients with good oral hygiene and can be highly retentive, particularly around the cervical margins of the teeth (Eriksen and Nordbo 1978). It sometimes occurs in patients with Mediterranean diets (see Figure 1.31).
- *Swimmers' calculus*. This is a yellow to dark-brown stain, which occurs on the facial and lingual/palatal surfaces of the anterior teeth of patients who swim and train extensively. Both primary and secondary dentitions are affected. It appears that prolonged exposure to pool water can cause stains to develop on swimmers' teeth. The stains can be accompanied by gingivitis (Rose and Carey 1995). The stains are easily removed by a professional oral prophylaxis.

CHEMICALS

Chlorhexidine

Mouthwash containing chlorhexidine causes superficial black and brown staining of the teeth (see Figures 1.32) (Addy and Moran 1985, Addy et al 1985a, b, Leard and Addy 1997, Eley 1999). The staining is enhanced in the presence of tea and coffee. It may be related to the precipitation of chromogenic dietary factors on to the teeth and mucous membranes (Addy et al 1985). It is probable that the associated cationic group attaches chlorhexidine to the tooth, while the other cationic group producing the bacteriocidal effect can attach the dietary factors, such as gallic acid derivatives (polyphenols) found in foods and beverages such as tea and coffee and tannins, from wine to the molecule and hence to the tooth surface (Leard and Addy 1997, Eley 1999).

Metals

Metals such as copper, nickel and iron can cause staining of teeth. Copper ions, when they occur in the water in certain areas can cause staining of teeth. Workers in the copper and nickel industries have also shown green staining on the teeth (Donoghue and Ferguson 1996). The combination of plaque occurring around metallic orthodontic brackets can cause green line staining. Excessive iron intake can cause cervical staining, usually dark-brown or black in colour. The taking of iron supplements can cause black staining of the teeth and tongue (Addy et al 1985); black stains have also been noted on the teeth of ironworkers.

Tannins and chromogens

Some stains are easier to remove by bleaching than others. Different stains require different approaches to removal (Nathoo 1997). Biological and environmental variables affect the tenacity of the different stains. Tannin stains from tea and coffee are more tenacious and may take three or four power bleaching sessions or a longer period of home bleaching to remove. Tannins are composed of polyphenols such as catechins and leucoanthocyanins and it is the gallic acid derivatives in the polyphenols that causes the yellow-brown stain. The tannins may also act as stain promotors (Eriksen and Nordbo 1978).

Classifications

Extrinsic stain can be classified as either metallic or non-metallic. However, this classification does not explain the mechanism of discoloration and since staining is multifactorial, not all metals cause discoloration. Nathoo (1997) has proposed a classification based on the chemistry of the discoloration. This theoretical classification does not explain stains on teeth that start off as extrinsic stain and become intrinsic stain, such as nicotine staining; however, it is worth setting out in what follows as an explanation of extrinsic staining alone.

The deposition of extrinsic stain depends on the attraction of materials to the tooth surface (Nathoo and Gaffar 1995). The attraction forces include long-range interactive forces such as electrostatic and van der Waals forces and short-range interactions such as hydration forces, hydrophobic interactions, dipole–dipole forces and hydrogen bonds (Nathoo 1997). These chemical attractive forces allow the chromogen (coloured material) and prechromogen (colourless material) to approach the tooth surface and determine if adhesion will occur. The chromogens penetrate into the enamel.

- **N1-type dental stain** (direct dental stain)
  The chromogen binds to the tooth surface to cause tooth discoloration (see Figure 1.1). The colour of the chromogen is similar to that of the dental stain. Examples of these direct dental stains are the bacterial adhesion to the pellicle and formation of salivary pellicle (Eriksen et al 1985) experienced with tea, coffee, wine and metals. These materials generate colour due to the presence of conjugated double bonds and are thought to interact with the tooth surface via an ion exchange mechanism. Enamel which is bathed in saliva has a negative charge which is counterbalanced by the Stern layer or hydration layer. The metal ions in this Stern layer are responsible for staining. These stains can be prevented by good oral hygiene and can be easily removed with prophylaxis paste or toothpaste.

- **N2-type dental stain** (direct dental stain)
  The chromogen changes colour after binding to the tooth. Examples of this stain are food that has aged and the age-related formation of yellowish discoloration on the interproximal or gingival areas and increases in brown pellicle. N1-type food stains are known to darken to N2-type stains. N2 stains are more difficult to remove and may require professional cleaning.

- **N3-type dental stain** (indirect dental stain)
  The prechromogen binds to the tooth and undergoes a chemical reaction to cause a stain. The chromogenic material of chlorhexidine stain contain furfurals and furfuraldehydes. These compounds are intermediate products of a series of rearrangement reactions between sugars and amino acids termed the Maillard non-enzymatic browning reaction (Eriksen et al 1985). Examples of this include browning of foods that are high in carbohydrates and sugars, such as apples and potatoes. Cooking oils also can cause browning of teeth. Furfurals are also found in baked products and fruit. Dental stain from therapeutic agents such as stannous fluoride can also be classified as N3-type stains. Discoloration is due to a redox reaction between stannous ions and the sulphhydryl groups in the pellicle proteins. These are the most difficult to remove and would probably require oxygenating agents such as carbamide peroxide.

It may be that tea and coffee in the freshly prepared state cause more staining of teeth and dental restorations than 'instant' brands (Rosen et al 1989). Tea stains glass ionomer restorations more than coffee does (Rosen et al 1989) and chlorhexidine in combination with tea may cause more staining than in combination with coffee.

CONCLUSION

Before commencing bleaching treatment is it essential to question the patient to determine the aetiology of the discoloration. In some instances, there may be a multifactorial component as the discoloration can be due to the accumulation of stain and dietary factors over many years.

REFERENCES

Abbot PV. (1997) Aesthetic considerations in endodontics: internal bleaching. *Pract Periodont Aesthetic Dent* 9(7):833–40.

Addy M, Moran J. (1985) Extrinsic tooth discoloration by metals and chlorhexidine. 2. Clinical staining produced by chlorhexidine, iron and tea. *Br Dent J* 159:331–4.

Addy M, Moran J, Griffiths AA, Wills Wood NJ. (1985a) Extrinsic tooth discoloration by metals and chlorhexidine. 1. Surface protein denaturation or dietary precipitation? *Br Dent J* 159:281–5.

Addy M, Moran J, Newcombe R, Warren P. (1985b) The comparative tea staining of phenolic, chlorhexidine and antiadhesive mouthrinses. *J Clin Periodontol* 22:923–8.

Atasu M, Genc A, Ercalik S. (1998) Enamel hypoplasia and essential staining of teeth from erythroblastosis fetalis. *J Clin Pediat Dent* Spring;22(3):249–52.

Baratieri LN, Ritter AV, Monteiro S, de Andrada MAC, Vieira LCC (1995) Non-vital tooth bleaching: guidelines for the clinician. *Quintessence Int* 26(9):597–608.

Bishop K, Kelleher M, Briggs P, Joshi R. (1997) Wear now? An update on the etiology of tooth wear. *Quintessence Int* 28(5):305–13.

Bowles WH, Bokmeyer TJ. (1997) Staining of adult teeth by minocycline: binding of minocycline by specific proteins. *J Esthet Dent* 9(1):30–4.

Dayan D, Heifferman A, Gorski M, Beigleiter A. (1983) Tooth discoloration – extrinsic and intrinsic factors. *Quintessence Int* 12(14):1–5.

Donoghue AM, Ferguson MM. (1996) Superficial copper staining of teeth in a brass foundry worker. *Occup Med (Oxf)* June;46(3):233–4.

Dzierkak J. (1991) Factors which cause tooth colour change. *Pract Periodont Aesthetic Dent* 3(2):15–20.

Eley BM. (1999) Antibacterial agents in the control of supragingival plaque – a review. *Br Dent J* 186:286–96.

Eriksen HM, Nordbo H. (1978) Extrinsic discoloration of teeth. *J Clin Periodontol* 5:229–36.

Eriksen HM, Nordbo H, Kantanen H, Ellingsen OO. (1985) Chemical plaque control and extrinsic tooth discoloration. A review of possible mechanisms. *J Clin Periodontol* 12:345–50.

Faunce F. (1983) Management of discoloured teeth. *Dent Clin North Am* 27(4):657–5.

Feinman RA, Goldstein RE, Garber DA. (1987) *Bleaching teeth*, 1st edn. Quintessence: Chicago.

Goldstein RE. (1998) *Esthetics in Dentistry*, 2nd edn. Vol 1: *Principles, communications, treatment methods*, Chapter 12: Bleaching discoloured teeth. BC Decker: Hamilton, London, Ontario; 245–76.

Greenwall LH. (1992) The effects of carbamide peroxide on tooth colour and structures: an *in vitro* investigation. MSc thesis, University of London.

Hattab FN, Qudeimat MA, al-Rimawi HS. (1999) Dental discoloration: an overview. *J Esthet Dent* 11:291–310.

Hayes PA, Full C, Pinkham J. (1986) The etiology and treatment of intrinsic discolorations. *J Can Dent Assoc* 52:217–20.

Haywood VB. (1997) Extended bleaching of tetracycline-stained teeth: a case report. *Contemp Esthetics Restor Pract* 1(1):14–21.

Jordan RE, Boksman L. (1984) Conservative vital bleaching treatment of discoloured dentition. *Compend Contin Educ Dent* V(10):803–7.

Kidd EAM. (1991) The caries status of tooth-coloured restorations with marginal stain. *Br Dent J* 171:241–3.

Kidd EAM, Joyston-Bechal S, Beighton D. (1995) Marginal ditching and staining as a predictor of secondary caries around amalgam restorations: a clinical and microbiological study. *J Dent Res* 74(5):1206–11.

Kleter GA. (1998) Discoloration of dental carious lesions (a review). *Arch Oral Biol* Aug;43(8):629–32.

Leard A, Addy M. (1997) The propensity of different brands of tea and coffee to cause staining associated with chlorhexidine. *J Clin Periodontol* 24:115–18.

Louka AN. (1989) Esthetic treatment of anterior teeth. *J Can Dent Assoc* 55(1):29–32.

Love RM, Chandler NP. (1996) A scanning electron and confocal laser microscope investigation of tetracycline-affected human dentine. *Int Endodont J* 29:376–81.

Marin PD, Bartold PM, Hiethersay GS. (1997) Tooth discoloration by blood: an in-vitro histochemical study. *Endodont Dent Traumatol* 13:132–8.

McCaslin A, Haywood VB, Potter BJ, Dickinson GL, Russel CM. (1999) Assessing dentin color changes from Nightguard Vital Bleaching. *J Am Dent Assoc* Oct;130:1485–90.

McKenna BE, Lamely PJ, Kennedy JG, Batten J. (1999) Minocycline-induced staining of the adult permanent dentition: a review of the literature and report of a case. *Dental Update* May;**24**(4):160–2.

Morley J. (1997) The esthetics of anterior tooth aging. *Curr Opin Cosmetic Dent* **4**:35–9.

Nathoo SA. (1997) The chemistry and mechanisms of extrinsic and intrinsic discoloration. *J Am Dent Assoc* Suppl;**128**(4):6S–10S.

Nathoo SA, Gaffar A. (1995) Studies on dental stains induced by antibacterial agents and rational approaches for bleaching dental stains. *Adv Dent Res* **9**(4):462–70.

Ness L, Rosenkrans D de L and Welford JF. (1977) An epidemiologic study of factors affecting extrinsic staining of teeth in an English population. *Commun Dent Oral Epidemiol* **5**:55–60.

Patel K, Cheshire D, Vance A. (1998) Oral and systemic effects of prolonged minocycline therapy. *Br Dent J* **185**(11/12):560–2.

Rose KJ, Carey CM. (1995) Intensive swimming: Can it affect your patients' smiles. *J Am Dent Assoc* Oct;**126**:1402–6.

Rosen M, Christelis A, Bow P, Cohen J, Becker PJ. (1989) Glass ionomers and discoloration: a comparative study of the effects of tea and coffee on three brands of glass ionomer dental cement. *J Dent Assoc South Africa* **44**:333–6.

Rotstein I. (1998) Bleaching nonvital and vital discolored teeth. In: Cohen S, Burns RC. *Pathways of the pulp*, 7th edn. Mosby: St Louis, 674.

Salman RA, Salman GD, Glickman RS, Super DG, Salman L. (1985) Minocycline induced pigmentation of the oral cavity. *J Oral Med* July–Sept**40**(3):154–7.

Shannon IL. (1978) Stannous fluoride: does it stain teeth? How does it react with tooth surfaces? A review. *Gen Dent* **26**(5):64–71.

Shaw L, Smith AJ. (1999) Dental erosion – the problem and some practical solutions. *Br Dent J* **186**(3):115–18.

Shearer AC. (1991) External bleaching of teeth. *Dental Update* **18**(7):289–91.

Solheim (1988) Dental colour as indicator of age. *Gerodontics* **4**:114–18.

Smith BGN, Knight JK. (1984) An index for measuring the wear of teeth. *Br Dent J* **156**(4):435–8.

Swift EJ. (1988) A method for bleaching discoloured vital teeth. *Quintessence Int* **19**(9):607–11.

Teo CS. (1989) Management of tooth discoloration. *Acta Med Singapore* **18**(5):585–90.

van der Burgt TP, Eronat C, Plasschaert AJM. (1986a) Staining patterns in teeth discoloured by endodontic sealers. *J Endodont* May;**12**(5): 187–91.

van der Burgt TP, Mullaney TP, Plasschaert AJM. (1986b) Tooth discoloration induced by endodontic sealers. *Oral Surg Oral Med Oral Pathol* **61**:84–9.

Van der Bijl P, Ptitgoi-Aron G. (1995) Tetracyclines and calcified tissues. *Ann Dent* **54**(1/2):69–72.

Watanabe K, Shibata T, Kurosawa T, et al. (1999) Bilirubin pigmentation of human teeth caused by hyperbilirubinemia. *J Oral Pathol Med* March;**28**(3):128–30.

Watson IB, Tulloch EN. (1985) Clinical assessment of cases of tooth surface loss. *Br Dent J* **159**:144–8.

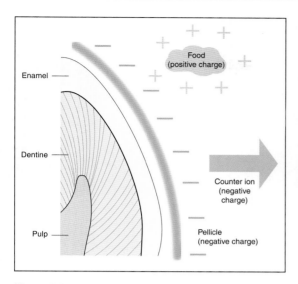

Figure 1.1

Nathoo classification N1-type mechanism: binding of food substances via ion exchange.

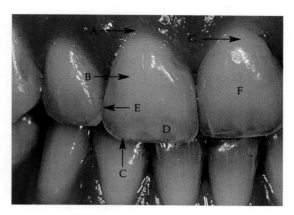

Figure 1.2

The colour of different areas of natural teeth. (A) The cervical margin; (B) the body of the tooth; (C) the incisal tip; (D) translucency; (E) the interproximal areas; (F) the enamel; (G) the dentine.

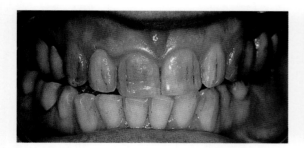

Figure 1.3

It is thought that this patient has **amelogenesis imperfecta.** All her posterior teeth have been crowned due to chipping and breakage of the enamel. The upper anterior teeth are hypoplastic and have longitudinal developmental ridges. The teeth have a brown discoloration. The lower anterior teeth are not as severely affected.

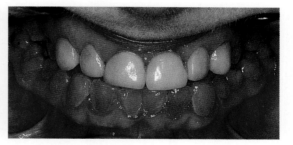

Figure 1.4

This patient has **dentinogenesis imperfecta.** She had porcelain-bonded veneers placed on the upper teeth to mask the opalescent dentine, which is visible on the lower teeth. These teeth have an amber-like colour due to the deposits of minerals within the dentinal tubules. There are some reports in the literature of successful bleaching with these types of discolorations.

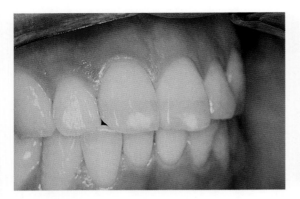

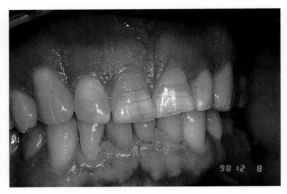

Figure 1.5

Enamel hypocalcification. White spots appear on the facial surfaces of the upper central incisors.

Figure 1.6

White developmental lines. This patient has white lines or stria on the upper central incisors and the incisal tips of the upper lateral incisors. This may have been caused by the presence of a high fever during chronological tooth development. There was a temporary disruption in enamel formation, as the other teeth were not affected. This can be called **chronologic hypoplasia** (Rotstein 1998).

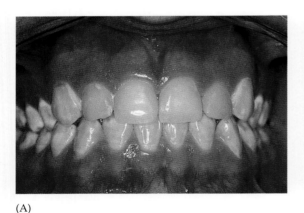

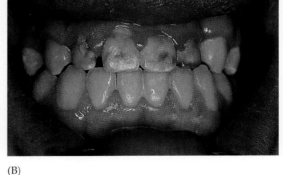

(A)   (B)

Figure 1.7

Fluorosis (A) This patient has mild generalized fluorosis on her teeth. The anterior teeth have composite bonded restorations placed to mask the discoloration when the patient was a teenager. It is thought this fluorosis is due to excessive use of fluoride supplement tablets ingested during odontogenesis. (B) More severe fluorosis stain. Brown discoloration is present on the upper four anterior teeth. It appears as irregular brown patches. The enamel surface is defective. (Courtesy of Dr M. Kelleher.)

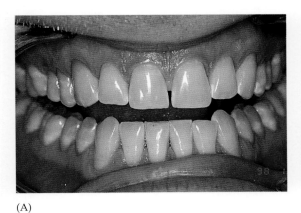 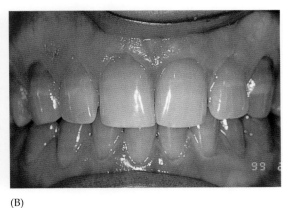

(A) (B)

Figure 1.8

Tetracycline staining has a variable nature due to many factors such as the type of tetracycline medication used and the duration and time of administration. (A, B) **First degree staining** shows mild tetracycline staining without banding, slight and uniformly distributed throughout the crown. This is amenable to bleaching.

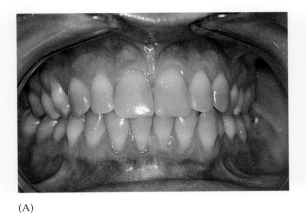 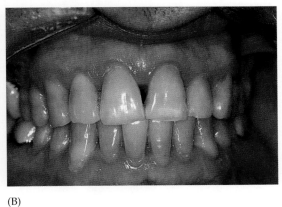

(A) (B)

Figure 1.9

(A, B) Tetracycline staining. **Second degree staining** shows stronger staining with a more yellow–grey appearance and banding. This may be amenable to home bleaching. It may be possible to try home bleaching first followed by combination bleaching with in-office visits if necessary.

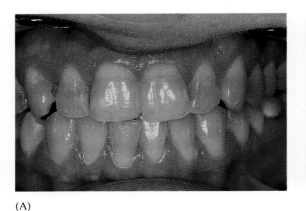

(A)

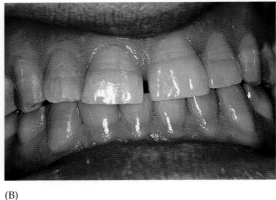

(B)

Figure 1.10

Tetracycline staining. **Third degree staining** (A) shows banding with grey–blue staining. This may be amenable to bleaching. However, patients need to be aware that it may take 3–6 months to achieve satisfactory lightening. (B) More pronounced banding in third degree staining.

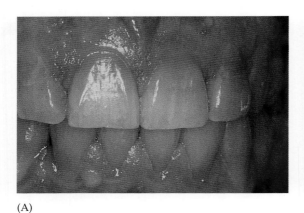

(A)

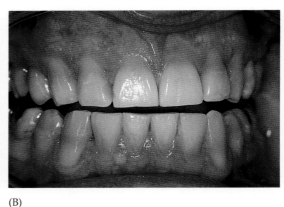

(B)

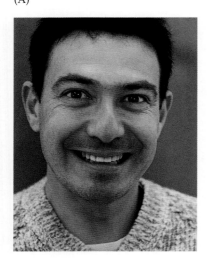

(C)

Figure 1.11

(A) This patient has third degree staining on his teeth. (B) The appearance of the teeth after 6 weeks of home bleaching. Note the appearance of the stained composite restoration is more noticeable following the whitening and lightening of the teeth. (C) The portrait of the patient after successful bleaching. The patient is delighted with the result.

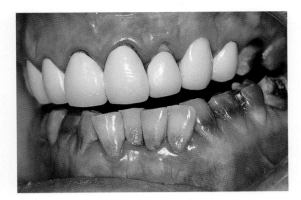

Figure 1.12

Fourth degree staining. The discoloration is so dark that it may not respond to bleaching. In this case the patient had the upper teeth crowned, 21 years previously. Besides crowning of the teeth the other realistic treatment options available at that time were intentional endodontic treatment and intracoronal bleaching. There are now further more conservative options, which would include bleaching followed by porcelain laminate veneers. Bleaching treatment can always be discussed with the patient. In this case the worst that can happen is no change in colour, but it is worth a try. Gingival recession has occurred around the crown margins and there are areas of cervical decay present. These restorations will need replacement.

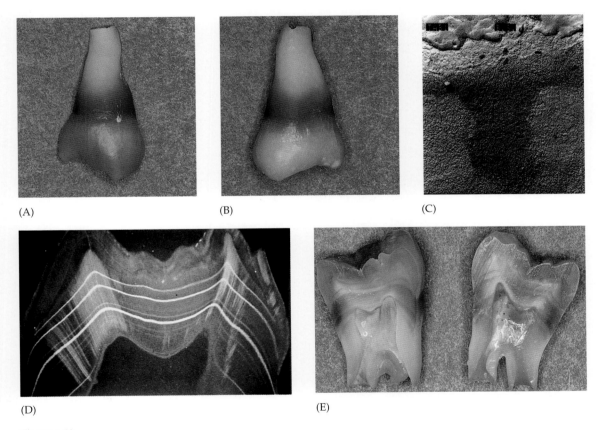

(A)   (B)   (C)

(D)   (E)

Figure 1.13

Tetracycline **staining on extracted teeth**. (A) This shows the characteristic banding on the teeth which occurs through the dentine. (B) This experimental tooth has been successfully lightened using a 10% carbamide peroxide material (from Greenwall 1992). (C) A scanning electron microscope view of the banded area of the tetracycline stained tooth at the junction of the enamel and the dentine (×120). The dentine in the affected band appears different to the surrounding dentine. The mineralizing front of the unaffected dentine is normal in appearance. The mineralizing front of the tetracycline-affected dentine band is devoid of calcospherite formation (Love and Chandler 1996). There are many surface defects. (D) Under fluorescent light the banding of tetracycline teeth becomes visible in the dentine layers. (Courtesy of Dr I. Rotstein.) (E) A tetracycline tooth in section showing the characteristic banding.

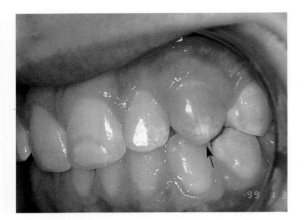

Figure 1.14

Pulpal changes. This patient's canine tooth (arrow) became non-vital following **trauma** sustained from a sporting injury. The tooth discoloured due to intrapulpal haemorrhage. The white hypoplastic lesion on the central tooth was removed using microabrasion. (See Fig. 10.8.)

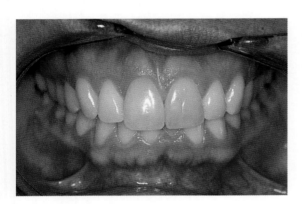

Figure 1.15

Pulpal changes. The two central incisors are darker than the other teeth due to **dentine hypercalcification** as a result of trauma sustained to the tooth 15 years previously.

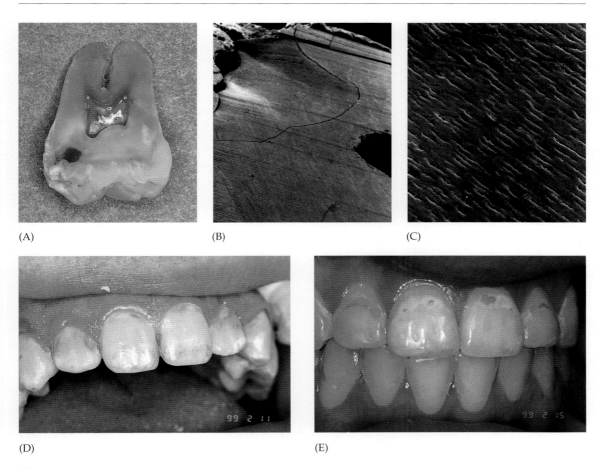

(A)   (B)   (C)

(D)   (E)

Figure 1.16

Dental caries. (A) This shows the tooth in longitudinal sections exposing a primary lesion within the dentin layers of the tooth. The caries is stained brown and has a white edge. The brown discoloration may be due to the initial products of the Maillard reaction, which are formed in the carious lesion (Kleter 1998). The carious lesion can take up food dyes making it become brown in colour and metal ions, which make it black. (B) Scanning electron micrograph of the carious lesion showing the shallow lesion (×40). (C) Scanning electron micrograph of the dentine showing the cleansing effect of the bleaching material on the caries. (D) This patient with haemophilia has stained teeth due to poor oral hygiene and precarious lesions. (E) This patient has brown staining which developed around orthodontic bands.

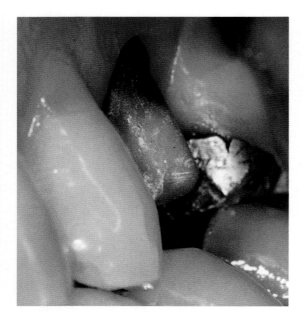

Figure 1.17

This discoloured non-vital tooth, which was endodontically treated, was prepared for a crown. The cervical neck is a black–brown colour. This is probably due to the intracanal medicament used during the root canal treatment. The medicaments penetrate into the dentinal tubules and discolor the dentine slowly.

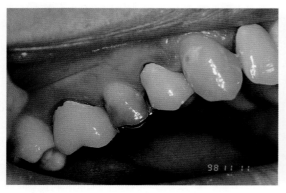

(A)

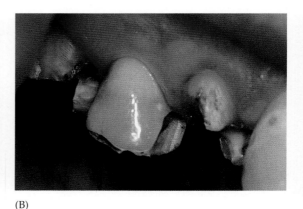

(B)

Figure 1.18

(A) This premolar tooth, which has a deep blue discoloration, has an amalgam core with a gold onlay over it. This patient's enamel is very thin and translucent. The discoloration is due to the amalgam core under the gold onlay. The blue stain is from the penetration of the dentine tubules by the metal compounds which may be aggravated by the galvanic reaction between the amalgam and the gold. There is also black staining around the crown of the adjacent premolar, due to marginal leakage where the crown margins are defective. There is also brown discoloration of the cervical area around the porcelain bonded crown on the molar tooth where there has been gingival recession, revealing that this tooth is non-vital. (B) Once the amalgam core was removed the staining disappeared from the tooth. The tooth was built up with a composite core to receive a porcelain-bonded crown. The leaking crowns on either side were removed and there was decay under the existing cores. These were rebuilt with glass-ionomer.

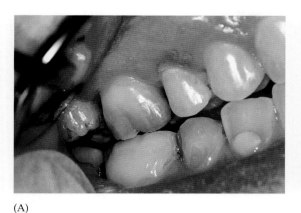 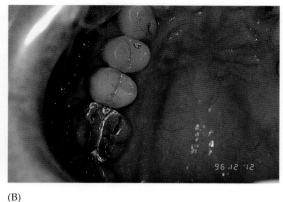

(A)   (B)

Figure 1.19

(A) This patient has discoloration on the lower half of the upper molar due to an old amalgam restoration. In the centre there is a red band which is probably secondary decay. However, the colour of the restoration is not normally a good indicator of the presence of secondary caries. The lower premolar has tooth wear from abfraction lesions and toothbrush abrasion. (B) Even replacing the existing restoration with a new restoration will not remove the grey staining.

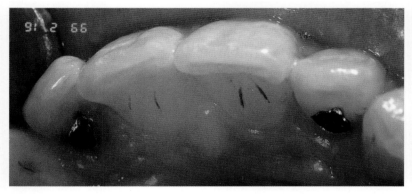

Figure 1.20

Discoloration due to amalgam restorations. (A) Palatally placed amalgam restorations often cause the tooth to appear grey because percolation of the metal salts through the tooth. (B) Even when the restoration is replaced with a tooth coloured composite restoration, the tooth still appears grey.

(A)

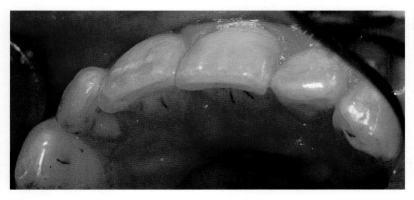

(B)

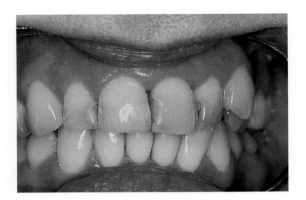

Figure 1.21

Discoloration due to composite restorations. This patient has large anterior composite restorations, which are leaking. There is brown marginal staining around the edges of the restorations where oral fluids, bacteria and food dyes can enter. The lower half of the tooth is more discoloured as it is exposed to the oral environment as the patient has a short lip, which does not sufficiently protect the enamel. It makes the tooth appear more yellow. There is white staining present, which is caused by secondary caries on the upper right central incisor. The central incisors are more translucent and the underlying dentine is demineralized and discoloured.

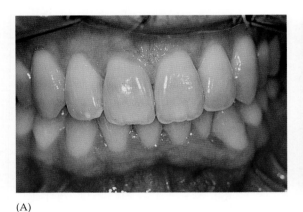

(A)

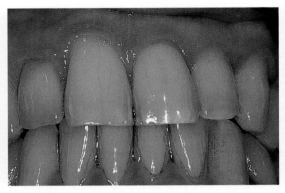

(B)

Figure 1.22

(A, B) Ageing produces colour changes in teeth that are the result of the thinning of the enamel, secondary deposition of the dentine, salivary changes and uptake of food substances within the enamel which make the teeth appear more yellow.

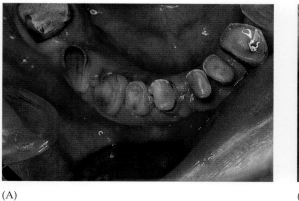 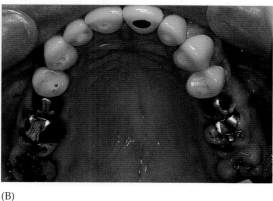

(A)   (B)

Figure 1.23

(A) This shows advanced **erosion** with dissolution of the enamel and the dentine is exposed underneath on the lower teeth. This advanced tooth wear is a contraindication to bleaching treatment. (B) The upper teeth of the same patient. Although the anterior teeth have been previously crowned, erosion has continued. This patient has tooth wear of unknown aetiology. The black staining may be due to nicotine as the patient is a heavy smoker. There is also staining around the cervical margins of the molar teeth, which cannot be removed by oral prophylaxis.

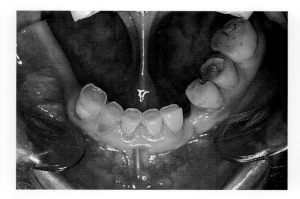 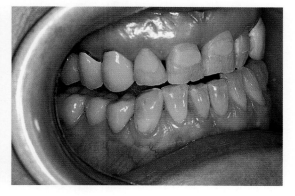

Figure 1.24

This patient has a combination of **attrition** on the incisal surfaces and erosion on the surfaces of the molar teeth.

Figure 1.25

Parafunctional changes have caused loss of the incisal edges of the upper and lower teeth. There are vertical white fracture lines present on the upper teeth.

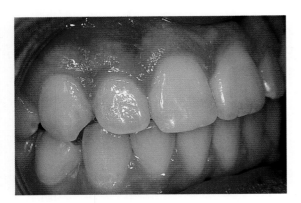

Figure 1.26

Plaque and pellicle on the facial surfaces of the teeth. This has a yellow colour. This is easily removed by tooth brushing. Toothpastes and whitening toothpastes are effective in removing this type of surface discoloration.

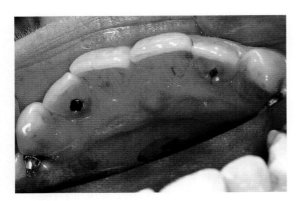

Figure 1.27

This patient reported drinking at least five cups of coffee per day. There is brown staining on the palatal surfaces of the teeth.

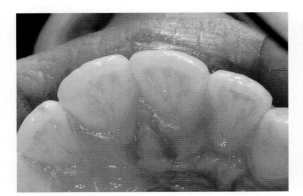

Figure 1.28

Tea staining. This patient has mild staining from tea, which was drunk without milk. As the tea was sipped very slowly there is more staining on the palatal than the buccal surfaces of the teeth.

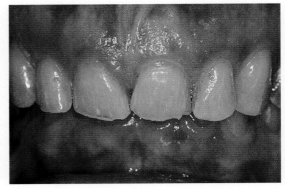

Figure 1.29

Green staining. Superficial staining from chromogenic bacteria in an older patient with poor oral hygiene methods.

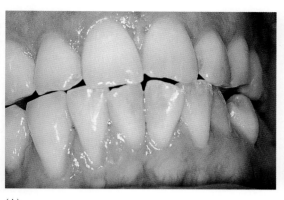
(A)

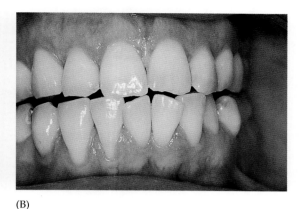
(B)

Figure 1.30

This patient reports that her teeth went yellow after use of two antibiotics used in combination for an upper respiratory tract infection. It may have been that during the illness the patient was unable to use good oral hygiene methods and hence the plaque adhered to the teeth more than usual. (B) The yellow stain is easily removable with an oral prophylaxis.

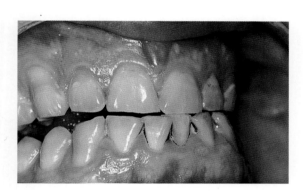

Figure 1.31

This patient who has mild tetracycline staining exhibits black staining around the cervical edges of the lower incisor tooth. This patient consumed a Mediterranean type diet. The black staining is easily removable with oral prophylaxis.

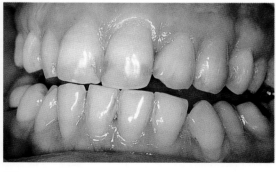
(A)

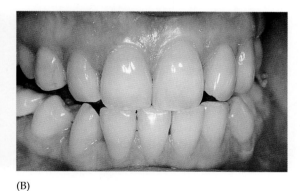
(B)

Figure 1.32

(A) This shows staining induced by use of a chlorhexidine containing mouthwash in a patient who has tetracycline staining. (B) The brown staining is easily removed with an oral prophylaxis.

2

A BRIEF HISTORY OF TOOTH BLEACHING

INTRODUCTION

Dentists have been perplexed by the problem of tooth discoloration for the last 200 years and have tried numerous chemicals and methods to remove the various types of discoloration. Many of the early attempts, although highly innovative in their time, were not successful and bleaching techniques were considered to be experimental and unpredictable. Colour regression was a problem (Kirk 1889). However, the technique of using 35% hydrogen peroxide to bleach vital teeth has been available for nearly 100 years. There was a great interest in aesthetic dentistry in the late 1880s which included recontouring of teeth, gold and porcelain inlays and bleaching of teeth (How 1886). All treatments were aimed at conserving natural teeth (Haywood 1992).

Attempts to bleach teeth started in earnest in the nineteenth century and have continued until successful bleaching techniques could be found. Numerous techniques have been tried including those for bleaching of non-vital teeth. It is the aim of this chapter to elaborate on the early history of bleaching vital and non-vital teeth and explain some of the origins of the bleaching techniques that will be discussed later in the book.

EARLY HISTORY

Most of the attempts to bleach teeth in the nineteenth century were tried on non-vital teeth but later dentists attempted to bleach vital teeth. The materials were quite caustic

and dangerous and had to be used with great caution. From the 1860s, one of the most effective early techniques for bleaching non-vital teeth was using chlorine produced from a solution of calcium hydrochloride and acetic acid; the commercial derivative was called Labarraque's solution (see Table 2.1), which was liquid chloride of soda.

THE LATE 1800S

Several oxidizing agents were used directly or indirectly to act upon the organic part of the tooth such as aluminium chloride, oxalic acid, pyrozone (ether peroxide), hydrogen dioxide (hydrogen peroxide or perhydrol) sodium peroxide, sodium hypophosphate, chloride of lime and cyanide of potassium. These materials were used for non-vital teeth. Sulphurous acid was a reducing agent that was often used. The most effective materials were considered to be pyrozone, superoxyl and sodium dioxide (Haywood 1992).

Bleaching agents were categorized according to which stains they were most effective in removing. Iron stains were removed with oxalic acid, silver and copper stains with chlorine, and iodine stains with ammonia. Stains from amalgam restorations were considered the most resistant to bleaching. Cyanide of potassium would remove metallic stains, but was not recommended as it was an active poison. Even in those days it was recognised that restorations were not affected by bleaching and that bleaching could remove the stains around margins that were leaking, giving them a longer life (Haywood 1992).

INTRACORONAL/INTERNAL BLEACHING

In the original technique to treat non-vital teeth, the bleaching agent was applied to the outside buccal surface of the tooth and was expected to penetrate through the enamel. This had limited success: it was only after the bleach was placed inside the tooth, making use of the pulp chamber, that the technique produced better results. Pearson in 1958 realised that the dentist could take advantage of the non-vital tooth's lack of pulp and place the bleaching material directly into the pulp chamber thereby expediting the lightening of the tooth (Goldstein and Garber 1995). Pyrozone (ether peroxide) continued to be used for bleaching non-vital teeth up to the 1950s and early 1960s. Spasser (1961) described a method of sealing a mixture of sodium perborate with water into the pulp chamber and leaving it in situ for 1 week. This technique became known as the '**walking bleach technique**'.

Nutting and Poe (1963, 1967) described a modified version using a combination of 30% hydrogen peroxide and sodium perborate sealed into the pulp chamber for a week. The two materials used in combination had a synergistic effect. This was known as the '**combination walking bleach technique**'. They advised that the gutta-percha be sealed before the procedure was initiated. Many modifications have been recommended for this technique. Problems of cervical resorption after internal bleaching were first reported by Harrington and Natkin (1979). Theories and reasons for this will be discussed in detail in Chapter 8. Although hydrogen peroxide and sodium perborate have been used successfully for 30 years, new bleaching materials are constantly being evaluated to improve bleaching efficacy (Rotstein et al 1991, Marin et al 1998).

The '**thermocatalytic technique**' (Stewart 1965) involves the placement of an oxidising chemical into the pulp chamber. This is followed by the application of a heating instrument either directly into the pulp chamber or the buccal surface of the tooth. Specially designed heating lamps were also used. The heat generated, in combination with the high concentration of hydrogen peroxide is thought to contribute to the possibility of developing cervical resorption and nowadays this technique is not used as frequently.

A new technique, using the open pulp chamber and 10% carbamide peroxide in a custom tray, has been recommended. This is called the '**inside/outside technique**' (Settembrini et al 1997, Carrillo et al 1998). The patient applies the bleaching material directly into the pulp chamber with a syringe and then the bleaching tray is seated in to the mouth. This way the tooth is bleached from the inside as well as the outside at the same time. Further information on this technique is given in Chapter 9.

HOME BLEACHING MATERIALS

It was an incidental finding and a chance discovery in the 1960s that led to the successful technique of home bleaching as we know it today. In this technique, the bleaching material, which is usually 10% carbamide peroxide, is placed in a custom-fitted tray. The patient places the tray with the material in the mouth and wears the tray for several hours or overnight while the teeth lighten within a few days, weeks or months (for tetracycline staining), depending on the nature of the discoloration. Dr Van Haywood and Dr Harald Heymann published the original technique, called Nightguard Vital Bleaching, in an article in 1989. The continued scientific research into this technique has demonstrated its safety, efficacy and success, leading to its acceptance in mainstream dentistry.

Hydrogen peroxide mouthwashes (such as Gly-oxide and Proxigel) were available as antiseptics for gum irritation and soft tissue inflammation since the 1960s. The initial findings were the result of astute dentists who noticed tooth lightening after use of these mouthwashes in a tray. Dr Klusmier, an orthodontist, used Gly-Oxide in an orthodontic

Table 2.1 History of tooth bleaching (adapted from data in Haywood 1992)

Date	Name	Material used	Discoloration
1799	Macintosh	Chloride of lime is invented; called Bleaching Powder	
1848	Dwinelle	Chloride of lime	Non-vital teeth
1860	Truman	Chloride and acetic acid Labarraque's solution (liquid chloride of soda)	Non-vital teeth
1861	Woodnut	Advised placing the bleaching medicament and changing it at subsequent appointments	
1868	Latimer	Oxalic acid	Vital teeth
1877	Chapple	Hydrochloric acid, oxalic acid	All discolorations
1878	Taft	Oxalic acid and calcium hypochlorite	
1884	Harlan	Uses the first hydrogen peroxide (called hydrogen dioxide)	All discolorations
1893	Atkinson	3% pyrozone used as a mouthwash which also lightened teeth 25% pyrozone was the most effective	
1895	Garretson	Chlorine applied to the tooth surface	Non-vital teeth
1910	Prins	30% hydrogen peroxide on to teeth	Non-vital and vital
1916	Kaine	18% hydrochloric acid (muriatic acid) and heat lamp	Fluorosed teeth
1918	Abbot	Discovers a high intensity light that produces a rapid temperature rise in the hydrogen peroxide to accelerate chemical tooth bleaching	
1924	Prinz	First recorded use of a solution of perborate in hydrogen peroxide activated by a light source	
1942	Younger	5 parts of 30% hydrogen peroxide heat lamp, anaesthetic	
1958	Pearson	Used 35% hydrogen peroxide inside tooth and also suggested 25% hydrogen peroxide and 75% ether which was activated by a lamp producing light and heat to release solvent qualities of ether	Non-vital teeth
1961	Spasser	**Walking bleach technique** Sodium perborate and water is sealed into the pulp chamber	Non-vital teeth
1965	Bouschar	5 parts 30% hydrogen peroxide, 5 parts 36% hydrochloric acid, 1 part diethyl ether	Orange coloured fluorosis stains
1965	Stewart	**Thermocatalytic technique** Pellet saturated with superoxyl inserted into pulp chamber and heated with hot instrument	Non-vital teeth
1966	McInnes	Repeats Bouschar's technique using controlled hydrochloric acid–pumice abrasion technique	Predictable?
1967	Cohen and Parkins	35% hydrogen peroxide and a heating instrument	Tetracycline stains
1967	Nutting and Poe	**Combination walking bleach technique** Superoxyl in pulp chamber (30% hydrogen peroxide)	Non-vital teeth
1968	Klusmier	Home bleaching concept started-incidental finding 10% carbamide peroxide in an custom fitted orthodontic positioner Gly-Oxide used	Vital teeth
1972	Klusmier	Used the same technique with Proxigel as it was thicker and stayed in the tray longer	

Table 2.1 Continued

Date	Name	Material used	Discoloration
1975	Chandra and Chawla	30% hydrogen peroxide 18% hydrochloric acid flour of Paris	Fluorosis stains
1977	Falkenstein	1-minute etch with 30% hydrogen peroxide 10% hydrochloric acid 100 watt (104°F) light gun	Tetracycline stains
1979	Compton	30% hydrogen peroxide heat element (130–145°F)	Tetracycline stains
1979	Harrington and Natkin	Reported on external resorption associated with bleaching pulpless teeth	
1982	Abou-Rass	Recommended intentional endodontic treatment with internal bleaching	Tetracycline stains
1984	Zaragoza	70% hydrogen peroxide + heat for both arches	Vital teeth
1986	Munro	Used Gly-Oxide to control bacterial growth after periodontal root planning. Noticed tooth lightening	Vital teeth
1987	Feinman	**In-office bleaching** using 30% H_2O_2 and heat from bleaching light	Vital teeth
1988	Munro	Presented findings to manufacturer resulting in first commercial bleaching product: White + Brite (Omnii Int.)	
1989	Croll	**Microabrasion technique** 10% hydrochloric acid and pumice in a paste	Vital teeth, superficial enamel discoloration, hypocalcification extrinsic stains
1989	Haywood and Heyman	**Nightguard Vital Bleaching** 10% carbamide peroxide in a tray	All stains, vital and non-vital teeth
1990		Introduction of commercial **over-the-counter** bleaching products (a controversy)	Vital teeth
1991		Bleaching materials were investigated while the FDA called for all the safety studies and data. After 6 months the ban was lifted	
1991	Numerous authors	**Power bleaching** 30% hydrogen peroxide using a light to activate bleach.	All stains, vital teeth
1991	Garber and Goldstein	**Combination bleaching** Power and home bleaching	
1991	Hall	Recommends no etching teeth before vital bleaching procedures	
1994	American Dental Association	Safety and efficacy established for tooth bleaching agents under the ADA seal of approval	
1996	Food and Drug Administration	FDA approve ion laser technology. Argon and CO_2 lasers for tooth whitening with patented chemicals	
1996	Reyto	**Laser tooth whitening**	Vital teeth
1997	Settembrini et al	**Inside/outside bleaching**	Non-vital and vital teeth
1998	Carrillo et al	Open pulp chamber 10% carbamide peroxide in custom tray	
Present day		• Plasma arc and light activated bleaching techniques • Power gels for-in-office bleaching • Laser activated bleaching • Home bleaching available in different concentrations and flavours	

positioner for a patient who had received an injury to the mouth. While the gum healed well, he also noticed that the teeth had got lighter. Treatment was continued until a satisfactory amount of lightening had been achieved. Dr Klusmier began offering this treatment to his patients and family. He noted that it took 6 months to lighten the teeth and that the mandibular arch was less favourably bleached (Haywood 1991a).

It was through the local dental study group meeting that Dr Jerry Wagner, a paedodontist, learnt about the technique (Haywood 1997). He used it on his 12–15-year-old patients who were leaving his practice. He had not heard of any long-term damage and reported that less than 10% of his patients had any resulting discomfort (Haywood 1991b). Dr Austin learnt the technique from a continuing education course given by Dr Wagner and he shared the technique with Dr Freshwater who tried it on his daughter and shared the technique with his local study club, the Coastal Dental Study Club in North Carolina. When Dr Haywood lectured at the study club the technique was shared with him. The study group asked him to do further research on the subject which he did. This resulted in the first article about Nightguard Vital Bleaching, published in 1989. Further research has subsequently been undertaken in many areas of vital bleaching.

Dr John Munro, who in 1986 used the technique to control bacterial growth after root planing, also noticed that the teeth lightened. He presented his findings to a manufacturer who developed the first commercial product for the Nightguard Vital Bleaching technique. This product was called White & Brite (Omnii International, St Petersburg Florida, USA). It was a 10% carbamide peroxide solution and sold as a daytime-use bleaching product (Haywood 1991a).

There are therefore two avenues through which the profession was introduced to the current tooth lightening techniques. The first was through study clubs and dentists sharing information, then through scientific literature. The second was through the manufacturers and their promotional efforts through advertising and marketing their products. More than 30 years on, it is clear that the technique works on most people.

The Food and Drug Administration (FDA) in 1991 began investigating tooth bleaching because of concerns about possible damage to teeth from the over-the-counter bleaching kits that required an acidic pre-rinse. The FDA considered reclassifying tooth bleaching chemicals as drugs, but eventually decided against this action (Haywood 1993). In 1994 the American Dental Association (ADA) established safety and efficacy guidelines for tooth bleaching agents under a 'seal of approval' Acceptance Program. At present there are six agents which have ADA approval. These products have gone through rigorous testing and assessment by the ADA.

The ADA recognised three types of dental product containing hydrogen peroxide and intended for home use:

1   Oral antiseptic agents available over the counter and intended for short-term use.
2   Whiteners or bleaching agents containing 10% carbamide peroxide (3% hydrogen peroxide) which may be prescribed by a dentist for home use or may be available over the counter.
3   The over-the-counter (OTC) dentifrices with low concentrations of hydrogen peroxide or calcium peroxide (Dunn 1998).

Guidelines for the ADA seal of approval require manufacturers to submit results of scientific studies showing that their bleaching product when used as directed is not harmful to hard or soft tissues and will effectively bleach teeth as shown in human clinical studies (Dunn 1998). The guidelines also require that the patients be followed for a period of 6 months post-treatment to determined shade change and post-treatment side effects (Leonard 1998). New materials are being introduced that do not contain hydrogen peroxide as their bleaching agent (Perry et al 1998). Further studies will be needed on these products.

In the UK in 1998, a bleaching manufacturer took the Department of Health and the Department of Trade and Industry to court as dentists were prohibited from using the bleaching products. The judge in the case conceded that the bleaching products were not cosmetics, but medical devices, because the colour change was more permanent (Tiernan 1998). Dentists in the UK were thus allowed to use bleaching products provided that they had a CE (Communite European) Safety Mark. However, that decision has been overturned and at present UK dentists are prohibited from supplying these products to patients. The bleaching manufacturer has made an appeal to the Law Lords at the House of Lords. The Law Lords have agreed to hear the case again. In September 2000, a German Law Court stated that the Opalescence Bleaching Material was authorized as a medical device under the law and the CE marking was valid (Butterfield 2000). The German authorities had questioned the validity of the CE marking of the bleaching material as a medical device.

IN-OFFICE POWER BLEACHING

There were numerous attempts to discover a bleaching material that was powerful enough to bleach teeth at the dentist's chairside. Probably the first attempt was in 1918 when Abbot discovered that a high intensity light would produce a rapid increase in temperature to increase the efficiency. This technique has been available for nearly a century. It normally involves the patient sitting for many hours with a rubber dam on the teeth to protect the mucosa and gingivae, with 35% hydrogen peroxide bleaching material on the teeth, under a heated bleaching lamp (Zack and Cohen 1965). This was very laborious for the patient and dentist. The patient's teeth were not anaesthetized so that the patient's tolerance for high temperatures on the teeth could be monitored. It was unpredictable, had a faster regression rate and often resulted in more tooth sensitivity due to the extreme heat of the lamp. It required numerous sessions to be successful. However, the successful bleaching of those patients who had had tetracycline staining led the technique to become more widespread.

The introduction of the faster and safer light-activated units for power bleaching has popularised this in-office technique. Many light units do not generate heat: the halogen curing light, plasma arc or xenon power arc light activates the bleach on the teeth. This power bleaching material is normally more concentrated (35% hydrogen peroxide or 35% carbamide peroxide) than the home bleach material. However, further research in this area is needed to prove that it is better or safer than the home bleaching technique. Lasers have also been advocated for chairside bleaching, but the American Dental Association does not approve their use as yet.

SUMMARY

Materials for bleaching teeth have evolved over the last 200 years. Dentists tried numerous chemicals in their quest to help patients remove the discoloration from their teeth. There was a certain fashion element in the choice of materials at the time. Dentists experimented with the materials that were available at the particular time in history, to see if they might bleach teeth. Some of the bleaching materials, although of very high concentrations and caustic, were successful but caused side effects. Some were briefly successful and some, due to continued clinical research, have been proved to be successful, almost all of the time. The chapters that follow will describe the bleaching techniques and materials in detail.

REFERENCES

Butterfield D. (2000) Tooth bleaching–The whole sad truth and nothing but the truth (letter to the editor). *Dentistry* **5 October**:16–17.

Carrillo A, Arrendo Trevino MV, Haywood VB. (1998) Simultaneous bleaching of vital teeth ad an open chamber non-vital tooth with 10% carbamide peroxide. *Quintessence Int* Oct;**29**(10):643–8.

Chapple JA. (1877) Restoring discoloured teeth to normal. Hints and queries. *Dental Cosmos* **19**:499.

Dunn JR. (1998) Dentist-prescribed home bleaching: current status. *Compend Contin Educ Dent* Aug;**19**(8):760–4.

Dwinelle WW. (1850) Ninth Annual Meeting of the American Society of Dental Surgeons – Article X. *Am J Dent Sci* **1**:57–61.

Goldstein RE, Garber DA. (1995) *Complete dental bleaching*, Chapter 1. Quintessence Publishing Company: Chicago; 1–23.

Hall DA. (1991) Should etching be performed as part of vital bleaching technique? *Quintessence Int* **22**:679–86.

Harlan AW. (1884) The removal of stains caused by the administration of medicinal agents and the bleaching of pulpless teeth. *Am J Sci* **18**:521.

Harrington GW, Natkin E. (1979) Cervical resorption associated with bleaching of pulpless teeth. *J Endodont* **5**:344–8.

Haywood VB. (1991a) Nightguard Vital Bleaching, a history and products update: Part 1. *Esthet Dent Update* Aug;**2**(4):63–6.

Haywood VB. (1991b) Nightguard Vital Bleaching, a history and products update: Part 2. *Esthet Dent Update* Oct;**2**(5):82–5.

Haywood VB. (1992) History, safety and effectiveness of current bleaching techniques and application of the nightguard vital bleaching technique. *Quintessence Int* **23**(7):471–88.

Haywood VB. (1993) The Food and Drug Administration and its influence on home bleaching. *Curr Opin Cosmetic Dent* 12–18.

Haywood VB. (1997) Historical development of whiteners: clinical safety and efficacy. *Dental Update* April; **24**:98–104.

Haywood VB, Heymann HO. (1989) Nightguard Vital Bleaching. *Quintessence Int* **20**(3):173–6.

How WS. (1886) Esthetic dentistry. *Dental Cosmos* **28**:741–5.

Kirk CE. (1889) The chemical bleaching of teeth. *Dental Cosmos* **31**:273–83.

Leonard RH. (1998) Efficacy, longevity, side effects and patient perceptions of Nightguard Vital Bleaching. *Compend Contin Educ Dent* Aug;**19**(8):766–81.

Marin PD, Heithersay GS, Bridges TE. (1998) A quantitative comparison of traditional and non-peroxide bleaching agents. *Endodont Dent Traumatol* **14**:64–7.

Nutting EB, Poe GS. (1963) A new combination for bleaching teeth. *J South Calif Dent Assoc* **31**:289–91.

Nutting EB, Poe GS. (1967) Chemical bleaching of discolored endodontically treated teeth. *Dent Clin North Am* **10**:655–62.

Pearson HH. (1958) Bleaching of the discoloured pulpless tooth. *J Am Dent Assoc* **56**:64–5.

Perry R, Kugel G, Kastali S. (1998) Evaluation of a non-hydrogen peroxide at home bleaching system. *J Dent Res* **77B**:957[Abstr].

Reyto R. (1998) Laser tooth whitening. *Dental Clin North Am* **42**(4):755–62.

Rotstein I, Zalkind M, Mor C, Tarabeah A, Friedman S. (1991) In vitro efficacy of sodium perborate preparations used for intracoronal bleaching of discoloured non-vital teeth. *Endodont Dent Traumatol* **7**:177–80.

Settembrini L, Glutz J, Kaim J, Schere W. (1997) A technique for bleaching non-vital teeth: inside/outside bleaching. *J Am Dent Assoc* **128**:1283–4.

Spasser HF. (1961) A simple bleaching technique using sodium perborate. *NY Dent J* **27**:332–4.

The Concise Columbia Electronic Encyclopedia, 3rd edn. Copyright 1994. Columbia University Press.

Tiernan J. (1998) Bleaching–is the future brighter? *The Dentist* **November**:75–6.

Woodnut C. (1861) Discoloration of dentine. *Dental Cosmos* **2**:662.

Zack L, Cohen G. (1965) Pulp response to externally applied heat. *Oral Surg* **19**:515–30.

Zaragoza VMT. (1984) Bleaching of vital teeth. *EstoModeo* **9**:7–30.

THE BLEACHING MATERIALS

INTRODUCTION

In the decade since home bleaching materials were introduced, there have been numerous changes to the materials. The first-generation materials were in a liquid form. These materials did not remain in the trays for long and needed more replenishment over time. The second generation materials that are currently available are more viscous and in a gel form. This is to stop the materials leaching out of the tray and causing soft tissue irritation. The second-generation materials also contain differing concentrations of active ingredients. The third-generation materials differ in their vehicle and colour. In general, quality control by the manufacturers and dental companies has improved, together with changes in the packaging and patient instruction, to make them more patient-friendly. The fear of adverse side effects has disappeared as scientific research has replaced early theories (Christensen 1997).

Table 3.1 Constituents of the bleaching gels

- Carbamide peroxide
- Hydrogen peroxide and sodium hydroxide (Li 1998)
- Non-hydrogen peroxide containing materials i.e. Sodium perborate
- Thickening agent – Carbopol or Polyx
- Urea
- Vehicle – glycerine, dentifrice, glycol
- Surfactant and pigment dispersants
- Preservatives
- Flavourings
- Fluoride (in some recent products to reduce sensitivity)

CONSTITUENTS OF THE BLEACHING GELS

CARBAMIDE PEROXIDE

Carbamide peroxide ($CH_6N_2O_3$) in a 10% aqueous solution is used in most of the home bleaching kits. This breaks down to a 3.35% solution of hydrogen peroxide (H_2O_2) and 6.65% solution of urea (CH_4N_2O). A 15% and a 20% solution of carbamide peroxide are also available for the dentist supervised home-bleaching procedure. The 15% carbamide peroxide solution yields 5.4% hydrogen peroxide and the 20% one yields 7% hydrogen peroxide (Fasanaro 1992).

A 35% solution of carbamide peroxide is available as Quickstart (Den Mat Corp. Santa Ana, CA) and Opalescence Quick (Ultradent Products Inc., South Jordan, UT). This is marketed to be used by the dentist as an in-office procedure prior to the patient using the home kit. This 35% solution yields 10% hydrogen peroxide. It can cause soft tissue damage and so should be used with a rubber dam or soft tissue protectant. Differences in bleaching efficacy between bleaching treatments of different concentrations has not yet been fully studied (Haywood and Heymann 1991).

HYDROGEN PEROXIDE

Most of the bleaching agents contain hydrogen peroxide in some form. The hydrogen peroxide breaks down into water and oxygen. It is the oxygen molecules that penetrate the tooth and liberate the pigment molecule causing the tooth to whiten.

Non-hydrogen peroxide containing materials

These materials contain sodium perborate as the active ingredient. They are also reported to contain Hydroxylite™ (Hi Lite 2: Shofu Dental Corporation, Menlo Park, CA; Vitint System®: Dental Partners, Rotterdam, Netherlands), sodium chloride, oxygen and sodium fluoride and other raw materials. It is reported not to contain or produce hydrogen peroxide and to generate a negligible amount of free radicals unlike the 10% carbamide peroxide gel (Li 1998).

During the manufacturing process, an oxygen complex is created whilst eliminating sodium perborate. A peroxide-free gel is produced in its final state. The gel interacts with the moist tooth structure and is activated. The oxygen complex interacts with the tooth structure and saturates and changes the amino acids and double bonds of oxygen which are responsible for tooth discoloration. However, sodium perborate breaks down to give hydrogen peroxide, so it has not been fully ascertained if the manufacturer's claim is true.

Thickening agents

Carbopol (carboxypolymethylene). This is a polyacrylic acid polymer. Trolamine, which is a neutralizing agent, is often added to Carbopol to reduce the pH of the gels to 5–7.

1 The solutions containing Carbopol (e.g. Opalesence, by Ultradent Products, Utah) release oxygen slowly, while those without it are fast oxygen-releasing solutions. The rate of oxygenation affects the frequency of solution replacement during bleaching treatment. The fast oxygen-releasing solutions release a maximal amount of oxygen in less than 1 hour, while the slow solutions require 2–3 hours for maximal oxygen release, but remain active for up to 10 hours (Matis et al 1999).

2 The Carbopol enhances the viscosity of the bleaching material. The thixotropic nature of the Carbopol allows better retention of the slow-releasing gel in the tray. Less bleaching material is required for treatment (approximately 29 mL per arch). The viscosity also improves adherence to the tooth. The currently available formula of Opalescence has more Carbopol than previously.

3 Carbopol retards the effervescence because it retards the rate of oxygen release. The thicker products stay on the teeth to provide the necessary time for the carbamide peroxide to diffuse into the tooth.

4 The increased viscosity seems to prevent the saliva from breaking down the hydrogen peroxide which might achieve more effective results according to Haywood (1991c). The partial diffusion into the enamel may also allow the tooth to be bleached more effectively deeper within its enamel and dentine layers (Garber et al 1991).

Polyx. Polyx (Union Carbide, Danbury, CT) is the thickener used in the Colgate Platinum System. The composition of the Polyx is a trade secret (Oliver and Haywood 1999). The additive influences the activity of the material and the tray design.

Urea

Urea occurs naturally in the body, is produced in the salivary glands and is present in saliva and the gingival crevicular fluid (Moss 1999). Urea breaks down to ammonia and carbon dioxide either spontaneously or through bacterial metabolism. The effect on the pH depends on the concentration of the urea and the duration of its application.

Urea is used in the bleaching kits to:

• stabilise the hydrogen peroxide (Christensen 1997); it provides a loose association with the hydrogen peroxide which is easily broken down
• elevate the pH of the solution
• enhance other desirable qualities, such as anticariogenic effects, saliva stimulation, and wound healing properties (Archambault 1990).

VEHICLE

Glycerine. Carbamide peroxide is formulated with a glycerine base which enhances the viscosity of the preparation and ease of manipulation. However, this may dehydrate the tooth. Many dentists have reported that the tooth seems to lose its translucent appearance and this may be caused by dehydration. The dehydrating effect and the swallowing of the glycerine in the solution may be responsible for the sore throat which is sometimes reported as a side effect when using these agents.
Dentifrice. This is used as the vehicle for Colgate Platinum System.
Glycol. This is anhydrous glycerine.

SURFACTANT AND PIGMENT DISPERSANTS

The surfactant functions as a surface wetting agent which allows the hydrogen peroxide to diffuse across the gel–tooth boundary. A pigment dispersant keeps pigments in suspension (as in commercial water softeners). Gels with surfactant or pigment dispersants may be more effective than those without them (Feinman et al 1991, Garber et al 1991). This may allow a more active gel and dentists who prescribe these particular kits ('Nu-Smile' and 'Brite Smile') should caution their patients to adhere to the manufacturers' suggested wearing time (Feinman et al 1991).

PRESERVATIVES

All the solutions contain a preservative such as citroxain, phosphoric acids, citric acid or sodium stannate. These preservatives sequestrate transitional metals such as iron, copper, magnesium, which accelerate the breakdown of hydrogen peroxide. These acid solutions give the gels greater durability and stability. They therefore have a mildly acidic pH.

FLAVOURINGS

Flavourings are used in the bleaching materials to add to the choice of bleaching agent and to improve patient acceptability of the product (e.g. melon, banana and mint).

OVER-THE-COUNTER BLEACHING KITS

One of the controversies about bleaching is the availability of over-the-counter (OTC) bleaching kits. Such products, sold as cosmetics, have escaped rigorous legislation in America, the UK and Europe. They are freely available through pharmacies, stores, mail order and the Internet. This has caused many problems for patients, and also dentists who should be monitoring bleaching procedures carefully. These kits contain the following:

1 *Acid rinse.* This is usually citric or phosphoric acid which may be harmful to the dentition, as continued rinsing may cause tooth erosion. The potential for misuse may be considerable (Jay, 1990). The pH of this rinse is between 1 and 2.
2 *Bleaching gel.* This gel, applied for two minutes, has an acidic pH.
3 *Post-bleach 'polishing cream.'* This is a toothpaste containing titanium dioxide which may give a temporary painted-white appearance.

The efficacy and structural effects of these systems have not been evaluated in the literature (see Figures 3.1 and 3.2).

H₂O₂ STRIP SYSTEM

The hydrogen peroxide strip system is a trayless bleaching system that does not require any prefabrication or gel loading. The delivery system is a thin strip precoated with an adhesive 5.3% hydrogen peroxide gel (Haywood 2000, personal communication, Sagel et al 2000). The backing is peeled off and the strip placed directly to the facial/buccal surfaces of the six anterior teeth. Each strip is worn for 30 minutes, removed and discarded, and the procedure takes place twice a day for 14 days. The manufacturers (Proctor & Gamble, Cincinnati, OH) claim that the strip holds the gel in place to whiten the teeth both extrinsically and intrinsically and provides a uniform controlled application of gel. The material will initially be supplied to dentists and will then be available over the counter.

PROBLEMS WITH OTC BLEACHING KITS

Cubbon and Ore (1991) reported that the over-use of OTC bleaching agents caused erosion of the labial surfaces of the teeth, dissolution of the enamel and loss of anatomy. The exposed dentine appeared darker than the remaining enamel and patients over-used this agent to re-achieve the 'white' tooth colour. Dentists should be aware of these hazards when questioning patients who show evidence of tooth erosion of unknown aetiology (see Figures 3.3 and 3.12).

Patients may misdiagnose and self-prescribe the bleaching treatment which may be inappropriate for their dental condition. A patient may have pulpal pathology which may be exacerbated by this treatment. Finally, a patient determined to speed up the bleaching action may be overzealous in use of the product. Such abuse may lead to further problems and sensitivity (Fischer 2000a, b).

MECHANISM OF BLEACHING ACTION

Enamel is often thought of as impervious; in fact it should be considered a semipermeable membrane (Figure 3.15). Peroxide solutions flow freely through the enamel and dentine due to the porosity and permeability of these structures (McEvoy 1989). The free movement is due to the relatively low molecular weight of the peroxide molecule and the penetrating nature of the oxygen and superoxide radicals. It is difficult to set up barriers to prevent the rapid penetration.

The hydrogen peroxide acts as an oxygenator and an oxidant. Its bleaching effect has been attributed to both these qualities, although the exact mechanism of action is not fully understood. In general, however, the hydrogen peroxide oxidises the pigments in the tooth. The yellow pigments (xanthopterin) are oxidized to white pigments (leucopterin). The oxidants react with the chromophores which are the colour radicals to cleave the double bonds. The hydrogen peroxide must be in-situ long enough and frequently enough to release the pigment molecules from the tooth by oxidation.

Carbamide peroxide is a bifunctional derivative of carbonic acid. The hydrogen peroxide breaks down to water and oxygen and for brief periods forms the free radical $HO_2^.$ perhydroxyl. The free radical is very reactive and has a great oxidative power:

- It can break up a large macromolecular stain into smaller stain molecules, which are expelled to the surface by diffusion.
- It can attach to inorganic structure and protein matrix (Fasanaro 1992).
- It can oxidise tooth discoloration.

Carbamide peroxide eventually breaks down to water, oxygen and urea, carbon dioxide and ammonia. These breakdown by-products are of some concern because their effects are as yet relatively unknown.

RELATIVE MERITS OF H$_2$O$_2$ VS. CARBAMIDE PEROXIDE SYSTEMS

Which is best? Neither is best (Christensen 1997). Both systems contain hydrogen peroxide and work well. It appears that the H_2O_2 system may be faster than the carbamide peroxide solution (CPS) (Frysh et al 1991), with a faster treatment and exposure time. Concentration of the hydrogen peroxide is determined by the teeth, not by the soft tissues, as the hydrogen peroxide solution contains mucous membrane protectant. However, there is no scientific literature about this and these are purely manufacturers' claims. The H_2O_2 systems are aqueous gel based whereas the CPS systems are anhydrous gel based. Dehydration of the hard tissue is less likely to occur with hydrogen peroxide treatment. The CPS systems bleach more slowly and need longer exposure times. They do not contain a soft tissue protectant. There may thus be more soft tissue irritation, possibly due to the higher concentration of hydroxyl ion, acid, urea, ammonia or carbonic acid. There is no scientific evidence to prove this.

MOVEMENT OF CARBAMIDE PEROXIDE SOLUTION

The CPS moves freely through the tooth and can laterally diffuse through the tooth, or to distant sites (Haywood et al 1990; see Figure 3.4). This means that the CPS can be applied palatally to the tooth surface in order to bleach the colour beneath labially placed veneers. The transient pulpal sensitivity that some patients experience may be related to the rapid movement of urea and oxygen through the teeth (Haywood and Heymann 1991).

After 10 minutes of power bleaching it becomes evident that lightening starts around the edges of the incisal area and in the incisal corners. Lower teeth sometimes show a demarcation line during the first few days of the treatment. This effect is most commonly noticed on lower canines and patients are often concerned that their teeth are bleaching unevenly. They can be reassured that this demarcation line usually fades a few days of further bleaching. An in-vitro study was undertaken by Oliver and Haywood (1999) to see whether the use of shortened dental trays could cause a demarcation line, but this proved negative and the teeth bleached evenly.

TREATMENT TIMINGS

Some materials claim to need shorter daily contact time to minimize side effects (Christensen 1997). There are various concentrations of active ingredient which allow for individualized bleaching programmes for patients. It appears that there is no significant difference in the bleaching efficacy of different concentrations of the material, as long as the manufacturer's instructions are followed. However, studies have shown that the higher concentration materials may bleach the teeth faster. An in-vitro study by Leonard, Sharma and Haywood 1998, showed that a 16% solution of highly viscous materials (Nite White®, Discus Dental Inc., Los Angeles, CA) successfully obtained a 2 unit shade change more quickly than 5% and 10%. However, at the end of the two trial period, there were no statistically significant differences between the 5%, 10% or 16%. Lower concentration of carbamide peroxide will also work, but it will just take longer. The researchers observed that canines responded better to a 16% solution than did the central and lateral teeth. This would be beneficial for dentists who are treating an isolated dark tooth or darker canines (Leonard 1998).

PREFERRED REGIMES

Owing to the great variation in colour of the teeth being bleached, the bleaching times vary according to the existing shade of the teeth and the desired shade. There have been many differences of opinion about the length of time for which bleaching solutions should be used and replenished. At present most of the suggested wearing times are empirical (see Figures 3.5–3.7). In a randomized double-blind clinical trial (Cibirka et al 1999) tested two different 10% carbamide peroxide materials used overnight for 2 weeks to bleach the upper teeth and results showed a significant degree of lightening. There was no significant difference between the two materials tested, which were Opalescence (Ultradent Products Inc., South Jordan, Utah) and Nite White (Discus Dental Inc., Los Angeles, CA). In another clinical evaluation of two carbamide peroxide agents, both caused the teeth to lighten (Heymann et al 1998). The latter authors made the comment that the actual treatment time may not represent the active concentration time because the carbamide peroxide is decomposing relatively rapidly in the initial phase of any treatment.

Thirty-eight patients participated in a Nightguard bleaching study using two first-generation bleaching materials. Participants were instructed to wear the guard at night or during the day for 2–4 hours for 6 weeks total treatment time. Haywood et al (1994) reported that 92% experienced successful lightening of their teeth. There were several categories of patient: (1) aging/inherent discoloration, (2) trauma, (3) fluorosis, (4) tetracycline staining. Of the first category, 100% of patients experienced tooth lightening compared with 80% of those with brown fluorosis and 75% of the tetracycline patients. Successful results could be seen within 20 hours of treatment.

The application techniques relies on the mouthguard to keep the bleach in contact with the tooth so that the bleaching products can penetrate through the enamel. The bleaching process is thus dependent on the time that bleach is in contact with the tooth. Some manufacturers suggest that the solution be changed after 1 hour as it loses its effectiveness, however, this may increase the incidence of sensitivity (Leonard 1998).

Using Opalescence bleaching material, Matis and coworkers (1999) have shown carbamide peroxide degrades in an exponential manner after the first hour and that the degradation rate is higher in areas closer to the tooth structure. After 2 hours, 50% of the active ingredient of the bleaching material was available and 10% was still available after 10 hours (Matis et al 1999; see Figures 3.8 and 3.9). Longer treatment times may thus be advisable i.e. as the agent needs to be active for extended periods of time; to get maximum use out of the bleach it is preferable to sleep with the tray in position. Further research is needed to determine the level of active bleaching agent that is required for lightening to occur (Matis et al 1999). The bleaching potential of a material is thus an important factor to

consider. Once this level has been determined, tray wearing times can be scientifically calculated.

Patients who have tetracycline staining may need to bleach their teeth for 6 months or longer to achieve successful lightening. By extending the treatment time, the efficacy rate for patients with tetracycline staining improved to 90% (Haywood et al 1997).

HOME BLEACHING

PROPERTIES OF THE IDEAL AGENT

The ideal bleaching agent should:

- be easy to apply to the teeth for maximum patient compliance
- be non-acidic/have a neutral pH
- lighten the teeth successfully and efficiently
- remain in contact with oral tissues for short periods
- have adjustable peroxide concentration
- use the minimum quantity of the bleaching agent to achieve the desired result
- not irritate or dehydrate the oral tissues
- not cause damage to the teeth or the enamel to be etched
- be well controlled by the dentist to customise the treatment to the patient's needs.

RATE OF COLOUR CHANGE

This is affected by the:

- frequency that solutions are changed
- amount of time that the bleach is in contact with the tooth
- viscosity of the material
- rate of oxygen release
- original shade and condition of the tooth
- location and depth of discoloration (Howard 1992)
- degradation rate of the material (Matis et al 1999).

EFFECTS ON THE ENAMEL

SURFACE TEXTURE

Most scanning electron microscopy studies of enamel surfaces treated with CPS bleaching agents have shown little or no change in morphology (see Figures 3.16–3.18). It is thought that the enamel surface remains intact and unaffected by the CPS and the bleaching process (Haywood et al 1991) by scanning electron microscopy focal areas of shallow erosion developed in human teeth exposed to CPS, but did not find any changes in the composition of the enamel. One study, testing 16% and 35% CPS however, reported significant changes in the enamel, including loss of the aprismatic layer, exposure and demineralization of enamel prisms and pitting (Bitter 1995).

SURFACE HARDNESS AND WEAR RESISTANCE

Enamel surface hardness is apparently unaffected by the bleach (Zalkind et al 1996, Kelleher and Roe 1999). However a study using a bleaching/remineralization cycle showed that 10% carbamide peroxide treatment significantly decreased enamel hardness. The application of fluoride improved remineralization of enamel. The reduction of hardness may reflect the loss of mineral from enamel which could also result in reduced wear resistance (Seghi and Denry 1992). The researchers also showed that there was a change in the fracture toughness of the enamel (McCracken et al 1996).

CHEMICAL COMPOSITION

There may be loss of organic components from treated enamel surfaces – carbon, hydrocarbon and tertiary amine groups replaced by oxygen, calcium and phosphorus. The calcium/phosphate ratio of dentine was significantly decreased by bleaching with 30% hydrogen peroxide and 10% carbamide peroxide in a study by Rotstein et al (1996). These researchers recommended that dental bleaching agents be used with caution. In a study by McCracken and Haywood et al (1996) teeth exposed to CPS for 6 hours lost an average of 1.06 $\mu g/mm^2$ of calcium. This amount was significantly greater than the controls. However, this amount is small and may not be clinically significant. Drinking one can of a cola drink produced a comparable calcium loss of about 1 $\mu g/mm^2$. These results are consistent to calcium loss from enamel after 2-min exposures to carbonated cola, orange juice, apple juice or diet carbonated cola (Grobler et al 1990). The potential for remineralization occurs in vivo and may counteract these effects, but these have not been studied for CPS yet.

Some of the OTC bleaches have a very low pH (5.6) and this may cause erosion of the enamel and the toothpaste provided with the kit may be abrasive to the tooth surface (Jay 1990). There is the potential side effect that the teeth can be etch-bleached (Bartlett and Walmsley 1991).

EFFECTS ON DENTINE

Tooth colour is primarily determined by the dentine and can be changed by bleaching treatments. In an in-vitro study (McCaslin et al 1999), using 10% carbamide peroxide placed directly on to the enamel to validate the colour change in dentine and to assess whether dentine changed uniformly, it was noted that a colour change occurred throughout the dentine and the colour change was uniform.

Dentine bonding may be altered after bleaching (Della Bona et al 1992) and the smear layer may be removed (Hunsaker et al 1990). The bonding between glass ionomer and dentine may also be affected (Titley et al 1991). This may be due to the precipitate of hydrogen peroxide and collagen that forms on the cut dentine surface after tooth bleaching. It is suggested that adhesive dentistry be delayed for 2 weeks post-bleaching (Powell and Bales, 1991), see further below.

EFFECTS ON PULP

Pulp penetration during bleaching varies significantly among commercial 10% carbamide peroxide bleaching products (Thitinanthapan et al 1999), which may result in different levels of tooth sensitivity or bleaching efficacy. Pulp penetration can occur within 15 minutes according to studies by Cooper et al (1992). The potential for pulpal damage thus exists as a result of enamel and dentine penetration (Powell and Bales 1991). There appears to be less penetration into the pulp from carbamide peroxide than from hydrogen peroxide. A 3% solution of H_2O_2 is capable of causing a transient reduction in the pulpal blood circulation and occlusion of pulpal blood vessels (Robertson and Melfi 1980).

Although the pulp is highly resilient to indirect insult from restorative materials, there is a danger that patients who are overzealous to achieve a faster whitening may cause undesirable consequences. Those patients who increase the frequency of application within one day may experience increased sensitivity. The most common side effect experienced by patients using the home bleaching technique is transient, mild temperature sensitivity (Heymann et al 1998) during the first hour post-treatment. The sensitivity appears to be dose-related rather than pH-related. In a study by Scherer et al (1991) the patients who experienced transient tooth hypersensitivity after week 2 had overloaded their trays. Nathanson (1997) recommends careful treatment when patients have large restorations, cervical erosions and enamel cracks.

The studies appear to support the clinical observation that controlled home bleaching is safe to the pulp (Kelleher and Roe 1999, Li 1998).

EFFECTS ON CEMENTUM

It appears from recent studies that the cementum is not affected by the materials used for home bleaching (Murphy et al, 1992, Rotstein and Friedman 1991). A study by Scherer et al 1991 showed that the surface morphology of the cementum was unaffected using an admix type of home bleaching system.

Cervical resorption (Latcham 1986, Madison and Walton 1990) and external root resorption (Cvek and Lindvall 1985) have been reported in teeth bleached by the internal bleaching technique using 35% hydrogen peroxide. In the latter study most of the teeth were associated with previous trauma and it is not known whether the trauma predisposed the tooth to the resorption or whether it was caused by the effects of the bleach. pH measurements of the root surface have demonstrated cervical resorption occurring in those teeth that were not previously traumatised.

WHITER, BRIGHTER OR LIGHTER?

A change in colour is normally evident within two weeks of starting the bleaching procedure (Cibirka et al 1999), but whether this colour change is due to the tooth becoming whiter, lighter or brighter is not known at present.

There is often a decrease in the translucency of the tooth, which may contribute to the effect, appearing as an improvement in the 'brightness' (Lyons and Ng 1998) and 'whiteness' of the tooth. The whiteness may be that the tooth has become dehydrated (Darnell and Moore 1990) following the bleaching procedure. This may be a transient effect. The brightening effect usually regresses over time (Garber et al 1991). It is not apparent what effect or combination of effects is occurring. A brightness index derived from computer analysis of digitized images may be useful for monitoring effectiveness of bleaching (Bentley et al 1999).

PATIENT RESPONSE TO HOME BLEACHING

Appropriate patient selection and counselling is important for patient satisfaction. In a longitudinal study by Haywood et al (1994) at 1.5 years post-treatment, 74% of patients who had responded to home bleaching were satisfied with the shade of their teeth. At 3 years post-treatment 62% were satisfied with their colour. At 7 years post-treatment of the same patient pool, 35% were satisfied with the colour of their teeth. No one reported reversion to the original shade (Leonard et al 1998).

Patient perceptions of the whitening technique are positive. Ninety-five per cent of patients are genuinely glad they went through the procedure and 97% recommended the procedure to their friends (Leonard 1998). Of the patients surveyed in the latter study, 87% said they would undergo bleaching again.

COLOUR REGRESSION AND SHADE RELAPSE

Once bleaching has been terminated a slight relapse in colour occurs over the following 2 weeks. It has been hypothesized that the tooth is filled with oxygen from the oxidative process and this changes the optical qualities of the tooth to appear more opaque. After 2 weeks, the oxygen has dissipated and the tooth demonstrates the actual lightened shade. Patients should be informed of this phenomenon because they tend to think that the bleaching is regressing; in reality the teeth are equilibrating to the new actual shade (Haywood 1999b). Colour regression occurred within the first month after bleaching in a study by Matis and coworkers 1998.

The process of colour regression towards darker shades is poorly described and understood in the literature (Heymann et al 1998), but is thought to be the opposite of the whitening procedure. Regression occurs over a longer period because some of the previously oxidized substances may become chemically reduced and cause the tooth to reflect the old discoloration or the enamel may become remineralized with the staining molecule of the original stain (Lyons and Ng 1998).

A clinical trial (Leonard et al 1999) evaluating the colour stability after 54 months of tetracycline stained teeth that were treated with 10% carbamide peroxide and extended bleaching times, showed that it is possible for the colour to remain stable for 54 months post-bleaching treatment. The colour stability may be related to the extended treatment time of 6 months. This is the longest post-treatment clinical study published. During this time no patient had to have a crown or root canal treatment as a result of the bleaching treatment. No patient felt the need to have the teeth retreated as a result of colour regression.

A recordable colour regression was noticed in an in-vitro study on teeth that had been bleached by White + Brite and placed into distilled H_2O_2 (Bartlett et al 1991), however the effect of saliva in vivo may reduce such regression. A 4% colour regression after 6 months has been reported in non-vital bleaching (Ho and Goerig 1989). The considerable application time with home bleaching techniques may explain the minimal colour regression reported. Shade retention can be expected in up to 90% of patients at 1 year post-treatment, 62% at 3 years and at least 35% at 7 years (Haywood et al 1994). Patients in the latter study re-whitened on average at 25 months. The shade never reverts to the original shade.

The success rate for home bleaching using a viscous bleaching material for 7–10 days is about 95% (Haywood et al 1994). By changing the treatment time and/or concentration of the bleaching material the success rate for tetracycline teeth is 90%.

RESPONSE OF THE STAINS TO BLEACHING

The initial colour of the affected teeth seems to determine the success or failure of the technique (Arens 1989). It appears that the lighter the stain, the easier it is to bleach. Yellow stains are the easiest to bleach. Less responsive stains in order of decreasing responsiveness are: light grey, light brown, dark yellow, dark brown, grey or black (Swift 1988). Length of bleaching time is an important predictor of success in teeth that have fluorosis staining (Seale and Thrash 1985). They suggested that because of increased porosity, younger teeth would be easier to bleach than older ones.

EFFECTS ON RESTORATIVE MATERIALS

There are mixed reports on the effects of CPS on existing restorative materials in the mouth. Initially, no effects on restorative materials were reported (Haywood et al 1991a). Recent studies have shown surface effects may occur on existing restorative materials (such as composites, glass ionomers and luting cements). A recent in-vitro study of the effects of carbamide peroxide on provisional crowns showed that an orange discoloration occurred with those provisional materials containing methacrylate (Robinson et al 1997).

BOND STRENGTH TO THE ENAMEL

Bleaching is frequently used in combination with other forms of restorative dentistry that require bonding to enamel. These procedures may include replacement of existing restorations to improve shade matching, diastema closure and placement of veneers (see Chapter 11). All these techniques rely on an adequate adhesion of the composite to the enamel. Any factor compromising adhesion can effect the aesthetics and longevity of the bonded restoration (Cvitko et al 1991).

As we have seen, bleaching with peroxide reduces the bond strength of enamel. Studies by Torneck et al (1991) have shown that there is a reduced bond strength of composite to enamel immediately post-bleaching with a 35% solution of hydrogen peroxide. However, the bond strength will improve if etching and bonding is delayed for 1–2 weeks post-bleaching (Titly et al 1991, Godwin et al 1992). Waiting 2 weeks will also allow the colour to stabilize. Hydrogen peroxide appears to change the surface chemistry. Resin tags in bleached enamel are less numerous, less defined and shorter than those in unbleached enamel (Titly et al 1991). The residual oxygen in the bleached tooth surface, also inhibits the polymerisation of the composite resin (McGuckin et al 1991) and disrupts the surface (Haywood 1999a).

Studies using 10% CPS also showed that the bond strength of composite to etched enamel was reduced (Cvitko et al 1991). There were no significant differences in bond strength between the different bleaching gels.

The reduced bond strength is transient, diminished after 24 hours and disappears after one week (Della Bona et al 1992). The use of topical fluoride post-bleaching may help to regain the bond strength (Haywood 1991). The use of acetone- or alcohol-based adhesive systems or roughening the surface may counteract these effects of peroxides on bond strength. More conservative enamel removal may be sufficient to counteract these effects of peroxides on bind strength, but further research is needed.

Internal bleaching of endodontically treated teeth has been shown to result in greater leakage of composite restorations (Barkhorder et al 1997).

COMPOSITE MATERIAL

Reports on the effects of bleaching on composite resins are conflicting. Some studies have shown that composites are unaffected by the CPS (Haywood et al 1991, Baughan et al 1992, Machida et al 1992). Others have shown that surface hardness is altered (Bailey and Swift 1991, Friend et al 1991) while another study showed that surface hardness was unaffected by bleaching (Nathoo et al 1994). Surface roughening and etching may occur (Singleton and Wagner, 1992) and tensile strength is affected (Cullen et al 1992). However, these effects are unlikely to be clinically significant (Swift 1998).

Haywood and Heymann (1991) have noted no significant colour changes other than the removal of extrinsic around existing restorations. The effect is primarily the superficial cleansing of the restoration and a lightening of the underlying tooth structure and not an intrinsic colour change of the restorative material itself. Bleaching has been shown to increase the micro-leakage of existing restorations. Restorations may need to be replaced after bleaching owing to the colour change in the tooth.

Amalgam restorations

Although there have been few reports of effects on amalgam restorations, studies (Hummert et al 1992) suggest that there may be significantly more mercury released from amalgam restorations during the bleaching procedure. Rotstein and coworkers (1997) found than 4–30 times as much mercury was released from amalgams in vitro compared to saline controls. Further clarification of this is required. It appears that prolonged treatment with bleaching agents may cause micro-structural changes in amalgam surfaces and this may possibly increase exposure of patients to toxic by-products (Rotstein et al 1997). Existing amalgams may change colour from black to silver (see Figure 3.19). This effect is dependent on the type of dental amalgam used (I. Rotstein 1999, personal communication). However not all combinations of amalgam and bleaching agents result in higher mercury levels.

Other materials

Fired porcelain showed a slight change after being immersed in the bleaching gels for three 2-hour periods a day for 5 weeks (Hunsaker et al 1990). No effect on gold has been reported. Early reports on glass ionomers suggested that they may risk clinical failure when they were exposed to the CPS due to the increased water sorption and hydrolytic degradation (Kao and Lin 1992) but this has now been proven unfounded. There appears to an alteration in the matrix of the glass ionomer (Jefferson et al 1991). Other luting cements may also be affected. Analysis by scanning electron microscopy has revealed erosion of the matrix of the luting cement and there was some degree of crystalline formation (Jefferson et al 1991) of the zinc phosphate cement.

Provisional restorations such as those using intermediate restorative material (IRM) may be affected by hydrogen peroxide. Macroscopically, IRM exposed to hydrogen peroxide appears cracked and swollen,

whereas carbamide peroxide does not appear to have an effect (see Figures 3.20 and 3.21). Provisional crowns made from methyl methacrylate may discolour and turn orange. Polycarbonate crowns and bis-acryl composite temporary materials do not discolour (Robinson et al 1997).

OTHER PROPERTIES OF CARBAMIDE PEROXIDE

CPS is used in a variety of external OTC use products such as ear drops and hair dyes. Patients with known sensitivity or allergy to any of the contents of the ingredients should not use the bleach. Allergic symptoms have been reported, such as swelling of the lips (Goldstein and Garber 1995).

Oral uses and effects

Carbamide peroxide also has an antibacterial effect (Gugan et al 1996), reduces plaque adherence and accumulation and therefore it has been used for treatment of periodontitis, oral hygiene (Stindt and Quenette 1989), reduction of gingivitis, reduction of caries rate, and aphthous ulceration (Tse et al 1991). It has been used since 1960 for oral wound debridement (Fasanaro 1992). CPS has been incorporated into a chewing gum with inhibition of plaque formation (Moss 1999). It has also been tried for treatment of recurrent herpes labialis. It has been tested for use as an irrigant in root canals as an adjunctive to sodium hypochlorite or as a lubricant in root canals (Stindt and Quenette 1989). It was also used for postoperative rinsing following tooth extraction. The studies using CPS have shown promising results.

Systemic side effects

The only systemic effect that has been reported has been one case that produced a mild laxative effect, because of the glycerine

Table 3.2 Possible side effects with bleaching materials

Gingivae
 Tissue sloughing
 Minor gingival irritation and/or ulceration
 Change in gingival texture
 Gingival soreness

Teeth
 Bleaching occurs in an uneven manner
 White spots or banding within the tooth may be
   more noticeable
 A demarcation line may be visible between the
   colour on the incisal tip and the cervical neck

Oral mucosa
 Sore throat
 Unpleasant taste
 Burning palate

Pain and sensitivity
 The teeth may become sensitive
 The cervical area may become sensitive, especially in
   an area of gingival recession

Gastric irritation

base (Tse et al 1991). The product concerned was OTC Gly-Oxide (Haywood 1991c).

Owing to the possibility of over-use and abuse of the CPS by the patient at home, it is prudent to encourage the patient to refrain from smoking during treatment (Larson 1990). This would reduce the associated staining.

Conclusion

The majority of the literature and research indicates that the use of 10% carbamide peroxide for the dentist-monitored home bleaching is an effective and safe way to lighten discoloured teeth.

WHITENING TOOTHPASTES

Toothpastes have become more specialized and sophisticated in the last decade (Koertge et al 1998) with many designed to perform either therapeutic or cosmetic functions. The therapeutic function through the use of fluoride should be the reduction of caries incidence and cariogenic bacteria, plaque removal, prevention of calculus formation and the reduction of dentinal sensitivity (Koertge et al 1998). Cosmetically the function of the toothpaste should be to remove stain effectively and increase whiteness of the teeth (Sharif et al 2000).

The introduction of whitening toothpastes has been very rapid. There has not been that much clinical research conducted on these products, which concerns the American Dental Association Council on Therapeutics (1994). There are many questions about these products, particularly whether they are effective at maintaining a white smile after bleaching and delay the colour regression. The whitening toothpastes seem effective at removing surface stains on the teeth and may be useful to reduce extrinsic stains that occur from tea and coffee. They may be used to maintain white teeth after bleaching (Adams 1999).

The toothpastes can be classified according to their mechanism of action (Haywood 1996).

MORE ABRASIVE THAN USUAL

The abrasive toothpastes try to remove the surface staining by 'sanding' the teeth. The paste toothpaste is more abrasive than the gel toothpaste. The overzealous use of the abrasive toothpaste will cause the removal of enamel as well as the stain. This results in the tooth appearing more yellow because the enamel layer is removed and the dentine-to-enamel ratio is changed (Haywood 1996). The combination of a hard toothbrush and an abrasive toothpaste has been recognized as creating further tooth-wear problems.

CHEMICAL REMOVAL OF SURFACE PELLICLE

These toothpastes act to remove the surface pellicle which houses the surface stain. They act in a similar manner to the tartar control toothpastes which aim to prevent the build-up of tartar. Although these toothpastes may be effective against stain reduction, they do not change the internal colour of the teeth (Haywood 1996).

Some products in this category contain titanium dioxide, a white pigment found in paint. It acts by entering the surface irregularities of the tooth (Haywood 1995b) and gives the illusion of whitened teeth. Only a surface phenomenon, titanium dioxide does not penetrate internally and thus does not modify the internal colour or whiten teeth.

TOOTHPASTES CONTAINING PEROXIDES

This type of toothpaste may contain either hydrogen peroxide, calcium peroxide, sodium percarbonate or carbamide peroxide as active ingredients to lighten teeth. Some of the toothpastes contain the same concentration of peroxide as the home bleaching agents, while other toothpastes contain hydrogen peroxide in very low concentration (a 1.5% concentration may be too low to exert a bleaching effect). The mechanism of application does not seem sufficient to warrant a significant amount of tooth lightening. However, long-term use with peroxide-containing toothpastes has the potential to make some changes, but there is a question about their safety (Haywood 1996). They act to remove the discoloration of surface staining and there may also be some chemical effects on the surface stains (Lynch et al 1998).

PROPHYLAXIS PASTE CONTAINING HYDROGEN PEROXIDE

There are prophylaxis pastes on the market which contain hydrogen peroxide and pumice (such as Natural Elegance, Challenge Products, Inc., Osage Beach Missouri, USA). These products are supposed to lighten at the same time as cleaning the tooth during a professional prophylaxis by the hygienist. A preliminary in-vitro study to assess the effect on lightening of teeth by comparing a regular prophylaxis paste with the paste containing hydrogen peroxide, did show more lightening than the regular prophylaxis paste (Bowles et al 1997). It appears that the paste containing hydrogen peroxide lightens teeth by both chemical and abrasive action (Bowles et al 1997).

TOOTHPASTES CONTAINING SODIUM BICARBONATE

The small particle size of the sodium bicarbonate may allow the material to penetrate into the enamel and clean inaccessible areas (Kleber et al 1998). An in-vitro study showed that brushing with a bicarbonate toothpaste has the potential to cause tooth lightening. However, the whitening ability of sodium bicarbonate appears to be dependent on the concentration of sodium bicarbonate, up to a threshold concentration (over 45%). A 65% concentration may also contain other products sodium lauryl sulphate which may facilitate stain removal by sodium bicarbonate.

TOOTHPASTES CONTAINING ENZYMES

The enzymes, such as bromain and papain, remove the pellicle layer and slow down the development of plaque on the surface layer. The enzymes are incorporated into toothpastes to activate or accelerate the whitening potential of the toothpaste.

TOOTHPASTES WITH MULTIPLE COMPONENTS

Some of the whitening toothpastes contain up to 20 ingredients of which 14 are said to be active. Some also contain two or more oxidising agents. A spray product for mouth freshening contains the same ingredients in liquid form (McKenzie 2000).

CLINICAL STUDIES

In a clinical study to assess the stabilising effects of two toothpastes, 30 patients who had had their teeth lightened were randomly assigned to two groups to test two whitening toothpastes (Matis 1998). The results after 3 months showed that the toothpaste containing 10% carbamide peroxide was able to stabilise the tooth lightening effect of the bleaching gel better than the toothpaste containing 3% hydrogen peroxide. However, the hydrogen peroxide had a lower tooth sensitivity rating.

Another randomized, double-blind clinical study by Koertge et al 1998 evaluated the ability of a bicarbonate-containing whitening toothpaste to reduce existing levels of stain and increase whiteness of teeth as compared to a regular silica-based toothpaste. Results showed that although the whiteness was increased with the bicarbonate-containing toothpaste, the stain removal potential differed from the regular toothpaste only at proximal surfaces of the teeth. The effectiveness of the sodium bicarbonate toothpastes was not related to their abrasivity as they are less abrasive than silica-based products.

GENERAL ADVICE

If these whitening toothpastes help to encourage better oral hygiene, they will have a beneficial effect, even if only making patients more conscientious about their home care. It is always essential for the patients to have a regular oral health evaluation and professional oral prophylaxis to remove the surface staining (Haywood 1997c). Patients should be instructed in proper brushing techniques which not only clean the teeth, but also keep the gingiva healthy. Instruction should include selection of an appropriate soft toothbrush, avoidance of over-vigorous brushing of one particular area, and use of a pea sized amount of toothpaste. It may be wise to instruct patients to start on the side of their dominant hand to prevent recession and sensivity of one particular side (Haywood 1996).

BIBLIOGRAPHY

Adams M. (1999) Patient education from the hygienist's perspective. *Contemp Esthetics Restor Dent* June; **3**(1):Suppl 10.

American Dental Association Council on Therapeutics. (1994) Guidelines for the acceptance of peroxide containing oral hygiene products. *J Am Dent Assoc* **125**:1140–2.

Archambault G. (1990) Caution, informed consent remain important as home bleaching grows. *The Dentist* **68**(3):16 and 22.

Arens D. (1989) The role of bleaching in aesthetics. *Dent Clin North Am* **33**:319–36.

Bailey SJ, Swift EJ. (1991) Effects of home bleaching products on resin. *J Dent Res* **70**:570 [Abstract No. 2434].

Barkhorder RA, Kempler D, Plesh X. (1997) Effect on non-vital tooth bleaching on microleakage of resin composite restorations. *Quintessence Int* **28**:341–4.

Barnes DM, Kihn PW, Romberg E, et al. (1998) Clinical evaluation of a new 10% carbamide peroxide tooth whitening agent. *Compend Contin Educ Dent* **19**(10):968–78.

Bartlett DW, Walmslay AD, Rippin JW, Wilson SJ. (1991) Analysis of two home bleaching products. *J Dent Res* **70**:726.[Abstract No. 452].

Baughan L, Dishman M, Covey DA. (1992) Effect of carbamide peroxide on composite resin bond strength. *J Dent Res* **71**:281.[Abstract No. 1403].

Bitter NC. (1995) A scanning electron microscopy study of the long term effect of bleaching agents on the enamel surface in vivo. *Gen Dent* **46**:84–8.

Bowles WH, Frysh H, Baker FL, Browning J. (1997) Preliminary in-vitro evaluation of tooth-lightening prophylaxis paste. *J Esthet Dent* **9**(5):234–5.

Buyers Guide to Whitening Systems. (1998) *Dent Today* **17**(12):88–98.

Christensen GJ. (1997) Tooth Bleaching, state of art. *CRA Newsletter* **21**(4):1–3.

Cibirka RM, Myers M, Downey MC, Nelson SK, Browning WD, Dickinson GL. (1999) Clinical study to tooth shade lightening from dentist-supervised, patient-applied treatment with two 10% carbamide peroxide gels. *J Esthet Dent* **11**:325–31.

Cooper J, Bokmeyer TJ, Bowles WH. (1992) Penetration of the pulp chamber by carbamide peroxide bleaching agents. *J Endodont* **18**(7):315–17.

Cubbon T, Ore D. (1991) Hard tissue and home tooth whiteners. *CDS Review* **85**(5):32–5.

Cullen DR, Nelson JA, Sandvrik JL. (1992) Effect of peroxide bleaches on tensile strength of composite resin material. *J Dent Res* No. 1405:281.

Cvek M, Lindvall AM. (1985) External root resorption following bleaching of pulpless teeth with oxygen peroxide. *Endodont Dent Traumatol* 1:56–60.

Cvitko E, Denehy GE, Swift EJ, Pires JAF. (1991) Bond strength of composite resin to enamel bleached with carbamide peroxide. *J Esthet Dent* 13:100–2.

Darnell DH, Moore WC. (1990) Vital tooth bleaching: The White and Brite Technique. *Compend Contin Educ Dent* 11(2):86–94.

Della Bona A, Baghi N, Berry TG, Godwin JM. (1992) In-vitro bond strength testing of bleached dentine. *J Dent Res* 71:659.[Abstract No. 1154].

Fasanaro TS. (1992) Bleaching teeth: history, chemicals and methods used for common tooth discoloratons. *J Esthet Dent* 4(3):71–8.

Fay RM, Powers JM. (1999) Nightguard Vital Bleaching: a review of the literature 1994–1999. *J Gt Houston Dent Soc* 71(4):20–6.

Feinman R, Madray G, Yarborough D. (1991) Chemical, optical and physiologic mechanisms of bleaching products: a review. *Pract Periodont Aesthetic Dent* 3(2):32–7.

Fischer D (2000a) Is there a future for dentist supervised tray tooth bleaching? *Restor Aesthet Prac* 2(1):72–5.

Fischer D (2000b) The need for dentist supervision when tooth bleaching. *Restor Aesthet Prac* 2(2):98–9.

Friend GW, Jones JE, Wamble SH, Covington JS. (1991) Carbamide peroxide tooth bleaching: changes to composite resins after prolonged exposure. *J Dent Res* 70:570.[Abstract No. 2432].

Frysh H, Baker FL, Wagner MJ. (1991) Patients perception of effectiveness of 3 vital tooth bleaching systems. *J Dent Res* 70:570.[Abstract No. 2430].

Garber D, Goldstein R, Goldstein C, Schwartz C. (1991) Dentist monitored bleaching: a combined approach. *Pract Periodont Aesthetic Dent* 3(2):22–6.

Gerlach RW. (2000) Shifting paradigms in whitening: introduction of a novel system for vital tooth bleaching. *Compend Contin Educ Dent* 21(Suppl 29):4–9.

Godwin JM, Barghi N, Berry TG, Knight GT, Hummert TW. (1992) Time duration of dissipation of bleaching effects before enamel bonding. *J Dent Res* 71:179.[Abstract No. 590].

Goldstein RE, Garber DA. (1995) *Complete dental bleaching.* Quintessence Publishing: Chicago, Berlin and London.

Greenwall LH. (1992a) Home bleaching. *J Dent Assoc South Africa* 6:304–5.

Greenwall LH. (1992b) The effects of carbamide peroxide on tooth colour and structure: an in-vitro investigation. MSc Thesis. University of London.

Greenwall LH. (1999) Home bleaching: the materials. *Independent Dent* 4(5):70–7.

Grobler SR, Senekal PJC, Laubscher JA. (1990) *Clin Prevent Dent* 12(5):5–9.

Gugan S, Bolay S, Alacam R. (1996) Antibacterial activity of 10% carbamide peroxide bleaching agents. *J Endodont* 22(7):356–7.

Haywood VB. (1991a) Overview and status of mouthguard bleaching. *J Esthet Dent* 3(5):157–61.

Haywood VB. (1991b) Nightguard Vital Bleaching, a history and products update: Part 1. *Esthet Dent Update* 2(4):63–6.

Haywood VB. (1991c) Nightguard Vital Bleaching, a history and products update: Part 2. *Esthet Dent Update* 2(5):82–5.

Haywood VB. (1995a) Advice to patients on over the counter bleaching agents. *Esthet Dent Update* 6(3):73–4.

Haywood VB. (1995b) Update on bleaching: material changes. *Esthet Dent Update* 6(3):74.

Haywood VB. (1996) Achieving, maintaining and recovering successful tooth bleaching. *J Esthet Dent* 8(1):31–8.

Haywood VB. (1997a) Bleaching of vital teeth. Current concepts. *Quintessence Int* 28(6):424–5.

Haywood VB. (1997b) Nightguard Vital Bleaching: current concepts and research. *J Am Dent Assoc* 128:19S-25S.

Haywood VB. (1997c) Historical development of whiteners: clinical safety and efficacy. *Dental Update* 24(3):89–104.

Haywood VB. (1999a) Ask the experts. Self-cured composites and bleaching. *J Esthet Dent* 11(3):122–3.

Haywood VB. (1999b) Current status and recommendations for dentist-prescribed, at-home tooth whitening. *Contemp Esthet Restor Pract* 3(Suppl 1):2–9.

Haywood VB, Heymann HO. (1991) Nightguard Vital Bleaching: how safe is it? *Quintessence Int* 22(7):515–23.

Haywood VB, Robinson FG. (1997) Vital tooth bleaching with Nightguard Vital Bleaching. *Curr Opin Cosmetic Dent* 4:45–52.

Haywood VB, Houck VM, Heymann HO. (1991) Nightguard Vital Bleaching: effects of various solutions on enamel texture and color. *Quintessence Int* 22:775–82.

Haywood VB, Leech T, Heymann HO, Crumpler D, Bruggers K. (1990) Nightguard Vital

Bleaching: effects on enamel surface texture and diffusion. *Quintessence Int* 21(10):801–4.

Haywood VB, Leonard RH, Dickinson GL. (1997) Efficacy of six-months Nightguard Vital Bleaching of tetracycline-stained teeth. *J Esthet Dent* 9(1):13–19.

Haywood VB, Leonard RH, Nelson CF. (1994) Effectiveness, side effects and long term status of Nightguard Vital Bleaching. *J Am Dent Assoc* 125:1219–26.

Heymann HO, Swift EJ, Bayne SC, et al. (1998) Clinical evaluation of two carbamide peroxide tooth-whitening agents. *Compend Contin Educ Dent* 19(4):359–76.

Ho S, Goerig AC. (1989) An in-vitro comparison of different bleaching agents in the discoloured tooth. *J Endodont* 15(3):106–11.

Howard WR. (1992) Patient-applied tooth whiteners. *J Am Dent Assoc* 132(2):57–60.

Hummert T, Osborne JW, Godwin J. (1992) Mercury in solution following exposure of various amalgams to carbamide peroxides. *J Dent Res* 71:281.[Abstract No. 1407].

Hunsaker KJ, Christensen GJ, Christensen RP. (1990) Tooth bleaching chemicals - influence on teeth and restorations. *J Dent Res* 69:303.[Abstract No. 1558].

Jay AT. (1990) Tooth whitening: the financial rewards. *Dental Management* 30(12):28–31.

Jefferson KL, Zena RB, Giammara BT. (1991) The effects of carbamide peroxide on dental luting agents. *J Dent Res* 70:571.[Abstract No. 2440].

Kao EC, Lin PP. (1992) Hydrolytic degradation of composites and ionomer after exposure to bleach. *J Dent Res* 71:281.[Abstract No. 1406].

Kelleher MGD, Roe FJC. (1999) The safety-in-use of 10% carbamide peroxide (Opalescence) for bleaching teeth under the supervision of a dentist. *Br Dent J* 187(4):190–4.

Kleber CJ, Moore MH, Nelson BJ. (1998) Laboratory assessment of tooth whitening by sodium bicarbonate dentifrices. *J Clin Dent* 9(3):72–5.

Koertge TE, Brooks CN, Sarbin AG, Powers D, Gunsolley JC. (1998) A longitudinal comparison of tooth whitening resulting from dentifrice use. *J Clin Dent* 9(3):67–71.

Kowitz GM, Nathoo SA, Wong R. (1994) Clinical comparison of Colgate Platinum Tooth-whitening System and Rembrandt Gel plus. *Compend Contin Educ Dent Suppl* S646–51.

Larson TD. (1990) The effects of peroxides on teeth and tissue: review of the literature. *Northwest Dentistry* 69(6):29–32.

Latcham NL. (1986) Post-bleaching cervical resorption. *J Endodont* 12(6):262–4.

Leonard RH, Bentley C, Phillips C, et al (1997) ADA controlled clinical trial of a 10%

carbamide peroxide solution. *J Dent Res* 76:309.[Abstract].

Leonard RH, Haywood VB, Eagle JC, et al. (1999) Nightguard Vital Bleaching of tetracycline-stained teeth: 54 months post-treatment. *J Esthet Dent* 11(5):265–77.

Leonard RH, Knight A, Haywood VB, et al. (1998) Nightguard Vital Bleaching—stability and side effects, 82 months post-whitening treatment. *J Dent Res* 77(AADR Abstracts) no.1339.

Leonard RH, Sharma A, Haywood VB. (1998) Use of different concentrations of carbamide peroxide for bleaching teeth: an in-vitro study. *Quintessence Int* 29:503–7.

Leonard RH. (1998) Efficacy, longevity, side effects and patient perceptions of Nightguard Vital Bleaching. *Compend Contin Educ Dent* 19(8):776–81.

Li Y. (1998) Tooth bleaching using peroxide containing agents: current status of safety issues. *Compend Contin Educ Dent* 19(8):783–94.

Lynch E, Sheering A, Samarawhickrama DYD, et al. (1998) Molecular mechanisms of the bleaching actions associated with commercially available whitening oral health care products. *J Irish Dent Assoc* 41(4):94–102.

Lyons K, Ng B. (1998) Nightguard Vital Bleaching: a review and clinical study. *NZ Dent J* 94(417):100–3.

Machida S, Anderson MH, Bales DJ. (1992) Effect of home bleaching agents on adhesion to tooth structure. *J Dent Res* 71:600.[Abstract No. 678].

Madison S, Walton R. (1990) Cervical root resorption following bleaching of endodontically treated teeth. *J Endodont* 16(12):570–4.

Matis BA, Cochran MA, Eckert G, Carlson TJ. (1998) The efficacy and safety of a 10% carbamide peroxide bleaching gel. *Quintessence Int* 29:555–63.

Matis BA, Gaiao U, Blackman D, et al. (1999) In-vivo degradation of bleaching gel used in whitening teeth. *J Am Dent Assoc* 130:227–35.

Matis BA. (1998) Dentifrice whitening after professional bleaching. *J Indiana Dent Assoc* 77(3):27–32.

McCaslin AJ, Haywood VB, Potter BJ, Dickinson GL, Russel CM. (1999) Assessing dentin colour changes from Nightguard Vital Bleaching. *J Am Dent Assoc* Oct;130:1485–90.

McCracken MS, Haywood VB, et al. (1996) Demineralisation effects of 10 percent carbamide peroxide. *J Dent* 24:395–8.

McEvoy SA. (1989) Chemical agents for removing intrinsic stains from vital teeth. (ii) Current techniques and their clinical application. *Quintessence Int* 20(6):379–84.

McGuckin RS, Thurmond BA, Osovitz S. (1991) In vitro enamel shear bond strengths following vital bleaching. *J Dent Res* **70**:377.

McKenzie T (2000) Over the counter tooth whitening products. *Restorative and Aesthetic Practice* in press.

Moss SJ. (1999) Carbamide and food – a review of the literature. *FDI World* **3**:9–14.

Murphy A, Samarawickrama DYD, Lynch E. (1992) Microradiographic assessment of roots of teeth after home bleaching. *J Dent Res* **701**:540.[Abstract No. 201].

Nathanson D. (1997) Vital tooth bleaching: sensitivity and pulpal considerations. *J Am Dent Assoc* **128**(Suppl):41S-44S.

Nathoo SA, Chielewski MB, Kirkups RE (1994). Effects of Colgate Platinum Professional Tooth Whitening System on microhardness of enamel, dentin and composite resins. *Compend Contin Educ Dent* **15**:S627–S630.

Oliver TL, Haywood VB. (1999) Efficacy of Nightguard Vital Bleaching technique beyond the borders of a shortened tray. *J Esthet Dent* **11**(2):95–102.

Powell VL, Bales DJ. (1991) Tooth bleaching: its effect on oral tissues. *J Am Dent Assoc* **122**:50–4.

Reinhardt JW, Eivins SC, Swift EJ, et al. (1993) Clinical study of Nightguard Vital Bleaching. *Quintessence Int* **24**:379–84.

Robertson WD, Melfi RC. (1980) Pulp responses to vital bleaching procedures. *J Endodont* **6**:645–9.

Robinson F, Haywood VB, Myers M. (1997) Effect of 10% carbamide peroxide on colour of provisional restoration materials. *J Am Dent Assoc* **128**:727–31.

Rosenstiel SF, Gegauff AG, Johnston WM. (1996) Randomised clinical trial of the efficacy and safety of a home bleaching procedure. *Quintessence Int* **27**(6):413–24.

Rotstein CD, Friedman S. (1991) pH variation among materials used for intracoronal bleaching. *J Endodont* **17**(8):376–9.

Rotstein I, Cohenca N, Mor C, et al. (1995) Effects of carbamide peroxide and hydrogen peroxide on surface morphology and zinc oxide levels of IRM fillings. *Endodont Dent Traumatol* **11**:279–83.

Rotstein I, Dankner E, Goldman A, et al. (1996) Histochemical analysis of dental hard tissues following bleaching. *J Endodont* **22**:23–5.

Rotstein I, Mor C, Arwaz JR. (1997) Changes in surface levels of mercury, silver, tin and copper of dental amalgams treated with carbamide peroxide and hydrogen peroxide in vitro. *Oral Surg, Oral Med, Oral Pathol, Oral Radiol, Endodont* **83**:506–9.

Russel CM, Dickinson GL, Johnson MH, et al. (1996) Dentist-supervised home bleaching with ten percent carbamide peroxide gel: a six month study. *J Esthet Dent* **8**(4):177–82.

Sagel PA, Odioso LL, McMillan DA, Gerlach RW. (2000) Vital tooth whitening with a novel hydrogen peroxide strip system: design, kinetics and clinical response. *Compend Contin Educ Dent* **21**(Suppl 29):10–15.

Scherer W, Cooper H, Ziegler B, Vijayaraghaven TV. (1991) At-home bleaching system: effects on enamel and cementum. *J Esthet Dent* **3**:54–6.

Seale NS, Thrash WJ. (1985) Systematic assessment of color removal following vital bleaching of intrinsically stained teeth. *J Dent Res* **64**(3):457–61.

Seghi RR, Denry I. (1992) Effects of external bleaching on indentation and abrasion characteristics of human enamel in vitro. *J Dent Res* **71**:1340–1344.

Sharif N, MacDonald E, Hughes J, Newcombe RG, Addy M. (2000) The chemical stain removal properties of whitening toothpaste product studies in vitro. *Br Dent J* **188**(11):620–4.

Shearer AC. (1991) External bleaching of teeth. *Dental Update* **18**(7):289–91.

Singleton LS, Wagner MJ. (1992) Peroxide tooth whitener concentration versus composite resin etching. *J Dent Res* **71**:281.[Abstract No. 1404].

Small BW. (1994) Bleaching with 10% carbamide peroxide: an 18 month study. *Gen Dent* **42**(2):142–46.

Stindt DJ, Quenette L. (1989) An overview of glyoxide liquid in control and prevention of dental disease. *Compend Contin Educ Dent* **10**(9):514–19.

Swift EJ. (1998) A method for bleaching discolored vital teeth. *Quintessence Int* **19**(9):607–11.

Swift EJ, May KN, Wilder AD, et al. (1997) Six-month clinical evaluation of a tooth whitening system using an innovative experimental design. *J Esthet Dent* **9**(5):265–74.

Thitinanthapan W, Satamanont P, Vongsavan N. (1999) In vitro penetration of the pulp chamber by three brands of carbamide peroxide. *J Esthet Dent* **11**(5):259–44.

Titley KC, Torneck CD, Smith DC, Chernecky R, Adibfar A. (1991) Scanning electron microscopy observations on the penetration and structure on the resin tags in bleached and unbleached bovine enamel. *J Endodont* **17**(2):72–5.

Torneck CD, Titley KC, Smith DC, Adibfar A. (1991) Effect of water leaching on the adhesion of composite resin to unbleached and bleached bovine enamel. *J Endodont* **17**(4):156–60.

Tse SC, Lynch E, Blake DR, Williams DM. (1991) Is home bleaching gel cytotoxic? *J Esthet Dent* **3**(5):162–8.

Zalkind M, Arwaz JR, Goldman A, Rotstein I. (1996) Surface morphology changes in human enamel, dentin and cementum following bleaching: a scanning electron microscope study. *Endodont Dent Traumatol* **12**(2):82–4.

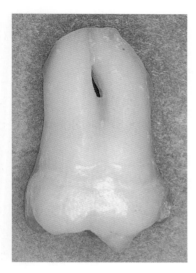

Figure 3.1

An experimental design for testing the bleaching material was devised. Teeth were discoloured artificially by spinning blood into them. The colour and appearance of a tooth is shown before bleaching with the OTC kit. (From Greenwall 1992.)

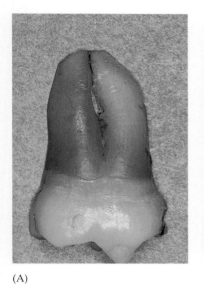

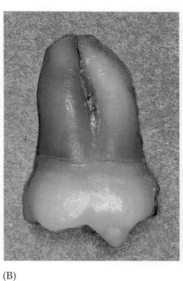

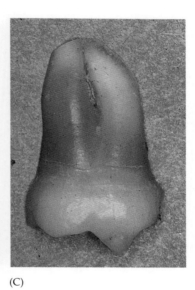

(A)   (B)   (C)

Figure 3.2

(A) After the discoloration by blood pigment, the tooth was sectioned and stored in artificial saliva. The appearance of the tooth after 3 days of bleaching. Note that although the bleaching material is placed onto the enamel surface only, the root surface is also getting lighter. (B) The appearance of the tooth after 7 days. (C) The appearance of the tooth after 28 days. Note the apex of the root has also lightened.

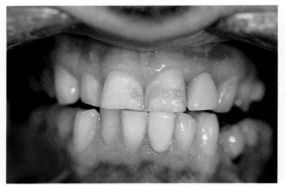

(A)

(B)

Figure 3.3

(A) This patient purchased an OTC bleaching kit to lighten his discoloured front teeth. It is not known if there was severe erosion before the kit was used, but this is the appearance of the teeth as he presented on his first visit to the practice. He reported that he tried bleaching his teeth at home for 3 weeks and stopped when he did not notice any change in the colour of his teeth. There is a porcelain bonded to a metal crown on the lateral incisor which does not change colour with bleaching in any event. In this case bleaching treatment is inappropriate and this highlights the problems associated with OTC kits. (B) The appearance of the teeth after crown lengthening surgery to reshape the gingival height of the right central and lateral incisors. Porcelain laminates were placed on these teeth and a new porcelain bonded to metal crown at the correct alignment and emergence profile. (C) The patient's smile after treatment.

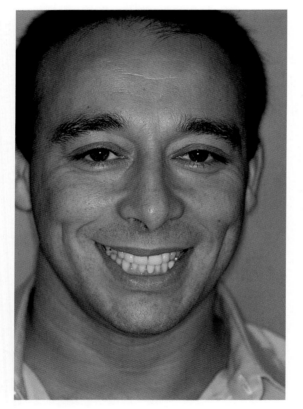

(C)

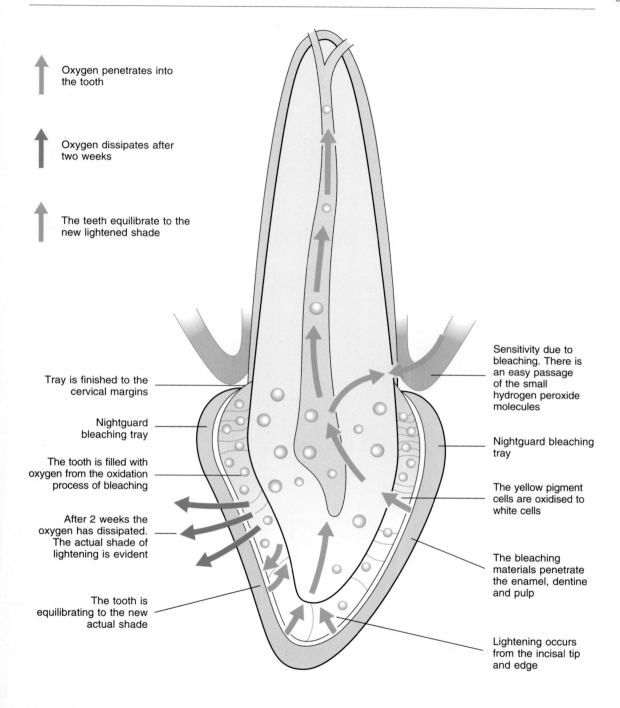

Figure 3.4

Movement of carbamide peroxide through the tooth.

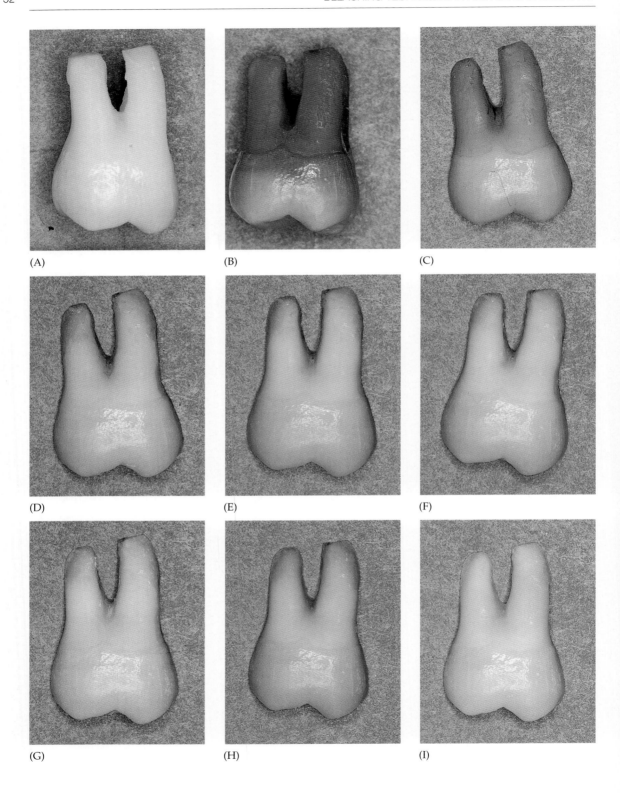

(A)

(B)

(C)

(D)

(E)

(F)

(G)

(H)

(I)

Figure 3.5

Teeth were discoloured artificially in vitro using the same technique as described in Figure 3.2 (Greenwall 1992). The teeth were stored in artificial saliva when not being bleached. The bleaching treatment was undertaken for two 90-min sessions per day. After the first session, new bleaching material was placed on the teeth. The specimen was treated with Rembrandt Lighten (10% carbamide peroxide solution) and the photo sequence demonstrates the lightening process as it took place. At the end of 28 days, the colour was lighter than the original colour before bleaching, as assessed by a panel of four independent assessors. (A) The colour of the tooth before bleaching. (B) The appearance of the tooth immediately after blood discoloration. (C) The appearance of the tooth after sectioning and bathed in artificial saliva. (D) The appearance of the tooth after 90 min of bleaching treatment with Rembrandt Lighten. (E) The appearance of the tooth after 3 hours of bleaching treatment. (F) The appearance of the tooth after 3 days of bleaching treatment. (G) The result after 7 days of bleaching treatment. (H) The result after 14 days of bleaching treatment. (I) The result after 28 days of bleaching treatment. Note the colour of the tooth is lighter than the original colour before bleaching treatment commenced.

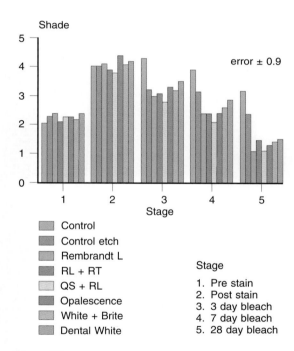

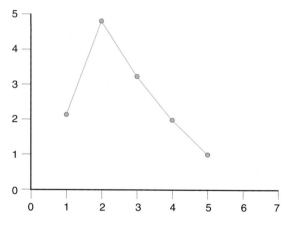

Figure 3.7

This shows the result of the bleaching treatment with Opalescence bleaching gel. The Carbopol enhances the bleaching action. The colour change is significant and the final shade of the bleached enamel is lighter than the original colour. The y-axis is the shade and the x-axis is the bleaching stage as in the key shown in Figure 3.6.

Figure 3.6

Although this was an in-vitro study, the results are demonstrated graphically. The stages of the bleaching treatment are itemized on the lower right-side key column. The shade was assessed by four independent assessors and a customized shade tab was used to assess shade differences. The shades are itemised as 1–5 from the lightest to the darkest colour. It is interesting to note that after 28 days of bleaching treatment, all teeth lightened, no matter what product was used. The control teeth also lightened, but this was not significant.

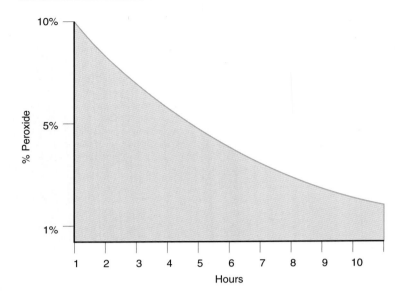

Figure 3.8

The breakdown of peroxide over time, with the Opalescence bleaching materials.

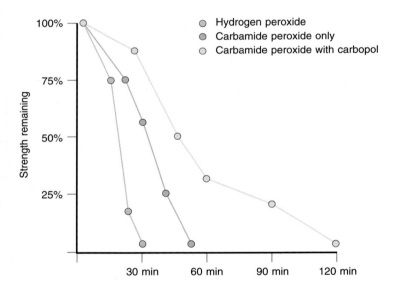

Figure 3.9

The difference in degradation rates of the different bleaching materials (courtesy of Dr I. Rotstein).

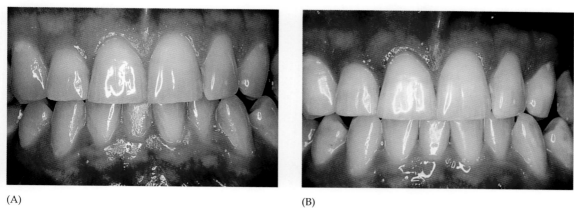

(A)   (B)

Figure 3.10

A middle aged male with ageing staining. A vital bleaching technique was used for 4 weeks. (A) This shows the appearance of the teeth before bleaching treatment. (B) After 4 weeks of bleaching treatment with Opalescence bleaching gel (Ultradent Products, Inc., South Jordan, Utah). (Courtesy of Dr V. Gordan.)

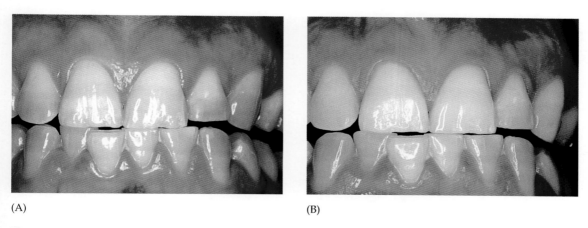

(A)   (B)

Figure 3.11

A 24-year-old female with mild tetracycline staining. Vital bleaching treatment with opalescence bleaching gel was used. (A) the appearance of the teeth before bleaching. (B) The appearance of the teeth after 6.5 weeks of bleaching treatment. (Courtesy of Dr V. Gordan.)

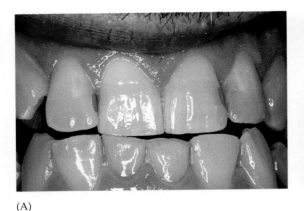

(A)

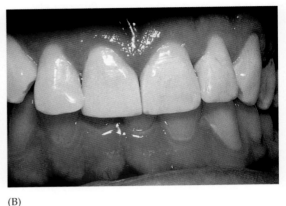

(B)

Figure 3.12

A middle-aged male with a combination of tobacco and ageing staining. Vital bleaching treatment was used for 3 weeks. The old composite restorations were replaced after bleaching treatment. (A) The appearance of the teeth before bleaching treatment. (B) The result after 3 weeks of home bleaching treatment. (Courtesy of Dr V. Gordan.)

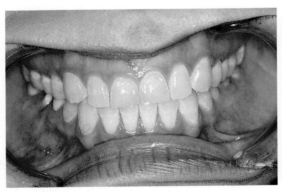

(A)

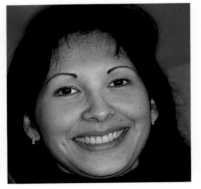

(B)

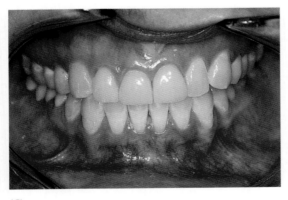

(C)

Figure 3.13

This patient noticed that her teeth were discoloured and purchased an OTC bleaching kit from an Internet mail order company. She used the bleaching material for 2 weeks before terminating the treatment as she felt it was unsuccessful. It is not known whether these teeth were eroded prior to commencing the OTC bleaching procedure. Bleaching treatment is inappropriate for this patient because there is erosive wear on the teeth. (A) Intra-oral view of the erosive wear on the labial surfaces of the upper central incisors and upper right lateral incisor. (B) The portrait of the patient after three porcelain laminates were placed on the eroded teeth. It is more appropriate to place porcelain veneers to protect the enamel from further wear and to improve the smile of the patient. (C) The intra-oral view of the patient after treatment.

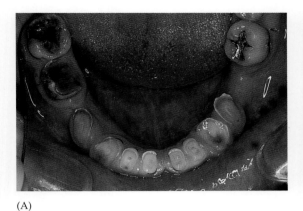

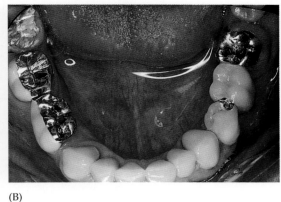

(A) (B)

Figure 3.14

This patient has severe tooth wear of unknown origin. (A) The teeth are discoloured due to erosion of the enamel. Bleaching treatment is not appropriate for this patient. (B) The result of the extensive restorative dentistry that was required to restore health and function to this patient.

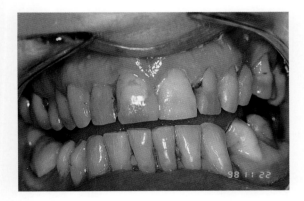

Figure 3.15

The anterior composite restorations are too large for an effective result with bleaching, however bleaching treatment can be performed first as an adjunct to treatment prior to placing porcelain laminates. The lightening helps to enhance the aesthetics of the laminates.

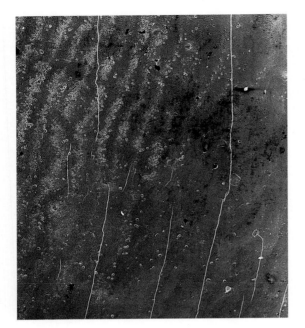

Figure 3.16

The normal appearance of non-bleached enamel under the scanning electron microscope. There is a great variation in the appearance of enamel and this is also related to the particular area chosen to view. The porosity of the enamel surface shows how the bleaching material can enter the tooth and travel along the prisms.

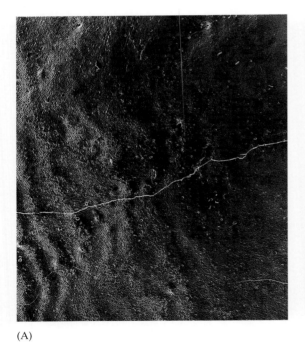

(A)

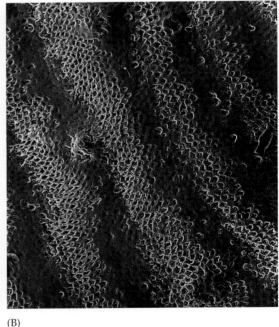

(B)

Figure 3.17

The appearance of enamel which was (A) bleached for 4 weeks with 10% carbamide peroxide (Opalescence bleaching material). The appearance is very similar to the appearance of unbleached enamel. (B) A closer view: the bleaching material travels along the interprismatic substance which acts like a wick to allow permeation of oral fluids.

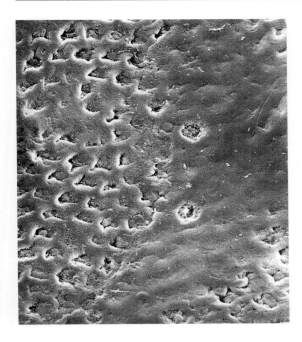

Figure 3.18

A close view of enamel which was bleached with a different 10% carbamide peroxide bleaching material (White + Brite). The appearance of the enamel is similar to that in Figures 3.16 and 3.17.

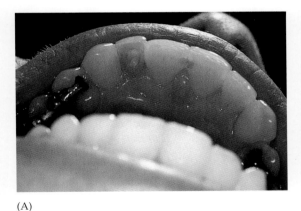

(A)

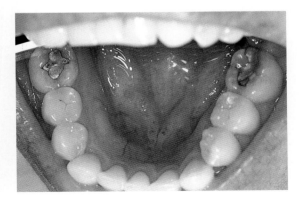

(C)

Figure 3.19

(A) The appearance of the amalgam restorations in a patient prior to bleaching treatment. The existing amalgam restorations are dark as they have been present for 15 years. (B) The same patient after bleaching treatment. The passivation layer of the amalgam restoration is removed and the surface of the restorations have been oxidised and appear much lighter in colour. (C) The posterior amalgam restorations on the lower teeth are also a lighter grey colour. After bleaching treatment and a period to let the colour settle, these restorations were replaced with composite restorations (see Figure 9.6).

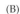

(B)

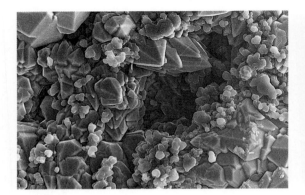

Figure 3.20

A scanning electron micrograph showing the appearance of 10% carbamide peroxide on intermediate restorative material (IRM). This material is sometimes used for barrier placement of non-vital bleaching. In view of this effect, it may be more appropriate to use glass ionomer material as an effective barrier instead. (By courtesy of Dr I. Rotstein.)

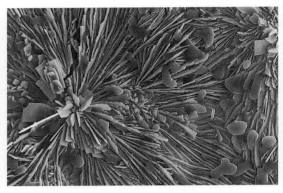

Figure 3.21

A scanning electron micrograph showing the effect of 10% hydrogen peroxide solution on IRM. This concentration of hydrogen peroxide is used in power bleaching procedures. (By courtesy of Dr I. Rotstein.)

4 TREATMENT PLANNING FOR SUCCESSFUL BLEACHING

INTRODUCTION

When planning treatment for bleaching and other associated aesthetic treatments it is essential to carefully understand the patients' needs, requirements and desires for their teeth. This can be achieved by undertaking a full and comprehensive dental and oral examination. This chapter will demonstrate methods of gathering useful information about patients, emphasizing the importance of medical and dental histories. Patient communication, methods for undertaking a smile analysis, managing patients' expectations, informed consent and planning fees for bleaching treatment will be discussed. Examples of questionnaires and forms are provided, which can be used in the information-gathering process.

PATIENT COMMUNICATION

Beauty is an abstract and subjective concept, but an essential and ineradicable part of human nature (Etcoff 1999). Culture, age, gender and time can influence perception of beauty. Because of this subjectivity, it is extremely important to establish good communication between the dentist and patient early on so that both can work towards the same goals. Excellent communication leads to treatment acceptance (Jameson 1994) with the patient understanding the benefits and risks, advantages and disadvantage of each treatment option that is available. This is particularly important when the patient's expectations exceed the reality of

what is possible to achieve (see Figure 4.17C). Studies have shown significant differences between dentists and patient preferences for aesthetic dentistry (Brisman 1980).

A questionnaire can be used to evaluate the patient's hopes and aspirations for his or her smile (see Figure 4.2). The questionnaire can include questions regarding the patient's self-perception of teeth and smile. Questions should be open-ended, allowing the patient to talk and express any concerns. Patients can be asked about shape, positioning, colour and proportion of teeth. The information gathered will establish a base for the clinician to interact, communicate and evaluate the patient's problems.

The individuality of each case makes aesthetic decisions more difficult, but also more interesting and challenging. Patients should be educated and questioned regarding their expectations and perceived final outcome. Before bleaching techniques can be undertaken it is essential to start with a comprehensive dental and oral health evaluation. It is useful to gather information with a checklist so that all the information that is necessary is received.

NEW PATIENT CHECKLIST

As with any normal new patient consultation, it is important to evaluate:

- medical history
- previous dental history: patient's attitude to dentistry, patient's previous experiences, patient's expectations (see Figure 4.2)

- extraoral examination: besides assessing for pathology and temperomandibular joint dysfunction, it is essential to do a smile analysis (see Figure 4.4)
- intraoral examination (Figure 4.3)
  - soft tissue examination
  - dental examination
  - periodontal examination
  - occlusal examination
  - assessment of the temperomandibular joint dysfunction
  - special considerations: vitality tests
- Other information: study models, facebow records, articulated study models.

Medical history

The patient's medical history should be carefully assessed. A specific bleaching questionnaire should be filled out with the patient (see Figure 4.1). Patients' smoking habits need to be assessed: they should not smoke and bleach their teeth. It is essential for those patients who smoke to stop or at least reduce the amount they are smoking before bleaching is undertaken. This can sometimes be used as an incentive for patients to stop smoking altogether. Allergies to plastic, peroxide or any of the other ingredients of the bleach should be noted. Patients' current medications need to be recorded on the medical history sheet, especially those preparations that cause a dry mouth such as antihistamines. Patients taking hormones sometimes have an exaggerated gingival response. Patients who are pregnant or breastfeeding should be excluded from bleaching procedures because there is lack of information concerning possible effects on the developing fetus (Haywood 1995a).

Dental history

The aetiology of the discoloration needs to be assessed because different causes (e.g. caries, internal resorption, trauma) necessitate different treatments. Extrinsic staining can usually be easily removed with a good dental cleaning and prophylaxis. Establish whether new patients are regular dental attenders or those who only visit the dentist when they have pain, as the latter type of patient may not comply with home bleaching instructions and may not follow the bleaching programme or return for review appointments when requested.

SMILE ANALYSIS AND AESTHETICS

What makes a beautiful smile? One definition is one in which the size, position, and colour of the teeth are in harmony, proportion and relative symmetry to each other and with the elements that frame them. Analysis, by definition means reduction of the component parts in order to discover the interrelationships (Ricketts (1968). The components of a smile consist of the facial components (the facial features, tooth visibility, age, upper lip curvature, negative space, smile symmetry and occlusal line) as well as the dental components (the dental midline, axial alignment, tooth arrangement, gradation, shape of the teeth, contact points, and the gingival morphology and contour) and the physical components (Rufenacht 1990). The teeth are only part of a greater picture that must be viewed within the frame of the gingival soft tissue, the interarch dark space, the lips (Moskowitz and Nayyar 1995) and the face (Paletz et al 1994).

Bleaching teeth alone may not solve patients' aesthetic requirements (see Figures 4.8F and 4.9). A smile analysis should be conducted prior to bleaching and should be included in the treatment planning stages. Smile analysis sheets can be used to determine the smile requirements and the patient's needs (see Figure 4.8). There are many factors to consider when conducting a smile analysis: the shape and length of the teeth; the lip line; the smile line, and the occlusal relationship of the teeth. Each element is an important feature, but all these features are interwoven to create aesthetic harmony (Moskowitz and Nayyar 1995).

Table 4.1 Treatment planning checklist[1]

Stage 1 Emergency treatment: elimination of pain
- Dressings.
- Emergency relief of pain-emergency root canal therapy.
- Extractions.
- Control of infections.
- Discuss possible treatment options, treatment implications, financial arrangements.

Stage 2 Elimination of active disease and achievement of oral stability: disease control
- Periodontal:
  - Assessment with indices
  - Oral hygiene instruction
  - Scaling and prophylaxis
  - Root surface debridement (root planning and curettage)
  - Surgery
  - Other treatment
- Caries control:
  - Use of fluorides: topical applications, mouthwash
  - Dietary counselling
  - Provisional restorations and simple restorations:
    Intracoronal restorations: glassionomers, composites, amalgams
    Extracoronal restorations: provisional veneers, crowns, bridges, prostheses
- Root canal treatment
- Extractions: routine, surgical
- Occlusal analysis and adjustment
- Orthodontics
- Referral for advice/treatment
- Other treatment: consider bleaching after elimination of active disease.

Stage 3 Definitive and restorations: once oral stability has been achieved
- Monitor periodontium
- Monitor caries (non-active lesions)
- Record indices as applicable
- Assess long-term implications with patient (costs, ability to maintain)
- Periodontal: monitoring, crown lengthening, other
- Bleaching
- Definitive restorations:
  - Veneers/laminates
  - Crowns
  - Bridges
  - Prosthesis
- Orthodontics
- Implant fixture placement
- Oral surgery
- Other (including post treatment photographs).

Stage 4 Maintenance and monitoring at monthly intervals
- Record indices
- Check radiographs
- Review preventive advice: dietary assessment, oral hygiene instruction, fluoride applications
- Oral prophylaxis
- Repeat aspects of Stage 2 and Stage 3 if applicable (such as implant abutment connection and implant prosthesis).

Administration
- Written treatment plan with financial responsibilities sent to patient.
- Estimated laboratory bill.
- Patient's written acceptance of treatment plan.
- Total time estimated.
- Appointments scheduled accordingly.
- Total fees earned.

[1]Adapted and modified from Eaton and Nathan (1998) with kind permission

COMPONENTS OF A SMILE

Three essentials of a smile involve the relationships between the three primary components (Garber and Salama 1996):

1 The teeth
- The shade and shape
- Position, length and axial alignment
- The tooth surface characteristics and morphology
- The shade and shape of the opposing dentition
- The occlusion and occlusal line
- The dental midline: this is an imaginary line that separates the two central incisors
- The surface texture: e.g. perikymata, stippling, rippling. The surface texture will not change with bleaching.

2 The lip framework
- The lip line: the amount of tooth exposed during a smile
- The smile line: a hypothetical curved line drawn along the edges of the four anterior maxillary teeth that should run parallel with the curvature of the inner border of the lower lip (Rufenacht 1990)
- The upper lip curvature: the position of the upper lip height relative to the teeth
- Negative space: the dark space that appears between the jaws between laughter and talking
- The smile symmetry: the symmetric placement of the corners of the mouth in the vertical plane (Figure 4.8B)

3 The gingival scaffold
- The gingival height of contour
- Appearance of the gingival tissues
- Symmetry of the heights of the central incisors (Figure 4.8F)
- Incisal and gingival embrasures.

THE GOLDEN PROPORTION

Artists, mathematicians and philosophers have been preoccupied with the relationship between beauty and harmony. Harmony in proportion has been regarded as the essential aesthetic principle. Nature has devised a complex mathematical formula (which was attributed to Pythagoras) which is the relationship of 1:1.618 (Levin 1978). Dr Eddie Levin has designed a golden mean gauge in the same proportion (see Figure 4.10). He discovered that the relationship between the widths of the central and lateral incisors were in the golden proportion and that the lateral negative space was in the golden proportion of one-half the width of the anterior segment. This golden mean gauge can help assess the harmony of the face and can help to determine the relationships of the teeth to the lips and to the face and of the teeth to each other. This gauge can help with planning treatment and lengths and shape of teeth for veneers after bleaching.

WHAT IS AN IDEAL SMILE?

Photographs of models in magazines and advertising always demonstrate the 'ideal smile'. The smile should be harmonious (see Figure 4.7).

The ideal smile is considered to be:

- Bright (Philips 1996).
- Vigorous.
- Youthful, regardless of age (Moskowitz and Nayyar 1995).
- Symmetrical teeth.
- Showing natural teeth.
- Light tooth shade (Dunn et al 1996).
- Healthy gingival colour, harmony and form (Garber and Salama 1996).
- Gingival line following upper lip contour.
- Incisal edge following lower lip contour.

Tooth shade was the most important factor in a study conducted by Dunn et al (1996) to assess patients' perceptions of dental attractiveness. This was followed in sequence by natural (unrestored) tooth appearance and the number of teeth showing. Bleaching is thus such an attractive simple option to lighten the appearance of natural teeth.

INTRAORAL EXAMINATION

The existing condition of the teeth and periodontium needs to be examined prior to bleaching. Defective restorations need to be noted these need to be discussed with patients prior to bleaching. The teeth need to be assessed for:

- Thickness of the enamel.
- Existing gingival/cervical recession.
- Existing sensitivity prior to bleaching needs to be noted on the patients dental charts.
- The translucency of the teeth: translucent teeth still retain their 'blackish' look after bleaching (Haywood 1995a). Patients need to be told of this consequence to avoid disappointment. Most patients are so happy with their new whiter smile that the existing translucency is of no concern.
- White spots or opacities: these do not disappear during bleaching and in the early stages of bleaching may become more visible. Patients need to be warned about this.
- Teeth that are banded due to tetracycline staining or desiccation still retain their banded appearance after bleaching. These aspects need to be discussed with patients prior to bleaching so the patient is not disappointed with the result after bleaching.
- Although bleaching teeth improves gingival health, bleaching treatment should not be attempted on teeth with surrounding gingivitis or more severe gingival problems (Small 1998).

SPECIAL TESTS

- *Vitality testing* of all teeth to be bleached should be undertaken. This can be done using the temperature tests such as heat or cold or through electric pulp testers. All tests need to be recorded on the patient's notes (see Figure 4.12).
- *Radiographs.* Recent radiographs need to be used to check for pathology, or existing decay of all teeth prior to bleaching. A single screening anterior periapical radiograph can be taken with the aid of a beam-aiming device, prior to bleaching (see Figure 4.13). However, it is better to have full mouth periapicals of all teeth to be bleached to ensure there is no previous or existing pathology. Problems have arisen when dentists have not taken an anterior periapical prior to bleaching. Teeth with existing periapical pathology can develop exacerbations which may be difficult to treat endodontically. Single dark teeth may be non-vital and these need to be checked prior to starting (see Figure 4.17B).
- *Diagnostic wax-up.* Sometimes it may be necessary to take study models and have the dental technician make a diagnostic wax-up of how the teeth will appear after the total treatment. As bleaching treatment may be followed by porcelain laminate veneers, the diagnostic wax-up will help the patient to see the final result before treatment commences (see Figure 4.17C).

PATIENTS WITH EXISTING RESTORATIONS IN AESTHETIC AREAS

It is essential to warn those patients with existing matching anterior composite restorations that as the shade of the teeth will change (Figure 4.16), they may require new composite restorations using a lighter shade composite after bleaching. The actual composite restorations do not change colour. Sometimes those composite restorations that have a black edge around them appear whiter because the black edge disappears. Those teeth with caries or defective, discoloured anterior restorations can be repaired after bleaching. The cariostatic action of the bleaching material will stop any progression of the lesion during bleaching. Patients should be aware that the restorations can only be replaced 2 weeks after the termination of the treatment, because bond strengths to enamel are weakened during bleaching (Figures 4.17J, K).

PATIENTS' EXPECTATIONS

It is fundamental, prior to commencing any bleaching procedure that the patient's expectations are assessed. A patient who expects pure white teeth is seldom satisfied (Haywood 1995a; see also Figure 4.16). Normally a colour change of two shades occurs; this can be demonstrated on a porcelain shade guide prior to bleaching. Patients need to be made aware that the worst that can happen is no shade change at all. Darker teeth take longer to bleach. Older patients' teeth respond well to bleaching, although the root surfaces do not bleach as well. These patients should thus be warned of this prior to commencing bleaching or that additional bonding procedure may be necessary to place composites at the neck of the roots.

Table 4.2 Factors that affect the amount of lightening

- The existing colour of the teeth.
- The amount of time the trays are replenished and the solutions are changed.
- The longer the bleaching materials are in contact with the teeth.
- The concentration of the bleaching material.
- The rate of oxygen release.
- The nature of the discoloration (e.g. tetracycline staining).

Photographs should be taken during the bleaching treatment, particularly 'before' and 'after' photos. Patients often forget how dark or discoloured the teeth were before commencing treatment and may be dissatisfied as they do not notice further shade changes. It helps to photograph the teeth with the baseline porcelain shade tab so that the patients can appreciate the degree of colour change when they see the colour change on the guide. That is why it is normally best to bleach only one arch at a time so that a direct colour comparison can be kept. Normally the upper arch is bleached first as patients notice this more. However, some patients who show more of the lower teeth may want to bleach these first. It is important to warn patients that the discoloration of worn lower incisors will

still appear discoloured; however, there is evidence that the dentine is also lightened during the bleaching treatment. (Haywood 1995b). Separate fees should be charged for the bleaching of the different arches.

TREATMENT PLANNING DISCUSSION AND INFORMED CONSENT

Prior to commencing any dental treatment it is essential to have a treatment planning discussion with the patient. During this appointment the patient's radiographs can be explained and discussed, as can treatment sequencing and any further treatment that may be required. Bleaching may not solve the patient's aesthetic requirements and all associated treatment needs to be discussed. At this time the patient can have the opportunity to ask further questions and gain clarification of what is involved in the proposed treatment, particularly regarding the dentist-prescribed home bleaching treatment. It is prudent to give the patient an informed consent form to sign. The benefits and risks need to be discussed as well as the advantages, disadvantages, and alternatives to bleaching and other treatment options (see Figure 4.17). Two copies should be signed; one is given to the patient and one is kept with the patient's dental records. Any expected or possible side-effects need to be mentioned (see Figure 5.1).

SUCCESS RATES OF BLEACHING

Although bleaching teeth as a dental treatment is now more predictable than ever, there is still no guarantee that the teeth will bleach to a lighter shade. The only way of knowing whether teeth will respond is to endeavour to undertake the treatment. Further treatment may be required to achieve an excellent smile such as composite bonding, porcelain laminates or full crowns (see Figures 4.9 and 4.17).

The success rates of bleaching have been published by numerous researchers. However, the success rates vary and there are numerous reasons for these differences.

Patients may often ask about the success rate and it is important to discuss these and be realistic with patients prior to commencing treatment of their teeth (Haywood 1995b). Not all teeth are responsive to treatment and not all teeth respond at the same rate. Some patients' teeth can whiten to the lightest shade on the shade guide, while others respond with a slight degree of lightening. The patient's smile though often appears brighter and this is an added benefit.

PHOTOGRAPHING TEETH DURING BLEACHING

It is often difficult to photograph and capture the slight differences of the shade changes during the bleaching treatment. There are many reasons for this (Figure 4.14):

- The lighting in the surgery may not be adequate.
- The reflectance of the operating light may distort the colour change.
- It is often difficult to record the same patient at the same distance so that the teeth appear the same size, with the same exposure.
- Metamerism (differences in the spectral characteristics of light reflected from natural teeth) may play a part.
- The flash of the camera may not fire at the same rate.

Photographs should include a shade tab (see Figure 4.17I) that closely matches a baseline colour of the teeth. The entire sequence of photographs should include this shade tab. Often the colour of the porcelain shade tab appears different due to variations in the reflecting light.

SHADE ASSESSMENT AND SELECTION

There are many ways of selecting the correct shade of the teeth prior to bleaching. The study of colour and shade taking is a vast subject in itself and will not be discussed in depth. Proprietary shade guides are normally used to determine the pre-operative shade. There can be variation between the individual shade guides (Miller 1987). Some bleaching kits have their own customized shade guides which can be used for the dentists and the patient as a reference. However, small changes in shade may be difficult to discern using these guides. Determination of the correct shade prior to bleaching, during bleaching and after bleaching is easier when the shade tabs are arranged according to value not hue (see Figure 5.5A). This helps particularly well when assessing small changes in colour after a few days of bleaching. A study trying to assess the viewer's perceived arrangement of value showed that none of the observers was able to arrange the shades as per the manufacturer's recommendations (Geary and Kinirons 1999). They also showed that some colour differences encountered by the observers may be too small to be noticed.

Selecting the appropriate shade has always been difficult as it is dependent on so many factors (see Figure 4.14). Shade selection is often subjective. Some surgeries are fitted with special colour-corrected bulbs in their fluorescent lights to help with shade determination.

FACTORS INVOLVED IN SHADE DETERMINATION

Factors that determine shade value:

- The amount of natural light in the area where the shade is taken.
- The hue of the tooth colour (yellow or blue range).
- The value of the colour, i.e. the lightness and brightness.
- Chroma: the strength or weakness of the colour.

There are three dimensions of colour: hue, chroma and value (Miller 1987). Hue is the pigment or most commonly called the 'colour'. Chroma denotes the strength or concentration of a hue and may also be referred as the colour saturation. Value is the relative whiteness or blackness of a colour and is a qualitative assessment of the grey component. Value is independent of hue or chroma and, in dental shade matching, it is the most important of the three dimensions of colour. Value should be selected first. Rearrangement of the colour guide from the lightest to the darkest shade is recommended to avoid distractions. Hue selection should be undertaken next. The basic hue can be best seen in the middle and cervical thirds. Chroma variations can be perceived within the same tooth. The cervical third usually presents higher chroma and a more saturated hue than the middle third. The incisal third often presents a lower value when compared with the middle and cervical thirds.

There have been great technical improvements to help dentists select shades. One innovation is the 3D Master Shade System. It is claimed that the systematic arrangement of the tabs within the guide in tri-dimensional colour space is designed to cover almost the complete range of naturally occurring shades. User instructions on shade-taking protocol suggest determination of each of the three elements separately. The initial step is the evaluation of colour value from five shades covering the lightest to darkest shades. This should be beneficial for assessing changes in shade which occur during bleaching.

As some teeth can bleach beyond the colour of the normal Vita Shade Guide, the manufacturers have introduced lighter porcelains to match the shade of the bleached teeth (see Figure 5.5C). This helps in the communication and treatment planning stage to show what may be possible. Some patients may not want the very white shade as they do not think it looks natural. Overbleached teeth may take on a very white opaque appearance.

After the shade has been selected a decision must be made if the discoloration or change in colour can be corrected. A guideline mentioned by Haywood (1999) states that if the sclera (white of the eye) is lighter than the existing shade of the teeth, the teeth can usually be lightened. If the colour of the

teeth is lighter than the sclera, it is probably going to be more difficult to achieve successful tooth bleaching (see Figure 4.14C).

PLANNING FEES FOR BLEACHING TREATMENT

It is essential during treatment planning that the correct fees for bleaching treatment are planned and assessed. Careful treatment planning includes careful planning of fees. The treatment planning stages and case presentation are demonstrated in Figures 4.17. Careful planning involves all members of the dental team and particularly the team member responsible for scheduling appointments and responsible for fee collection (Jameson 1996). Problems with patients could arise, if the correct fees are not quoted prior to commencing treatment. Some dentists quote a separate fee per arch and the first arch is normally more expensive that the second arch as it takes longer to assess and plan the first arch. Normally the upper arch is treated first.

FACTORS AFFECTING THE LEVEL OF FEES

1 Darker teeth will take longer to bleach. Thus they will requires more bleaching material. Should fees be assessed per arch or per the amount of materials used?
2 Those patients who sleep with the trays in their mouth may require less bleaching material (one application) than those who use it during the day (one or two applications).
3 Tetracycline-stained teeth will require extended treatment times and thus use more material. These patients should be charged for the additional amount of bleaching material used. This can be arranged as a monthly fee where they have an assessment and collect new material. Fees can be charged per visit, plus the bleaching materials, rather than per arch.
4 Those patients who wear a partial denture

will require two bleaching trays, one to wear during the day and one for night-time use and should be charged accordingly.

5 Fees should be quoted per arch, assuming a certain amount of bleaching material is used–let us say, x amount. If the patient requires $2x$ to bleach the teeth, charges should be made accordingly.

6 Fees will vary depending on the bleaching material used. Some are more expensive than other. Some products, e.g. Colgate, include the fee for making the bleaching trays in the whole kit, thus the costs to the dentist will be less.

7 Fees should be planned, discussed and written estimates given for those patients who will require additional treatment, such as the cost of replacing anterior composites to change them to a lighter shade.

8 The cost of further treatment should be discussed, written down and planned with patients such as those patients for whom bleaching will be done first then porcelain veneers or crowns on certain teeth.

Benefits of quoting fees per arch

1 Once the upper arch is bleached the patient may be satisfied with the result and not wish to continue to the lower teeth.

2 If one arch does not bleach or does not lighten satisfactorily, the fee for the other arch is avoided (Haywood 1995b).

3 If one arch will lighten, the other arch will lighten, although the lower arch does not lighten as well as the upper arch.

THE DENTIST'S COSTS

1 Surgery time; examination and discussion with patient, impression taking. Checking the fit of the trays, review and assessment time (3–5 appointments).

2 Laboratory costs for making the bleaching trays.

3 Material costs: bleaching material, bleaching toothpaste, appliance case.

4 Photography costs: developing of film or digital imaging.

5 Indirect costs of marketing the bleaching techniques to new and existing patients.

6 Overhead costs: running a surgery and employing staff.

A rider clause should be included on the estimate sheet to ensure that the patient be made aware of the following:

- the full fee is due at the impression appointment
- fees cannot be waived if the treatment is voluntarily discontinued or discontinued due to side effects
- there will be a replacement fee if the appliance is lost, worn or damaged
- further treatments may be necessary and these will be discussed with the patient prior to commencing
- separate fees will be quoted for in-office/power bleaching treatments.

Setting the appropriate fees for bleaching treatment within the practice is essential to the survival and profit of the dental practice (Lund 1997). Misunderstanding can be rectified before problems arise by the correct treatment planning, consent and appropriate fees for such treatment. Most dentists enjoy providing bleaching treatments for their patients as it is rewarding to see how patients are so delighted with the results of their whitened teeth and improved self-esteem (Small 1998).

BIBLIOGRAPHY

Brisman AS. (1980) Esthetics: a comparison of dentists' and patients' concepts. *J Am Dent Assoc* **100**:345-52.

Dunn WJ, Murchison DF, Broome JC. (1996) Esthetics: patients perceptions of dental attractiveness. *J Prosthodont* **5**(3):166-71.

Eaton K, Nathan K. (1998) The MGDS examination:

a systemic approach. 3. Part 2 of the examination: diagnosis, treatment planning, execution of treatment, maintenance and appraisal, writing-up log diaries. *Primary Dental Care* **5**(3):113-18.

Etcoff N. (1999). *Survival of the prettiest: the science of beauty.* Doubleday: New York.

Garber DA, Salama M. (1996) The aesthetic smile: diagnosis and treatment. *Periodontology 2000* **11**:18-28.

Geary LJ, Kinirons MJ. (1999) Use of a Common Shade Guide to Test the Perception of Differences in the Shades and Values by Members of the Dental Team. *Primary Dental Care* **6**(3):107-110.

Goldstein RE. (1998) *Esthetics in dentistry*, 2nd edn. Vol 1: *Principles, communications, treatment methods.* BC Decker: Hamilton, Ontario.

Haywood VB. (1995a) An examination for Nightguard Vital Bleaching. *Esthet Dent Update* **6**(2):51-2.

Haywood VB. (1995b) Nightguard Vital Bleaching: information and consent form. *Esthet Dent Update* **6**(5):130-2.

Haywood VB. (1999) Current status and recommendations for dentist-prescribed, at-home tooth whitening. *Contemp Esthet Restor Pract* **3**(Suppl 1):2–9.

Jameson C. (1994) *Great communication = great production.* Pennwell Books: Pennwell Publishing Company: Tulsa, Oklahoma.

Jameson C. (1996) *Collect what you produce.* Pennwell Books: Pennwell Publishing Company: Tulsa, Oklahoma.

Klaff D. (1999) Aesthetic dentistry for the millennium. *Restor Aesthet Prac* **1**(1):98-104.

Korson D (1990) *Natural Ceramics.* Quintessence Publishing Company: Chicago, IL.

Levin EI. (1978) Dental esthetics and the golden proportion. *J Prosthet Dent* **40**:244-52.

Lund P. (1997). *Building the happiness-centred business*, 2nd edn. Solutions Press: Capalaba, Australia.

McClean JW. (1979) *The science and art of dental ceramics*, Volume 1. Quintessence Publishing Company: Chicago, IL.

Miller L. (1987) Organizing colour in dentistry. *J Am Dent Assoc* (special issue): 26E-40E.

Miller LL. (1994) Shade selection. *J Esthet Dent* **6**:47-60.

Morris RM (1999) *Strategies in dental diagnosis and treatment planning.* Martin Dunitz: London.

Moskowitz ME, Nayyar A. (1995) Determinants of dental aesthetics: a rational for smile analysis and treatment. *Compend Contin Educ Dent* **16**(12):1164-86.

Paletz JL, Maktelow R, Chaban R. (1994) The shape of a normal smile: implications for facial paralysis reconstruction. *Plastic Reconstruct Surg* **93**(4):784-91.

Phillips E. (1996) The anatomy of a smile. *Oral Health* **93**(4):784-91.

Ricketts RM. (1968) Esthetics, environment and law of lip relation. *Am J Sci* **54**(4):272-89.

Rufenacht CR (1990) *Fundamentals of Esthetics.* Quintessence Publishing Company: Chicago, IL.

Salaski CG. (1972) Colour light and shade matching. *J Prosthet Dent* **27**:263-8.

Small BW. (1998) The application and integration of at-home bleaching into private dental practice. *Compend Contin Educ Dent* **9**(8):799-807.

Smiles so Bright. Manufacturer's Instructions Vitapan 3D Master. Paradent: London.

Smith BGN (1998) *Planning and Making Crowns and Bridges*, 3rd edn. Martin Dunitz Ltd: London.

Sproull RC. (1973) Colour matching in dentistry. Part 2: Practical applications for the organisation of colour. *J Prosthet Dent* **29**:566-66.

Tooth Bleaching Questionnaire

I understand that you are interested in having your teeth bleached. Please would you kindly complete the details below so that we can help you to achieve successful whitening of your teeth and a happy smile!

Medical History

	Yes	No
1. Are you allergic to plastics or peroxides?	....	....
2. Did you ever take tetracycline antibiotics for any period of time?	....	....
3. Are you taking drugs that dry the mouth?	....	....
4. Are you taking hormones that cause bleeding?	....	....
5. Do you ever have any of the following medical conditions?		
5.1 Any genetic diseases, cystic fibrosis, cerebral palsy	....	....
5.2 Kidney damage	....	....
5.3 Rocky Mountain spotted fever	....	....
5.4 Acne	....	....

As a child

6.1 Was there any Rh incompatibility when you were born?	....	....
6.2 Did you ever receive a head or neurological injury?	....	....
6.3 Did you ever take fluoride tablets?	....	....
6.4 Did you ever live in a high fluoride area?	....	....
6.5 Did you ever have a vitamin deficiency?	....	....
6.6 Did you ever have any blood diseases such as erythroblastosis fetalis, porphyria, haemolytic anaemia?	....	....
6.7 Did you ever have infant jaundice?	....	....

Do you smoke?

7.1 If yes how many?	....	....
7.2 How long have you smoked?	....	....
7.3 Have you ever smoked?	....	....

Dental History

1. Did you ever receive a blow to the face or teeth?	....	....
2. Did you ever have any accidents involving the teeth?	....	....
3. Have you ever bought any over-the-counter bleaching kits?	....	....
4. Are any of your teeth sensitive? Some?.............All?.............	....	....
4.1 Type of toothpaste used		
5. Have you been told or are you aware of any gum recession?	....	....
6. Do you use any mouthwashes on a regular basis?	....	....
7. Have you noticed that your teeth have become more yellow over the last few years?	....	....
8. Do you grind your teeth?	....	....
9. Do you suffer from facial pain?	....	....
10. Do you have temporo-mandibular dysfunction?	....	....
11. Do you wear a bite plate?	....	....

Diet

	Yes	No	Amount per day
Do you eat any of the following?			
1. Curry	....	....	....
2. Berries when in season	....	....	....
3. Fried foods	....	....	....
4. Which oil do you use to fry your food?	....	....	....
Do you drink any of the following?			
5. Coffee	....	....	....
6. Regular tea	....	....	....
7. Herbal tea	....	....	....
8. Coca-cola or Diet Coke	....	....	....
9. Red wine	....	....	....

Figure 4.1

Tooth bleaching questionnaire.

Patient:.. Date:..

Complains of

What can I do for you?: (main complaint)

Hopes and aspirations for dentistry:

What would you like from me?

Hopes to keep teeth:

Special dislikes/Worried about treatment:

Previous dental history

Last dental visit:...Regular attender:....................................

What was done:

Past experience: i.e. Why did you leave your last dentist?...

Pain: Nature of pain

Sensitivity from   Hot   Cold   Sweet   Pressure

Gingivae
Bleeding gums:
Other gum problems:
Calculus formation:

Smoker: How long?   Ex smoker:
Previous hygiene treatment: Interval
Disclosing   Brushing   Flossing   Diet sheets

Smile assessment
Are you happy with the colour of your teeth?
Are you happy with your smile? (Look at lip line and smile line):
What do you like most about your smile?
What do you like least about your smile?
If you could change anything about your smile what would you want to do?

Teeth
Root canal treatment:
Previous orthodontic treatment:
Teeth missing:
Teeth replaced: Fillings.........................Crowns/Caps.........................Bridges.........................
Migrating teeth/loose teeth:
Food impaction:
Wisdom teeth:
Temporomandibular joint
Clicking...................................Bruxing...................................Clenching....................................

Past experiences with local anaesthetic:
                            general anaesthetic:
Anything else:

Figure 4.2

New patient pre-examination questionnaire (modified from Dr C. Hall Dexter, with kind permission).

Date: Charting:

Stage 2																	
Stage 1																	
present																	
	8	7	6	5	4	3	2	1	1	2	3	4	5	6	7	8
present																	
Stage 1																	
Stage 2																	

Date:

8	7	6	5	4	3	2	1	1	2	3	4	5	6	7	8
8	7	6	5	4	3	2	1	1	2	3	4	5	6	7	8

Date:

8	7	6	5	4	3	2	1	1	2	3	4	5	6	7	8
8	7	6	5	4	3	2	1	1	2	3	4	5	6	7	8

Temporomandibular joint   Extra oral   Lymph nodes

Soft tissues   Tongue

Appearance of gums   Periodontal disease

Overhangs   Recession   Mobility

Occlusion type
Canine guidance: left   right   Group function: left   right
Lateral exclusions: right   left
Protrusion

Initial contact
Type of slide: Vertical   Horizontal   Amount

Condition of existing restorations   Tooth wear   Wear facets

Non-functional   Tilted   Over-erupted

Aesthetics

───────────────────────── Lipline ─────────────────────────

Figure 4.3

Intraoral assessment and charting form (modified from Dr. C Hall Dexter, with kind permission).

Date: _____

Patient's name: _____ Date of birth: _____
Patient's concerns and main complaint:

Assessment of the Face
Proportions: Forehead: _____ Midface: _____ Mandible: _____
Facial musculature: _____
Vertical dimensions: In proportion to face: _____ Overclosed: _____ Loss of occlusal vertical dimension: _____
Tooth visibility of smile: Maxillary _____ Mandibular _____
Lipline: High _____ Low _____ Other _____
Smile line: Broad _____ Narrow: _____
Type of smile: upper lip curvature: _____
Negative space: Lateral negative space   Present: _____ Absent: _____
Smile symmetry: _____

Assessment of the Teeth
Occlusion:
Skeletal pattern: Type 1 _____ Type 2 Division 1 _____ Type 2 Division 2 _____ Type 3 _____
Occlusal alignment:
Interferences: ICP=RCP   ICP RCP Slide type: Vertical _____ Horizontal _____
First point of contact: _____
Lateral guidance: Working side contacts _____ Non working side contacts: _____
Canine guidance: _____ Group function: _____
Dental midline: _____ Presence of diastemas: _____
Golden proportion: _____
Tooth Arrangement: _____ Axial alignment: _____
Arch type: Square: _____ Narrow: _____ Rounded: _____ Tapered: _____
Existing upper anterior tooth length: Centrals: _____ Laterals: _____
Tooth width: Centrals: _____ Laterals: _____
Contact points: _____ High: _____ Low: _____
Tooth wear: _____ Type: _____ Wear facets: _____
Existing tooth shade: _____

Tooth Morphology
Surface white spots: _____ Subsurface white spots: _____
Stains on teeth: _____ Brown areas: _____ Developmental defects: _____
Cracks: _____ Caries: _____ Exposed dentine: _____ Translucent teeth: _____

Gingival Morphology _____
Amount of attached gingivae: _____
Gingival health: _____ Gingival disease: _____
Colour of gingivae: _____
Recession: _____
Type of gingivae: Thick: _____ Thin: _____ Collagenous: _____

Planning
Diagnostic waxup needed: Yes: _____ No: _____
Mounted study models: _____
Bleaching alone will solve aesthetic requirements: _____ Further treatment: _____

Other

Patient Expectations
Patient understands treatment options: _____
Patient has reasonable success goals: _____
Patient understands responsibility for treatment: _____

Figure 4.4

Smile analysis assessment form.

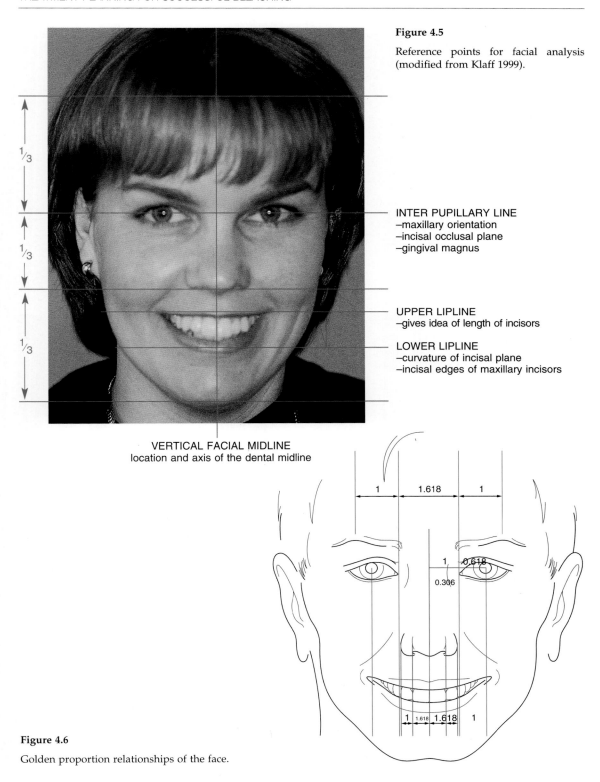

Figure 4.5

Reference points for facial analysis (modified from Klaff 1999).

INTER PUPILLARY LINE
–maxillary orientation
–incisal occlusal plane
–gingival magnus

UPPER LIPLINE
–gives idea of length of incisors

LOWER LIPLINE
–curvature of incisal plane
–incisal edges of maxillary incisors

VERTICAL FACIAL MIDLINE
location and axis of the dental midline

Figure 4.6

Golden proportion relationships of the face.

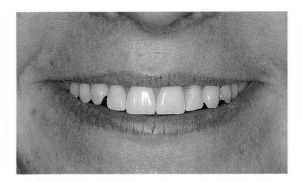

Figure 4.7

Smile analysis. Components of a smile such as the teeth, the lips and the gingival scaffold are all assessed: this includes the lipline and smile line. This patient has a broad smile and shows the upper molars when she smiles. Other factors such as interdental contacts, zenith points, incisal embrasures, texture of the enamel, tooth shape, size and alignment are all assessed.

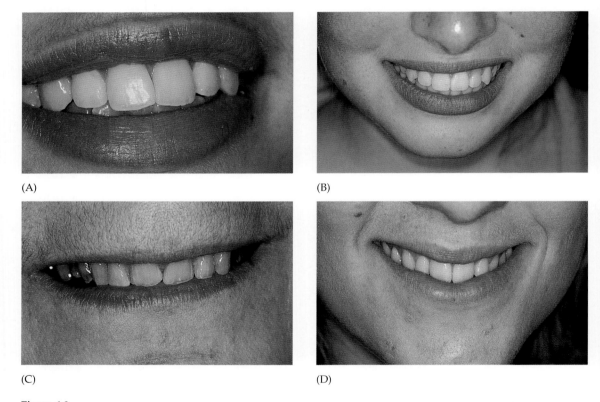

(A)   (B)

(C)   (D)

Figure 4.8

Smile variations. (A) This patient has a smile which only shows the central incisors. (B) This patient has asymmetry in the upper lip when she smiles. (C) This older patient has a low lipline. (D) It appears that this smile line is low on the central incisors, but high on the lateral incisors.

continued on the next page

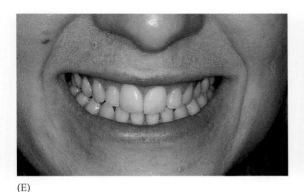

(E)

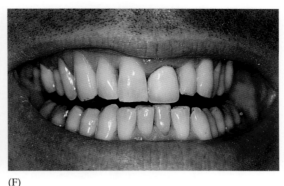

(F)

Figure 4.8 continued

(E) However, when the patient makes a broad smile the appearance of the smile changes. Dentists should be aware of this phenomenon as after bleaching treatment and other aesthetic dentistry, the patient may make a broader smile to show-off their new smile and reveal more teeth. (F) This patient has a high lipline which shows the discrepancy in the heights of the gingival scaffold around the central incisors. Merely changing the crown will not solve the aesthetic problem. It is better to do gingival contouring such as crown lengthening to give symmetry to the two central incisors.

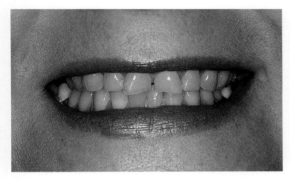

(A)

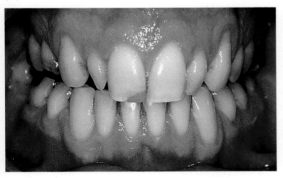

(B)

Figure 4.9

Bleaching alone will not solve the patient's aesthetic requirements (A) This patient has a low lipline. She has small teeth which have been worn down caused by occlusal problems on the molar teeth, a bruxing habit and erosive wear due to a health-orientated acidic diet. Bleaching alone will not solve the aesthetic problem. Detailed occlusal analysis is essential in this case to detect the discrepancy between the intercuspal position and the retruded contact position. Treatment here will require an occlusal splint, adult orthodontics followed by bleaching and full coverage crowns for the central incisor teeth. Bleaching treatment will form part of the treatment, but further treatment will be required to solve aesthetic and functional requirements. Patients need to be aware of the extent of treatment that is required to achieve health and stability. (B) Note the discrepancy in the small peg-shaped laterals and the well-shaped central incisors. The stained existing composite restoration will have to be replaced after bleaching treatment is completed.

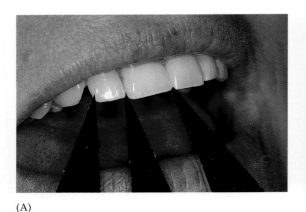
(A)

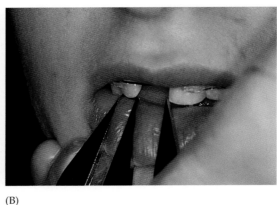
(B)

Figure 4.10

Assessment of Golden Proportion using the proportion gauge. (A) The Golden Proportion gauge has been made in the relationship 1:1.618. It is adaptable to many situations and can be used to measure the proportional relationship between the central and lateral incisors. (B) The gauge is also used to measure the relationship of the edentulous space to the incisor. The orthodontist waits for the opinion of the restorative dentist prior to completing the necessary orthodontic treatment. The gauge helps to accurately measure these proportions.

Figure 4.11

Intraoral evaluation. This patient presented with an existing crown that was 10 years old which was mismatched with the surrounding dentition. The patient had been treated for periodontal disease which was now stable and she was well maintained. She enquired about lightening her yellow teeth and replacing the existing crown. Treatment options were discussed with the patient which included orthodontic correction to align the anterior incisors in a better, more aesthetic position the teeth; replacement of the existing crown. As the patient was concerned about the appearance of the existing crown, the crown was removed and a provisional metal composite crown was placed for the duration of the orthodontic treatment. This would facilitate bonding of the orthodontic brackets. Following realignment, bleaching treatment for the upper teeth only was provided. A period of 6 weeks was allowed prior to commencing the definitive stage of the treatment. Thereafter a new, definitive porcelain crown was placed. (A) Appearance of the teeth prior to commencing treatment. (B) Appearance of the teeth during orthodontic alignment. The existing crown was removed and a provisional metal/composite crown placed. The crown is well fitting around the margins, but the patient was finding it difficult to keep the teeth clean with the brackets on the teeth. The staining is from a chlorhexidine mouthwash to improve the upper gingival inflammation. (Orthodontist, Dr Brian Miller.) (C) Appearance of the teeth following orthodontic treatment. Inflammation is generally resolved. There is still a little inflammation as orthodontic retainer is worn all the time as the patient is concerned that the teeth will move back to their original position. Bleaching treatment was commenced. The patient was instructed to alternate wearing the bleaching trays with the retainer. (D) Result after bleaching. (E) The final result with new porcelain crown.

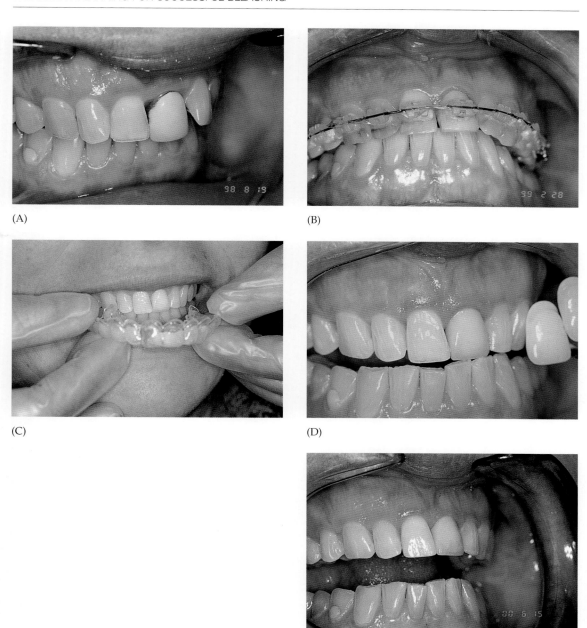

(A)

(B)

(C)

(D)

(E)

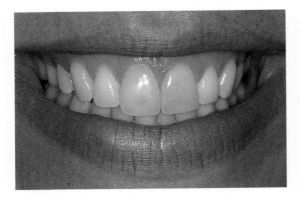

(A)

Figure 4.12

(A) This patient was concerned about the appearance of her discoloured central incisors. She was not sure why these teeth had discoloured. When questioned about trauma she vaguely remembered an incident of mild trauma to the front teeth. It was not sure whether these teeth were vital or non-vital. The patient has a high smile line showing the upper gingivae when she smiles, so making the discoloured teeth more noticeable. (B) Vitality testing was undertaken using two methods. A cold chemical spray was placed onto the teeth to see if the patient could feel the cold sensation; both teeth tested positive to the cold spray. A periapical radiograph of the central incisors showed that the walls of the pulp chamber and canal had narrowed owing to secondary dentine formation which was deposited to protect the tooth from the resulting trauma. An electric pulp tester was then used to check the responses of all the six upper anterior teeth. Toothpaste was placed onto the teeth to act as a conductor for the electrical current. The teeth responded well to testing and it was thus determined that although discoloured they were still vital. (C) It was decided to bleach the upper teeth using the dentist-prescribed home bleaching technique. Other treatment options such as porcelain laminates were discussed with the patient. No guarantees were given as to the amount of lightening that could be achieved. Bleaching trays were made for the upper teeth. The patient was instructed to place the bleaching material in the tray and wear the tray overnight. The pre-operative shade was taken. (D) The result after 1 week showed that considerable lightening was possible. The patient was motivated to continue bleaching treatment until further whitening had taken place. For the second week, the patient was encouraged to place the material only on to the two central incisors to try to achieve a match between the central and lateral incisors.

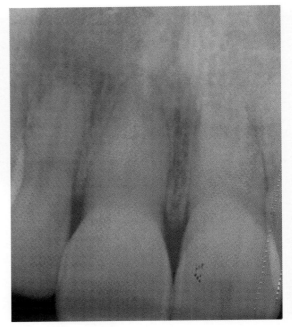

(B)

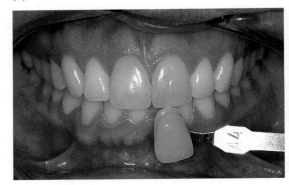

(C)

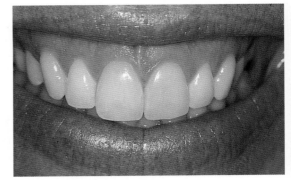

(D)

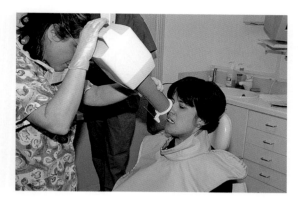

Figure 4.13

Radiographic analysis. Beam aiming devices using the paralleling technique are used to take accurate radiographs of the teeth.

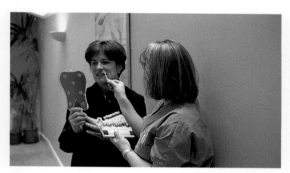

(A)

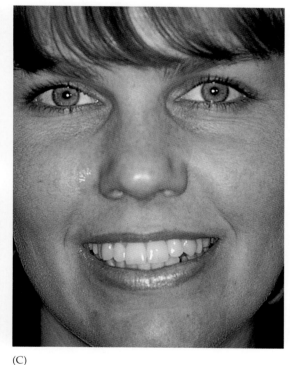

(C)

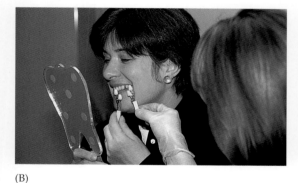

(B)

Figure 4.14

Shade assessment. **Different surroundings** affect the colour selected for teeth. The amount of **natural light** is important. When taking shades, it is essential to use natural light where possible. In the treatment room there are many sources of light that contribute to the shade assessment, such as the dental light which is a low-voltage halogen light. There are also overhead lights from the ceiling. Colour-corrected bulbs can be used to prevent any distortion of the natural light. (A) The shade can be taken in a place where there is more natural daylight from skylights. The colour of the walls may have an effect on the selection of the shade. (B) The patient checks the shade which has been chosen. (C) There is an interesting relationship between the colour of the whites of the eyes and the colour of the teeth. When assessing a patient, it is useful to use this relationship to determine whether bleaching will be successful. If the white of the eye is a similar colour to the teeth, successful bleaching may not be achievable. However if the white of the eye is lighter than the existing shade of the teeth, as is the case here, bleaching is likely to be successful.

continued on the next page

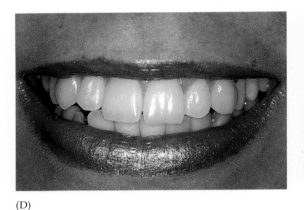

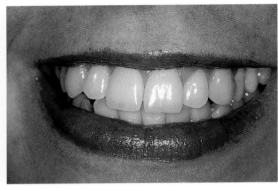

(D)   (E)

Figure 4.14 continued

(D) The colour of the lipstick also plays a part in the colour of the teeth. Lighter shades of lipstick will make the teeth appear more pale, while an orange-brown lipstick makes the teeth look more yellow. (E) The patient should choose a lipstick with a more blue tone in it to allow the teeth to appear whiter. These factors are important to discuss with the patient prior to commencing bleaching.

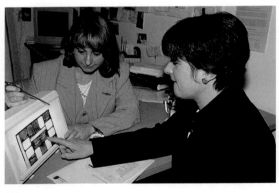

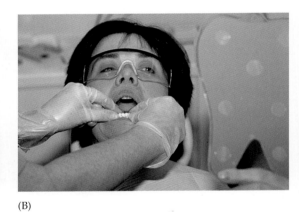

(A)   (B)

Figure 4.15

The stages in the treatment planning discussion. Prior to the patient's treatment planning appointment, the dentist discusses the sequence of treatment with the practice manager and treatment co-ordinator. The treatment plan is written-up and the dentist checks that it is correct. Any other possible options for treatment are discussed. (A) The treatment planning discussion appointment. The dentist conducts a tour of the X-rays to demonstrate what is present and what problems have been detected. Possible treatment options are discussed using models and other photographs of similar cases. The sequences of treatment are discussed and the patient is given the treatment plan. After the discussion any changes in the proposed treatment are discussed with the treatment co-ordinator. The treatment co-ordinator then makes financial arrangements that are comfortable for the patient and schedules the appropriate appointments for treatment to commence. The consent form is signed by the patient prior to commencing any treatment. (B) The placement of the bleaching material is demonstrated to the patient, and the patient observes in the mirror how the bleaching tray is placed in the mouth and how the excess is removed.

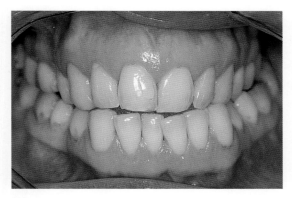

(A)

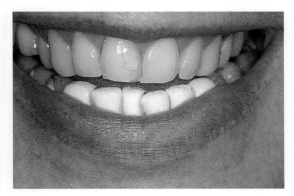

(B)

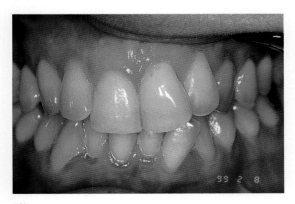

(C)

Figure 4.16

Patient expectations. Some patients need to be made aware that they will require replacement of discoloured composite restorations after bleaching treatment is completed. There are also often existing anterior composite restorations that will require replacement and the patient needs to know this also prior to commencing bleaching treatment, as well as the costs involved. Orthodontic treatment (which is extensive for some patients) should be completed prior to commencing bleaching treatment. Sometimes the retainer can act as the bleaching tray and this needs to be discussed with the patient's orthodontist prior to removing the braces. Patients with multiple aesthetic requirements need especially careful treatment planning. One option is to bleach the teeth to lighten the existing veneers using the access cavities from the endodontic treatment. The patients need to be aware that this is possible and the bleaching will be staged into the appropriate part of the complex aesthetic dentistry: bleaching alone will not solve all aesthetic requirements. (A) This patient is not happy with her smile. She has an anterior open bite, with thin enamel. A diagnostic wax-up was made to show the patient a possible way of correcting some of the aesthetic problems. During this discussion it became obvious that the patient's expectations of what could be achieved were vastly different to what the dentists could achieve or what was possible. Two different diagnostic wax-ups were made. The patient requested several corrections to these wax-ups. Although the dentist thought that the teeth should be lengthened to correct the open bite and the natural curvature of the lips, the patient requested that the incisor teeth be shortened. It was decided that aesthetic treatment was not to be undertaken at present. It is better not to provide treatment for patients with unrealistic expectations of what can be achieved. (B) Bleaching treatment was demonstrated to the patient using the lower bleaching tray. The toothpaste-like bleaching material is applied to the lower teeth for demonstration purposes. (C) This patient is not concerned about the discoloured canine tooth but rather the crowded appearance of the rest of the teeth. It is essential that these concerns are assessed prior to planning treatment for the patient.

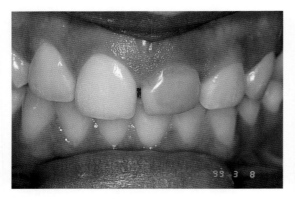

(A)

Figure 4.17

The importance of treatment planning prior to commencing bleaching treatment. This patient presented with a single dark tooth which was unsightly. The tooth had been involved in a traumatic incident at the age of 11 years and needed to have a root canal treatment. As a result of this, the tooth discoloured. The gingival margin did not mature around this central tooth and the adjacent tooth. Just treating the single dark tooth by bleaching would not be sufficient to solve the patient's problem as the gingival contours were different on the upper left central and lateral incisor tooth. Treatment options included bleaching the upper left central incisor, crown lengthening the left central, and lateral incisors to correct the gingival heights, and then a full porcelain crown, a porcelain veneer, or composite bonding. It was decided to opt for bleaching of the dark central incisor followed by a porcelain laminate since the existing tooth was short and required too much correction to achieve good alignment, by just using composite bonding. (A) Close-up of the appearance of the central incisor prior to treatment. Note also the difference in heights of the gingival contour of the right and left side. (B) The periapical X-ray showed that there was an excellent root canal treatment with a hermetic seal and no evidence of apical pathology. (C) The diagnostic wax-up of the proposed treatment. Discussions were held about keeping the midline diastema, trying to close it or closing the diastema between the central and lateral incisor. A second wax-up to close the midline diastema did not prove satisfactory, as the central incisor would appear too wide and would be out of proportion with the rest of the teeth. The diagnostic wax-up presented here shows the midline diastema placed with the corrected height of the gingival contours on the upper left central and later incisor.

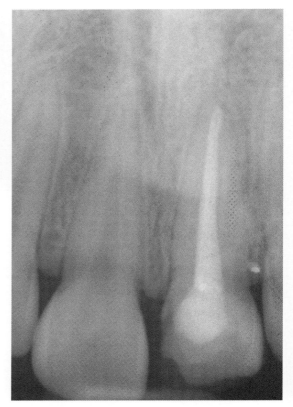

(B)

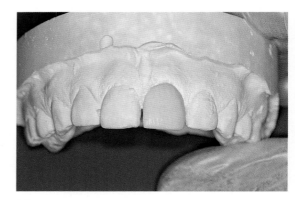

(C)

continued on the next page

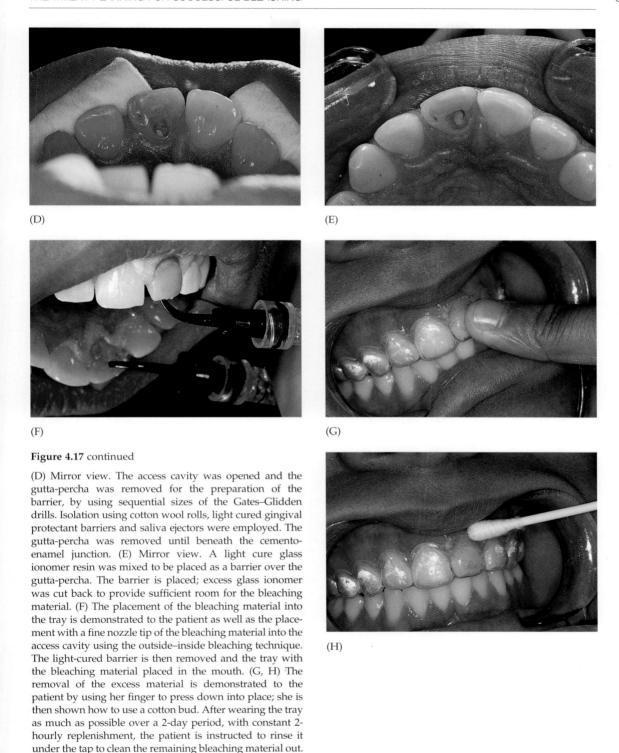

(D)

(E)

(F)

(G)

(H)

Figure 4.17 continued

(D) Mirror view. The access cavity was opened and the gutta-percha was removed for the preparation of the barrier, by using sequential sizes of the Gates–Glidden drills. Isolation using cotton wool rolls, light cured gingival protectant barriers and saliva ejectors were employed. The gutta-percha was removed until beneath the cemento-enamel junction. (E) Mirror view. A light cure glass ionomer resin was mixed to be placed as a barrier over the gutta-percha. The barrier is placed; excess glass ionomer was cut back to provide sufficient room for the bleaching material. (F) The placement of the bleaching material into the tray is demonstrated to the patient as well as the placement with a fine nozzle tip of the bleaching material into the access cavity using the outside–inside bleaching technique. The light-cured barrier is then removed and the tray with the bleaching material placed in the mouth. (G, H) The removal of the excess material is demonstrated to the patient by using her finger to press down into place; she is then shown how to use a cotton bud. After wearing the tray as much as possible over a 2-day period, with constant 2-hourly replenishment, the patient is instructed to rinse it under the tap to clean the remaining bleaching material out.

continued on the next page

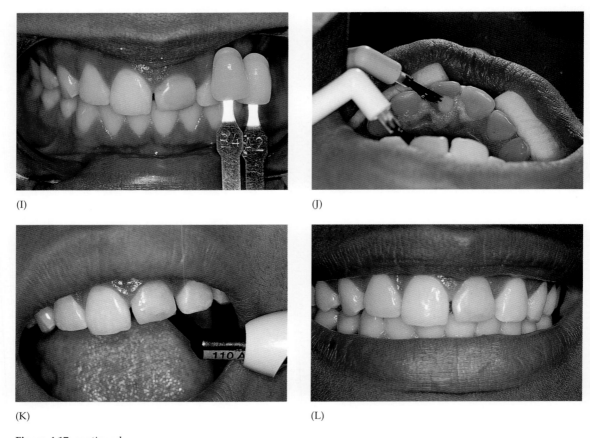

(I)

(J)

(K)

(L)

Figure 4.17 continued

(I) Pre-operative assessment of the existing and proposed shades prior to commencing bleaching treatment. (J) Mirror view. After 2 days, the access cavity is rinsed, disinfected and a glass ionomer restoration is placed immediately. While the glass ionomer material is setting, a light-cured, glaze or unfilled resin is placed over the restoration. A brush is used to apply the glaze. The patient continued to bleach the tooth in the bleaching tray for a further week. (K) After 3 weeks, the glass ionomer is cut back and a composite resin restoration is placed using a lighter shade of composite than the bleached tooth to allow for light reflecting through the tooth. The existing composite resin placed on the incisal edge is noticeable darker compared to the new bleached shade. (L) The appearance of the tooth after bleaching and after crown lengthening. The colour of the central incisor now matches the rest of the dentition. The height of the gingival contour is now symmetrical on left and right sides. A period of 12 weeks was left for the margins to settle prior to bleaching the porcelain laminate veneer.

continued on the next page

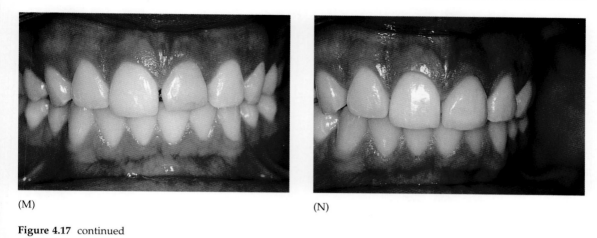

(M) (N)

Figure 4.17 continued

(M) The results 12 weeks after crown lengthening. (N) The porcelain laminate veneer just after cementation. (The tooth is still a little dry from the isolation.)

5 THE HOME BLEACHING TECHNIQUE

INTRODUCTION

Home bleaching is a simple technique whereby, after an initial consultation with the dentist, a mouthguard or tray is made for the patient to bleach the teeth at home. The patient is given the bleaching materials (normally 10% carbamide peroxide) to take home together with a bleaching protocol. The patient applies the bleaching material into the tray. The tray with the material is worn for several hours during the day or at night depending on the patient's schedule, while the teeth lighten. It is a predictable technique and has a success rate of 98% for non-tetracycline stained teeth and 86% for tetracycline stained teeth (Leonard 2000). The introduction of Nightguard Vital Bleaching in 1989 revolutionized bleaching technology, as the technique was simple and dentists could provide treatment easily for patients. The overall cost was reduced and the technique has become extremely popular, enabling millions of people around the world to benefit from bleaching treatment. It is the aim of this chapter to describe the home bleaching technique and protocol in detail, so that successful bleaching treatments can be achieved.

TERMINOLOGY

Many names have been used for home bleaching. The original term used was 'Nightguard Vital Bleaching', as patients bleached the teeth at night while they slept with the tray in their mouths (Haywood and Heymann 1989).

'Home bleaching', some may argue, does not distinguish the procedure from patients that buy the over-the-counter kits and self-prescribe the bleaching treatments. However, the term will be used for simplicity. Names associated with home bleaching are:

* Nightguard Vital Bleaching
* Matrix bleaching
* Dentist-assisted/prescribed home-applied bleaching
* Dentist-supervised at-home bleaching
* At-home bleaching

THE PROS AND CONS OF HOME BLEACHING

Advantages
* It is simple and fast for patients to use (Christensen 1997).
* It is simple for dentists to monitor without extended clinical time.
* It is cost effective (Greenwall 1992).
* The laboratory fees for making the bleaching tray are not expensive.
* It is not usually a painful procedure.
* Patients can bleach their teeth at their convenience, according to their personal schedule.
* Patients can see the results relatively quickly.
* Patients are normally delighted with the result!

Disadvantages
* Patients need to participate actively in their treatment (Miller 1999).

- The colour change is dependent on the amount of time that the trays are worn. If patients do not wear the bleach in the trays for the specified amount of time, changes in tooth lightening will be slow.
- Some patients cannot be bothered with applying the bleach in the trays every day. The drop-out rate of home bleaching may be as much as 50% according to anecdotal feedback (Miller 1999). Some patients may need further motivation and encouragement to continue the programme by office assisted programmes or power bleaching.
- The system may be open to abuse by using excessive amounts of bleach for too many hours per day (Garber 1997).
- It is difficult for patients who retch easily to tolerate the bleaching trays in their mouth.

INDICATIONS FOR USE

The home bleaching agents (Greenwall 1999b) can be used for:

- Mild generalized staining (combination of factors, Greenwall 1992)
- 'Age yellowing' discolouration (see Figure 5.18)
- Mild tetracycline staining
- Very mild fluorosis (brown or white) (see Figure 5.19)
- Acquired superficial staining
- Stains from smoking tobacco
- Absorptive and penetration stains (tea and coffee).
- Colour change related to pulpal trauma or necrosis
- Patients who desire a minimal amount of dental treatment to achieve a colour shift
- Young patients with an inherited grey or yellow hue to the teeth who are unhappy about this.

CONTRAINDICATIONS FOR USE

There are many contraindications for home bleaching (Greenwall 1999b). Home bleaching agents should not be used for:

- severe tetracycline staining
- severe pitting hypoplasia
- severe fluorosis stain
- discolorations in the adolescent patient with large pulps (Haywood 1995)
- patients with unrealistic expectations about the anticipated aesthetic result (Wise 1995)
- teeth with inadequate or defective existing restorations (these should be temporarily blocked before bleaching)
- teeth with tooth surface loss due to attrition, abrasion and erosion
- teeth with insufficient enamel to respond to bleaching (i.e. pitted teeth, defective enamel); however, this might be acceptable as it is the dentine which is important for determining the shade colour (Bentley et al 1999)
- teeth with deep and surface cracks and fracture lines
- teeth with large anterior restorations (see Figure 5.18)
- teeth with pathology such as a periapical radiolucency
- teeth that are fractured or maligned may be better treated with other treatments such as porcelain veneers or orthodontics
- patients who demonstrate a lack of compliance through inability or unwillingness to wear appliance for the required time (Garber et al 1991)
- patients who are pregnant or lactating – at this stage, the effect of the bleach on development of the fetus is unknown (Garber et al 1991)
- patients who smoke – patients cannot smoke and bleach their teeth at the same time as this may enhance the carcinogenic effect of the smoking
- teeth exhibiting extreme sensitivity to heat, cold, touch and sweetness.

Although the last point is not strictly a contraindication, bleaching teeth can sometimes cause transient sensitivity. It may be better to treat the sensitivity first with fluoride applications, a bonding agent or a bonded restoration prior to bleaching. It may also be necessary to protect any erosion or abrasion area (Greenwall 1999a).

ALTERNATIVES

The alternatives to home bleaching may involve:

- In-office bleaching, such as power or laser bleaching
- Porcelain veneers
- Composite veneers
- Composite bonding
- Crowns: all porcelain crowns or porcelain bonded to metal crowns
- Further restorations
- Combinations of treatments.

Most of the above options are more invasive and destructive than home bleaching. The preparation of crowns (particularly the new all porcelain crowns) require removal of tooth tissue of at least 1 to 1.5 mm (even 2 mm).

THE PROTOCOL

Once a patient has expressed an interest in having his or her teeth lightened, there are several aspects which need to be discussed, prior to the first bleaching visit. After assessing the patient's medical history, it may be useful to ask the patient to complete a tooth discoloration questionnaire to ascertain which foods or drinks are causing the staining. Patients should reduce the intake of foods that are causing the staining of the teeth prior to commencing bleaching treatments. Patients should be warned of the possibility of experiencing caffeine withdrawal symptoms if they stop drinking coffee, tea etc. immediately.

The dentist needs to assess whether the patient is taking any medication that can affect bleaching treatment such as antihistamines which make the mouth dry (see Chapter 4). Any allergies to components in the bleach, such as glycerine, flavouring agents or preservatives or the bleaching tray components need to be checked (see Figure 5.3). Patients who smoke should be counselled to stop smoking prior to providing any bleaching treatments. Patients are advised that they should not bleach their teeth if they

are smoking. They should stop smoking at least a week before, not smoke during the bleaching treatment, which could take up to one month, and not smoke for at least a month after.

INITIAL CONSULTATION

The initial discussion with the patient should address:

- the advantages and disadvantages of tooth bleaching
- alternatives to bleaching treatments
- any side effects that may be experienced (such as sensitivity, gingival irritation)
- the risks and benefits of the procedures and obtainment of the patient's informed consent
- all treatment options, including the possibility that more than one bleaching treatment may need to be undertaken
- the duration of treatment
- further aesthetic treatment that may be needed
- further dental treatment such as replacing stained and leaking composites.

It is essential to set bleaching goals prior to treatment. Use the appropriate procedures for diagnosis, treatment planning and evaluating the teeth which were discussed in Chapter 4.

CLINICAL EXAMINATION OF ALL TEETH

A comprehensive examination should assess the oral environment (Fischer 2000b), soft tissues, mucosae, teeth gingivae and oral health status of the patient. Check the integrity of the existing restorations. Check recent X-rays for dental disease, periapical radiolucencies (Haywood 1997a). The size and vitalities of the pulps of the teeth can be assessed on X-rays to predict sensitivity levels (see Figure 5.4). The vitality of the teeth should be tested, particularly single discoloured teeth. Teeth that are non-vital should be root-treated with a good apical seal,

Table 5.1 The Vita value-orientated Shade Guide with 16 shades ranked from lightest colour on left to darkest colour on the right

B1/	A1/	B2/	D2/	A2/	C1/	C2/	D4/	A3/	D3/	B3/	A3,5/	B4/	C3/	A4/	C4
1-	2-	3-	4-	5-	6-	7-	8-	9-	10-	11-	12-	13-	14-	15-	16-

Lightest .... Darkest

prior to commencing bleaching treatment. Cervical recession, periodontal health and any cracking of the anterior teeth should be assessed. Measure translucency, as highly translucent teeth do not bleach as well; they sometimes appear greyer rather than whiter. Patients should be informed that translucent teeth do not bleach as well.

PRE-EXISTING SHADE EVALUATION

Discuss with the patient the possible shade lightening that can be achieved, prior to commencing treatment. This is normally two shades lighter on a normal porcelain shade guide or 1–3 shades on a value-orientated shade guide. Shade taking can be via the normal methods, i.e. using the porcelain shade guide or via the shade guide supplied with the bleaching kit (see Figure 5.5). The patient should be fully involved in the shade taking process and should acknowledge the pre-operative shade that was taken and may sign in the notes for verification.

PLANNING THE TREATMENT

It is normally advisable to bleach only one arch at a time so that the patient has the opportunity for a comparison. Patients who bleach both arches at the same time stand an increased chance of developing side effects and occlusal problems. Often the patient forgets how dark the teeth were to begin with and wants to carry on with the treatment, perhaps unwisely. Both arches can be done when time is short, such as for a forthcoming wedding celebration.

It is also essential to discuss with patients that their existing composite restorations may not match after bleaching and that it may be necessary to replace these composites with lighter ones after the bleaching procedures. Photographs together with the existing shade tab of the teeth are taken. Intraoral photos can also be taken. These images can be enhanced so that the patient can see the possible outcome prior to commencing treatment, but no guarantees are given if the images are enhanced.

Table 5.2 Factors that have a guarded prognosis for home bleaching success

- A history or presence of sensitive teeth
- Extremely dark gingival third of tooth visible during smiling
- Extensive white spots are present and very visible
- Presence of TMJ dysfunction or bruxism
- Translucent teeth
- Excessive gingival recession and exposed root surfaces

IMPRESSION TAKING

Excellent impressions reproducing the surfaces of the upper and lower teeth should be taken so that bleaching trays can be made. Alginate or another accurate material can be used. When mixing the materials, attempts should be made to eliminate as many air bubbles as possible (see Figure 5.6). Alginate mixing machines can be used to reduce air bubbles. A small amount of alginate can be rubbed on to the occlusal surface of the teeth to achieve good detail. Closed mouth techniques are used to eliminate the possibility of distortion of the mandible. Alginate impressions should be poured and cast very soon to prevent distortion of the casts. Bleaching trays are made from these impressions (see Chapter 6).

Selecting the appropriate bleaching material

There is a vast array of bleaching materials available. It is important to select the appropriate material for the particular patient. The greater the concentration of carbamide peroxide, and the thicker the material, the quicker the bleaching will take place and the less the trays will need to be worn. Some systems have graded concentrations of active agent such as 5%, 10%, 15% and 20%, or even 35%, to enable the patient to get used to bleaching without causing tooth sensitivity. Studies comparing bleaching agents have shown that they all work and there is minimal difference among them (Lyons and Ng 1998). There is an inverse relationship: if the concentration of the bleaching agent is decreased, the treatment time must be increased.

The choice of which bleaching agent to use depends on:

- **The discoloration**
  - The source of the discoloration
  - The form, shape, depth (whether superficial or deep) and extent of the discoloration
  - The existing colour, as darker teeth will take longer to bleach
  - The location of the staining i.e. within the enamel or dentine (Touati et al 1999)
- **The bleaching material**
  - The cost of the material (is the cost of the tray fabrication included?)
  - CE mark (type and classification)/ADA Seal of Approval
  - Chemical constituents of the base material (hydrogen peroxide, carbamide peroxide or perborate)
  - Mode of action: pH values?
  - Dispensing method
  - Tissue tolerance
  - Safety studies: have the products been evaluated by the Food and Drug Administration?
  - Suggested wearing times
  - Patient friendly, clear instruction sheets
  - Ease of use, application
  - The flavour
- **Patient factors**
  - Existing tooth sensitivity
  - Lifestyle
  - Personal schedule
  - Patient dexterity
  - Goals for whitening

Bleaching introduction

It is customary to provide an oral prophylaxis prior to any bleaching procedure. This may be done by the hygienist or the dentist. However, a study (Knight et al 1997) showed that those patients who experience sensitivity after an oral prophylaxis are more prone to experience sensitivity and other side effects during bleaching. Leonard (1998) advised to wait 2 weeks after an oral prophylaxis before beginning the whitening procedure. Written home bleaching instructions are explained to the patient. The bleaching record sheet (see Figure 5.1) is completed and the patient signs the consent form. A power bleach session can be done to initiate the bleaching at the chairside or to motivate the patient into continuing bleaching at home, but there would be increased cost for this additional procedure.

Seating the tray

For a full arch

The bleaching trays are checked for correct fit, retention and over-extension on the gingival area. The trays can be trimmed back if they are over-extended by using a small sharp scissors. The rough edge is then polished with a rubber wheel or flame smoothed. The aim is for the tray to fit well, to keep the bleaching material in contact with the teeth but not to impinge on the gingivae. The amount of bleaching material to be used can be demonstrated to the patient and the patient is helped to insert and remove the trays (see Figure 5.7). The patient is instructed to place enough material to fill the tray with minimal excess (Leonard et al 1999). A demonstration of how to remove the excess bleaching material from the soft tissue can be undertaken.

Instruct the patient not to swallow the excess but to remove it first using a cotton wool roll, finger or toothbrush. Patients are instructed to brush and floss their teeth and then to apply the tray with the bleaching material in their mouth. They can choose to either bleach their teeth while they sleep or to apply the tray during the day, depending on their schedule.

Supply the bleaching material, a few cotton rolls, cotton buds and the bleaching tooth-paste (not mandatory) in a home kit. Document the amount of bleaching material given to the patient as well as the name of the bleaching agent used on the bleaching record sheet (Fascanaro 1992) (Figure 5.1). A patient bleaching log (see Figure 5.2) is supplied for the patient to document the use of the materials, sensitivity levels and the amount of time the trays are worn. Instruct the patient to telephone the practice if any adverse reactions are experienced, particularly sensitivity to hot and cold. Normally it is best to start with the bleaching of the maxillary teeth first as these bleach quicker. This is thought to be due to better retention of the upper tray, the effects of gravity and the reduced effects of salivary flow compared to the mandibular arch.

For single teeth

Full arch trays are constructed, but patients are instructed to only place the bleaching material in the location of the dark tooth. To help patients identify where to place the bleaching material, a small notch can be cut into the tray above the tooth (Small 1998). After the teeth are all the same value, the entire arch can be bleached. This could be achieved the other way, by bleaching all the teeth first and then titrating the shade by bleaching only the single dark tooth.

DISCUSSION OF TREATMENT REGIMEN

The decision about when and how long to keep the trays in the mouth depends on the patient's lifestyle, preference and schedule. Bleaching times will vary according to the patient's schedule. It is useful for the patient to document wearing times in order to modify wearing times if necessary. Some patients titrate and/or adjust the amount of bleach used for certain teeth as they notice some teeth lightening more than others. Some patients report slower bleaching of the canine teeth so they sometimes selectively bleach only the canines for 1 week until the colour is the same in all the teeth. This is particularly the case in teeth with multiple shades and combination bleaching takes place. Higher concentrations of bleach, e.g. 15% or 20%, can be used on these canine teeth to bleach them to a similar level as the other teeth.

Some patients prefer to bleach during the day. Wearing the tray during the day allows replenishment of the gel after 1–2 hours for maximum concentration. Occlusal pressure and increased salivary flow dilute the gel (Dunn 1998). Overnight use may decrease loss of the material from the tray due to decreased salivary flow and reduced occlusal pressure. For maximum benefit per application and compliance for long-term treatment, the bleaching trays should be worn at night (Haywood 2000).

BLEACHING REVIEW

It is best to review the patient 1–2 weeks after wearing the trays. Monitor the oral environment, the soft tissue, mucosae, gingival health and teeth for any adverse reactions. Discuss length of time patient has been wearing the trays and any problems that were encountered. Review patient's logs. Give the patient a new log sheet and retain the old one to document the clinical notes. Modify any timing of tray wearing if necessary. Check the mouth for gingival irritation. The tray may need to be modified (see Figure 5.9). Take the new shade. Take photographs with the new and old shade tabs to evaluate the shade change. Supply the patient with more bleaching material if necessary. Patient compliance is normally better with those patients wearing

Table 5.3 Bleaching schedule

Type of staining	Materials used	Time	Duration
Moderate age-yellowed	10% CPS	1–2 h (d)	
		6–8 h night	2–3 weeks
Moderate tetracycline	10% CPS	3–4 h (d)	6 months
		8–10 h (n)	
	15–20%	same duration 4 months	
Dark canines			
Canines only first	15–20%	3–4 h (d)	1 week
Other teeth	10%	1–2 h (d)	2 weeks
		6–8 h (n)	
Sensitive teeth	5%	0.5–1 h (d)	1 week
		2 h (n)	1 week
if no sensitivity after 1 week	10%	1–2 h (d)	2 weeks
		6–8 h (n)	2 weeks
if no sensitivity	15%	as above	2 weeks
if no symptoms	20%	until bleaching ended	
Darker age-yellowed teeth	20%	3–4 h (d)	2 weeks
No previous sensitivity		6–8 h (n)	2 weeks
Review, re-evalute	20%	same	4 weeks
Single dark tooth	10, 15, or 20%	2–4 h (d)	2 weeks
		6–8 h(n)	2 weeks
		8–10 h (n)	2 weeks
Only bleaching one tooth in tray			
Other teeth age yellowed	10% all teeth	1–2 h (d)	2 weeks
		6–8 h (n)	2 weeks
Non-vital tooth			
Outside/Inside technique	10% in tray single tooth	6–8 h (n)	2 weeks
		dressing changed every 2h	2 days
Close access cavity			
Other teeth yellow	10% all teeth	1–2 h (d)	2 weeks
		6–8 h (n)	2 weeks
Fluorosis			
First try	10% all teeth	3–4 h (d)	3 weeks
		8–10 h (n)	3 weeks
Re-evaluate	Microabrasion	2 chairside appointments	
White spots on front teeth			
First try microabrasion	Microabrasion	2 appointments	
Then try bleaching	10% all teeth	1–2 h (d)	1–2 weeks
		6–8 h (n)	

d, day; n, night.

the bleaching trays at night than during the day (Hattab et al 1999).

Accurately measure bleaching progress after a further fortnight and review as above (Figure 5.7). If the teeth are two shades lighter the patient may wish to stop now, and bleaching treatment of the lower arch can be started.

An important aspect of the dentist-prescribed home bleaching is recalling the patient until it is determined that the current bleaching treatment is complete (Dunn 1998). Review the colour change and do a five or six week assessment, if necessary. Eventually there is a reduction in the rate of colour change and a stage is reached beyond which not much further whitening occurs. At this stage the bleaching treatment should be terminated. Ask the patient to return the trays to protect the patient from over-bleaching the teeth. Patients can become obsessed with achieving a whiter-than-white colour change on the teeth and may continue to over-bleach them. It is important to establish the end point and collect the trays back from the patient. The trays can be re-used for touch up bleaching treatment a few years later if required.

FURTHER TREATMENT

Patients who have bleached their teeth are normally delighted with the results. They often elect to have further aesthetic dentistry undertaken (Figure 5.11). Renewing any necessary composites can be undertaken 2 weeks after cessation of bleaching, once the enamel bond strength has returned. Cosmetic contouring can be undertaken straight away (see Figure 5.10). Preparation of anterior crowns or porcelain veneers should be delayed for at least one month to allow the shade to settle and to allow for any rebound shade shift which may be one shade difference on the value orientated shade guide. It is important to wait prior to making any new crowns as the teeth appear whiter and also brighter. The shade may change and settle very slightly, one week after bleaching has ceased (see Chapters 11 and 12).

MAINTENANCE AFTER TOOTH BLEACHING

Once the light colour has been achieved and the patient is satisfied with the colour, bleaching treatment is terminated. The trays are returned and kept at the dental office. It should be explained that patients should continue their regular maintenance visits which includes periodic oral health evaluation and visits to the dental hygienist. The advantage of home bleaching is that should the teeth darken slightly, re-bleaching is easy, providing the trays still fit correctly and do not distort. Additional re-bleaching or 'top-up' bleaching can be done every three to four years if necessary. Re-bleaching is normally achieved within a week and is not as expensive because the patient just pays for the supply of the bleaching material. However, if the bleaching tray is damaged due to a bruxing habit, it may be necessary to make a new tray. The dentist would continue to monitor the patient's oral health during this time.

TREATMENT OF ADVANCED CASES WITH DENTIST-PRESCRIBED HOME BLEACHING

TETRACYCLINE STAINED TEETH

There is great variation in the appearance of teeth that are stained with tetracycline antibiotics. The intensity and pattern of discoloration are dependent upon the dosage, duration and type given, as well as the calcification activity of the teeth (Leonard et al 1999). Staining can be generalized or localized in horizontal bands within the tooth (Chapter 3). Originally it was thought that tetracycline stained teeth would not be good candidates for the home-bleaching technique. However, several successful studies (Haywood 1997b, Haywood et al 1997) have shown that home bleaching works more slowly than for age-yellowed teeth, but successful lightening and whitening can be achieved over an extended period (from 3 to 6 months). Home bleaching treatment for tetracycline staining is the same as detailed in the protocol above, but the duration is extended until successful lightening has been achieved. Dentists should continue to monitor teeth and other tissues during this 6-month period (Fischer 2000a). Monitoring of the changes in the colour of the teeth needs to be undertaken on a monthly basis. Patients need to be compliant and the monthly review sessions will motivate the patient to continue treatment (see Figures 5.12 and 5.13).

Method of action

The tetracycline is tightly bound-up inside the dentine. This binding makes the discoloration difficult to remove, but it is achievable after a long time. The colour of the dentine is changed as well as the colour of the enamel.

Patients who had tetracycline stained teeth who participated in a longitudinal clinical bleaching study, and underwent dentist-prescribed home bleaching, were overwhelmingly positive about the procedure in terms of shade retention and lack of post-treatment side effects (Leonard et al 1999). Of these patients, 86% reported shade changes. The mean shade change from C4 to B1 was significant ($p < 0.005$) and 80% experienced side effects, namely sensitivity and gingival ulceration. These side effects were sporadic and often disappeared spontaneously. After nearly 1000 hours of bleaching the teeth over a 6-month period, the teeth were examined by scanning electron microscopy which showed no damage to the enamel from the extended bleaching time (Haywood et al 1997).

Payment for bleaching

Payment for extended bleaching can be calculated on a monthly basis, so the patient would pay for the monitoring session and the materials required for bleaching for one month. There can be an initial charge which is slightly higher than the regular monthly bleaching, and an additional fee for each monthly recall visit. This can be similar to other maintenance schemes. The amount of material used per month depends on the arch size, the tray design and the patient's application technique (Haywood 1999). Owing to the extended nature of the bleaching treatment, it is not sure exactly how long bleaching may take. Therefore, it is better for patients to pay month by month, because as soon as the desired colour is reached, bleaching treatment can be terminated. The dentist and patient can agree on continuation of treatment at each recall visit, or agree that bleaching can be terminated.

TEETH WITH MULTIPLE DISCOLORATIONS

Some patients have multiple discolorations in the same mouth. One tooth may become non-vital due to tooth decay, another may be discoloured due to large composite restorations and there may be naturally dark canines in the same mouth. All teeth do not respond to the bleaching material at the same efficacy rate (Leonard et al 1999). Teeth with lighter extrinsic stains respond better than those with darker stain (Leonard et al 1999). It is thus difficult to achieve even bleaching and lightening in a patient who has multiple discolorations. It may be best to adjust the amount of material applied to the teeth of darker discolorations. Normally, bleaching material can be applied evenly to all the teeth for a 2-week period to assess the amount of lightening that can be achieved. However, at the reassessment appointment, it may be appropriate to discuss with patients how to apply the material to certain teeth and not others. This titrating of the doses can be done for a further 2 weeks. Teeth that are darker in the same mouth, such as canines, may need higher concentration of the doses (see Table 5.3). This titrating of the doses can be done for two more weeks to achieve an even whitening colour. It is important to motivate the patient by continual review and assessment, as they may be despondent by the slower pace necessary to achieve a good colour.

TROUBLESHOOTING: SIDE EFFECTS AND PROBLEMS

Patients should be reassured that side effects are minor and transient and normally disappear soon after bleaching treatment is completed (Leonard 1998).

1. *Gingival irritation*. Patients may complain of painful gums after a few days of wearing the trays. It is important to check that the tray is fitting correctly and not impinging on the gingivae. The trays may need to be adjusted, trimmed back, polished or flamed.

2. *Soft tissue irritation*. Some of the patients develop soft tissue irritation (Garber 1997) which may be from overwearing the trays or applying too much bleach to the trays. Check with the patients how much bleach they should be applying (Garber 1997).

3. *Altered taste sensation*. Some patients report a metallic taste sensation immediately after removing the trays, but this normally disappears after a few hours.

4. *Tooth thermal sensitivity*. This is the most common side effect. It normally occurs about two or three days after wearing the trays. Some patients report sensitivity immediately after removing the trays in the morning, which disappears after about four hours. Patients should be advised to discontinue wearing the tray if it is uncomfortable and if tooth sensitivity is severe and to follow the treatment of sensitivity advice (see below). Question the patient about sensitivity. If this has occurred reassure the patient that it is a common side effect and that it will disappear after bleaching. Research has shown that sensitivity disappears following bleaching cessation and after 7 years no patients had sensitivity related to bleaching treatment.

SENSITIVITY ELIMINATION OR REDUCTION

Sensitivity is a common side effect when bleaching teeth (Haywood 1999). About 67% of patients may experience some type of sensitivity at some stage during bleaching (Haywood et al 1994, Nathanson 1997). Different levels of sensitivity may be experienced (Thitinanthapan et al 1999, Albers 2000). Normally patients do not experience any sensitivity for the first three or four nights. It is not known what determines whether or not a patient will experience sensitivity. In a study conducted at the University of North Carolina School of Dentistry, Leonard and coworkers (1997) found that of those patients who changed the solution more than once per night, 55% had sensitivity. This factor was found to be significant ($p < 0.02$). Two-thirds of the patients who demonstrated tooth characteristics such as gingival recession, defective restorations and enamel–cementum abrasion reported sensitivity, but when these characteristics were statistically evaluated, they were not found to be statistically significant risk factors. No statistical relationship existed between age, sex, allergy, bleaching solution used, tooth characteristics or dental arch lightened and the development of side effects.

ORIGIN OF SENSITIVITY

The yellow colour of dentine contributes to the overall colour of the tooth. Dentine consists of millions of round tubules (see Figure 5.14). Movement of fluid in the dentinal tubules is detected by the pain fibres. The movement is triggered by temperature changes, differences in osmotic pressure between different oral solutions and tactile pressure acting on the exposed dentine surface (Bartlett and Ide 1999). The sensitivity of dentine occurs when the dentinal tubules are open and exposed to the oral cavity. The presence of open tubules has been related to increased activation of the pain fibres within the pulp by cold stimuli when applied to tooth surfaces (Bartlett and Ide 1999). These factors may suggest why patients experience sensitivity during tooth bleaching treatment. Treatment is aimed at blocking the tubules.

There are two methods to consider for the treatment of sensitivity during bleaching treatment. The *passive* method consists of altering the bleaching time, frequency or concentration to find a comfortable solution for the patient (see below). The *active* method employs either the use of fluoride or potassium nitrate applied to the tray as a pretreat-

Table 5.4 Possible causes of tooth sensitivity and gingival irritation

- Addition of Carbopol and other thickening agents
- Age of the patient: patients under 40 experience more side effects.
- Anhydrous-based whitening products
- Chemical byproducts of carbamide peroxide
- Chemical interaction of the tray
- Concentration of whitening solution
- Dissolving media
- Exposure time
- Flavours added to the whitening solution
- Frequency of application
- Inherent patient sensitivity
- Medical status of the patient
- pH of the whitening solution
- Sex of the patient: women appear to experience more side effects than men
- Tray material used
- Tray rigidity

Data from Leonard (1998); findings of a study by Knight et al (1997)

ment or at the onset of symptoms. The use of fluoride and potassium nitrate to treat bleaching sensitivity has been clinically researched and seems to work well (Haywood 1999) (see Figure 5.12). The fluoride reduces sensitivity by blocking the tubules. This restricts the ingress of fluids according to the hydrodynamic theory of pain (Bartlett and Ide 1999). A neutral fluoride has been recommended for treatment use such as Prevident 5000 Plus (Colgate Pharmaceuticals). The potassium nitrate reduces sensitivity via chemical interference that prevents the pulpal sensory nerve from repolarizing after initial depolarization (Leonard 1998), or it aids the release of nitric oxide (Haywood 1999). Either way, the effect is directly on the nerve, resulting in a calming effect on the tooth. Many desensitizing toothpastes contain potassium nitrate. Brushing with the desensitizing toothpaste will reduce sensitivity after 2 weeks. The FDA allows 5% potassium nitrate as the maximum concentration. Some patients may experience a tissue burn as a side effect of placing the desensitizing toothpaste in the tray.

Options for treatment of sensitivity during bleaching

Active treatment
For patients with normally sensitive teeth:

- Fluoride toothpaste can be placed in the trays and worn on alternate nights. (Some bleaching agents contain fluoride within the bleaching material to reduce the likelihood of sensitivity, e.g. Opalescence F by Ultradent.)
- A desensitizing toothpaste can be brushed on the teeth or massaged into the cervical margins. Or a specific sensitivity reduction material (such as products by Ultradent and Den-Mat), which contains potassium nitrate, is placed in the bleaching tray and is worn for 1–2 hours, depending on the amount of sensitivity, or applied in the tray for 10–30 minutes before or after whitening.
- The patient can also use a neutral sodium fluoride gel in the trays overnight.
- A specifically manufactured potassium nitrate–fluoride gel for use in the tray can be applied when needed or alternated with the whitening treatment.

For patients with a history of sensitive teeth:

- Two weeks prior to commencing bleaching, the patient can brush regularly with desensitizing toothpaste (e.g. Sensodyne Gentle Whitening, which in the UK contains potassium chloride instead of potassium nitrate).
- Neutral fluoride in the bleaching trays can be applied to the teeth 3 weeks prior to commencing bleaching treatment to reduce sensitivity.
- A patient can begin to wear the empty tray at night for a few nights, then slowly increase the wear time from 1 hour a day for the first week to overnight on the second week or later (Haywood 1999).

Passive treatment
The bleaching technique can be modified:

- Ensure that all excess material is removed.
- Patient can use a bleaching gel with a

lower concentration. If using a 20% carbamide peroxide gel the patient can change to a 15%, 10% or 5% gel.
- Patient can reduce daily treatment time (Leonard 1998) or bleach every other night.
- Patient should not replenish the bleaching solution more than once.
- Patient can use less bleaching material in the tray and not overfill it, to avoid extrusion of excess gel.
- Dentist can ensure that the tray is trimmed back further so that it is not impinging on the gingiva.
- Patient can apply the bleaching treatment every second or third night.

Single tooth sensitivity

The type of sensitivity associated with bleaching treatment is different from single tooth sensitivity. If a patient presents with sensitivity from a single tooth, simple measures can be applied directly to the tooth such as a bonding agent (Bartlett and Ide 1999), fluoride varnish, hema or oxylate preparations, or if necessary the restoration can be replaced. These approaches will help only if sensitivity can be isolated to one accessible area. It is thus best for the dentist to supervise bleaching and to determine the best approach to deal with sensitivity should it arise.

CONCLUSION

Home bleaching is successful in 9 out of 10 cases. The colour duration is 1–3 years or longer. The treatment should be prescribed by the dentist, monitored and supervised by the dentist to ensure a successful and rewarding outcome.

BIBLIOGRAPHY

Albers HF. (2000) Dentine and sensitivity. *Adept Report* **6**:4,10–11.
Bartlett DW, Ide M. (1999) Dealing with sensitive teeth. *Primary Dental Care* **6**(1):25–7.
Bentley C, Leonard RH, Nelson CF, Netley CA. (1999) Quantification of vital bleaching by computer analysis of photographic images. *J Am Dent Assoc* **130**:809–16.
Christensen GJ. (1997) Bleaching teeth: practitioner trends. *J Am Dent Assoc* **128**:16S–18S.
Dunn JR. (1998) Dentist-prescribed home bleaching: current status. *Compend Contin Educ Dent* **9**(8):760–4.
Fasanaro TS. (1992) Bleaching teeth: history, chemicals and methods used for common tooth discolourations. *J Esthet Dent* **4**(3):71–8.
Fischer D. (2000a) Is there a future for the dentist-supervised tray tooth bleaching? *Restor Aesthet Pract* **2**(1):72–5.
Fischer D. (2000b) The need for dentist supervision when tooth bleaching. *Restor Aesthet Prac* **2**(2):98–9.
Garber DA. (1997) Dentist-monitored bleaching: a discussion of combination and laser bleaching. *J Am Dent Assoc Suppl* **128**(4): 26S–30S.
Garber D, Goldstein R, Goldstein C, Schwartz C. (1991) Dentist monitored bleaching: a combined approach. *Pract Periodont Aesthetic Dent* **3**(2):22–6.
Goldstein RE. (1998) *Esthetics in dentistry*, 2nd edn. Vol 1: *Principles, communications and treatment methods*. Part 2(12) *Bleaching discoloured teeth*. 245–76.
Goldstein RE, Garber DA. (1995) *Complete dental bleaching*. Quintessence Publishing: Chicago, IL.
Greenwall LH. (1992) Home bleaching. *J Dental Assoc South Africa* **June**: 304–5.
Greenwall LH. (1999a) Step-by-step home bleaching. *Independent Dentistry* **4**(2):70–4.
Greenwall LH. (1999b) To bleach or not to bleach. Indications for bleaching. *Independent Dent* **4**:60–3.
Hattab FN, Qudeimat M, Al-Rimawi HS. (1999) Dental discolouration: an overview. *J Esthet Dent* **11**:6291–310.
Haywood VB. (1995) Update on bleaching: material changes. *Esthet Dent Update* **6**(3):74.
Haywood VB. (1997a) Nightguard Vital Bleaching: current concepts and research. *J Am Dent Assoc* **128**:19S–25S.
Haywood VB. (1997b) Extended bleaching of tetracycline-stained teeth: a case report. *Contemp Esthet Restor Prac* **1**:14–21.
Haywood VB. (1999) Current status and recommendations for dentist-prescribed, at-home tooth whitening. *Contemp Esthet Restor Prac* June;**3**(Suppl 1):2–9.
Haywood VB. (2000) The current status of Nightguard Vital Bleaching. *Compend Contin Educ Dent.* **21**(Suppl 28)S18–S27.

Haywood VB, Heymann HO. (1989) Nightguard Vital Bleaching. *Quintessence Int* **20**(3):173–6.

Haywood VB, Leonard RH, Dickinson GL. (1997) Efficacy of six months Nightguard Vital Bleaching of tetracycline stained teeth. *J Esthet Dent* **9**(1):13–19.

Haywood VB, Leonard RH, Nelson CF, Brunson WD. (1994) Effectiveness, side effects and long term status of Nightguard Vital Bleaching. *J Am Dent Assoc* **125**:1219–26.

Knight MC, Leonard RH, Bentley C, et al. (1997) Safety issues of 10% carbamide peroxide in clinical usage. *J Dent Res* **76**[IADR Abstracts No. 2366].

Leonard RH. (1998) Efficacy, longevity, side effects and patient perceptions of Nightguard Vital Bleaching. *Compend Contin Educ Dent* **9**(8):766–81.

Leonard RH. (2000) Nightguard Vital Bleaching: dark stains and long-term results. *Compend Contin Educ Dent* **21**(Suppl. 28):S18–S27.

Leonard RH, Haywood VB, Phillips C. (1997) Risk factors for developing tooth sensitivity and gingival irritation associated with Nightguard Vital Bleaching. *Quintessence Int* **28**(8):527–34.

Leonard RH, Haywood VB, Eagle JC, Garland GE, Caplan DJ, Matthews KP, Tart ND. (1999). Nightguard Vital Bleaching of tetracycline-stained teeth: 54 months post treatment. *J Esthet Dent* **11**(5):265–77.

Lyons K, Ng B. (1998) Nightguard Vital Bleaching: a review and clinical study. *New Zealand Dental Journal* **94**:100–5.

Miller MB. (editor) Reality (1999 and 2000). *Reality: the information source for esthetic dentistry*. Vols. 13 and 14. Reality Publishing: Houston, Texas.

Nathanson D. (1997) Vital tooth bleaching: sensitivity and pulpal considerations. *J Am Dent Assoc* **128**:41S–44S.

Small BW. (1998) The applications and integration of at-home bleaching into private dental practice. *Compend Contin Educ Dent* **9**(8):799–807.

Touati B, Miara P, Nathanson D. (1999) *Esthetic dentistry and ceramic restorations*. Martin Dunitz: London.

Thitinanthapan W, Satamanont P, Vongsavan N. (1999) In-vitro penetration of the pulp chamber by three brands of carbamide peroxide. *J Esthet Dent* **11**(5):259–63.

Wander P, Gordon P. (1987) *Dental photography*, 1st edn. BDJ Publications: London.

Wise MD. (1995) *Failure in the restored dentition: management and treatment*. Quintessence: London. 397–412.

Name——————————————————————————— Age: ———————————
Patient's main complaint ————————————————————————————————
Discoloration type: ——————————————————————— Mismatched tooth colours: ————
Special colorations: ———————— Incisal third variation: ———————— Middle third variation: ————
Gingival third variation: ——————————————————————————————
Date bleaching commenced: ——————————————— Preoperative shade ————————————
Shade guide used ————————————————— Patient's desired colour————————————

Informed consent: The patient is informed that there are no guarantees as to the amount of lightening that can be achieved with bleaching treatment. Further dental treatment may be required to bleach the teeth. These options may include microabrasion, bonding, porcelain laminate veneers, crowns or combinations of the above. The patient is instructed to discontinue treatment should any problems occur.

Patient's Signature: ———————————————————————— Date: ———————————

Bleaching Method
❏   Non vital tooth: tooth number.................................. Root canal treatment present..
     Patency of apical seal.. Radiograph checked ....
     Bleaching method: walking bleach........................... Inside/Outside technique...
     Bleaching material used:... Concentration ....

❏   Power bleach:................................... Upper teeth.................................. Lower teeth...............................
     Bleaching material:...Concentration ....
     Radiographs checked..

❏   Home bleach:...................................Upper teeth.................................. Lower teeth................................
     Presence of anterior composites............................... Patient informed they may need to be replaced............
     Bleaching material used:...Concentration ....

Bleaching Audit

Appointment date	Arch	Bleach used	Amount dispensed	Problems
1.				
2.				
3.				
4.				
5.				
6.				
7.				
8.				
9.				
10.				

Post Operative Assessment
Shade preoperative ——————————————————— Shade post operative ————————————————
Recommended rebleaching ————————————————————————————————
Problems encountered ——————————————————————————————————

Maintenance —————————————————————————————————————

Further Aesthetic Treatment ————————————————————————————————

Figure 5.1

Patient bleaching record sheet (modified from Fasanaro 1992).

BLEACHING LOG SHEET

Name: Date:

Present shade of teeth: Desired shade:

Date bleaching started: To bleach upper/lower/both

Day   Date   Amount of hours trays worn   Upper/lower/both   Sensitivity Y/N

Please complete this log while you are bleaching your teeth at home and bring it to each appointment so that we can see the amount of progress you are making. Store it together with your kit for ease of access. If you have any untoward problems, please call the practice. You will be asked to return the trays once bleaching is completed.

Figure 5.2

Bleaching log sheet which the patient has to complete during bleaching at home so that the dentist can monitor the patient's progress and make any recommendations for timing of treatment. The patient should fill these in every day while bleaching. The log sheet should be brought to every appointment so that treatment times can be modified if necessary. Patient compliance can also be assessed.

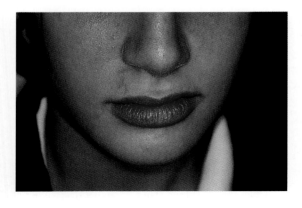

Figure 5.3

Allergic response during home bleaching. This patient successfully bleached her upper teeth with no problems. One week after commencing the bleaching treatment for the lower teeth, she called to say that she awoke during the night and her face and lower lip were swollen. Her teeth were painful. When she attended the practice, it was noted also that there was redness and oedema around the perioral tissues. An allergy to the peppermint flavouring in the bleaching agent was suspected and the patient was referred for further allergy testing on the components of the bleaching materials and plastics.

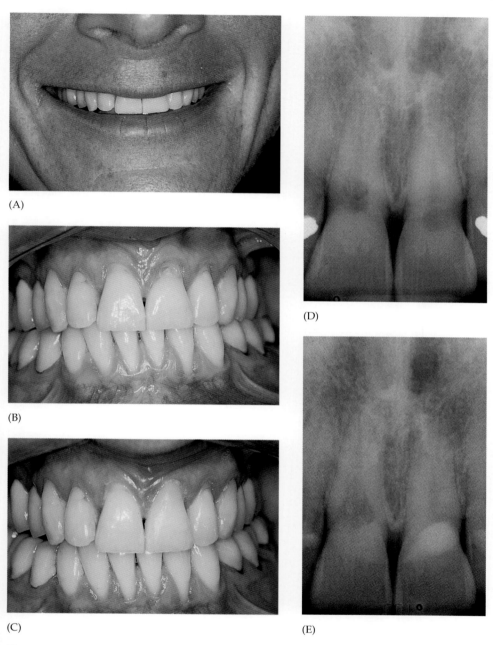

Figure 5.4

(A) This patient appears to have an aesthetic smile and teeth suitable for bleaching. (B) Clinical investigation reveals a missing restoration at the cervical margin. This restoration should be replaced prior to commencing bleaching as it may contribute to sensitivity. (C) The cavity is restored with a compomer restoration (a light-cured glass-ionomer). (D) Radiographic investigation reveals the presence of internal resorption in the pulp chamber. The patient gives a history of the tooth going 'numb' 20 years previously after completing orthodontic treatment. The tooth still responds to vitality testing. (E) Further radiographic investigation 2 years later reveals enlargement of the internal resorption area. Endodontic treatment will have to be commenced. Bleaching is contraindicated in this patient at the present time.

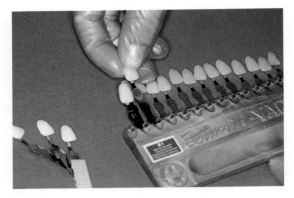

(A)

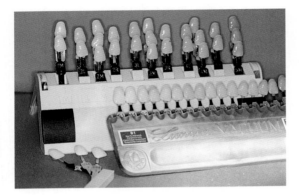

(B)

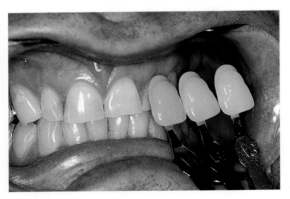

(C)

Figure 5.5

Shade determination. The existing shade is determined using the porcelain shade guide, which can be arranged according to value to help detecting the smaller shifts in shade as the bleaching progresses. It is a good idea to keep two shade guides: one for restorative dentistry for selecting shades of teeth for crowns, bridges and veneers; and one solely for bleaching work. (A) The Vita Classical shade guide is here being arranged according to value, with B1 as the lightest shade. The success of bleaching has allowed teeth to lighten so much that the colour can go beyond the Vita Shade guide. Bleaching shade tabs have been introduced so that porcelain restorations can be matched to the new bleached shade. The bleaching shade guide is placed next to the classical shade guide. (B) The Vita Master Shade Guide offers more selection in shade choice. This figure shows the choice of shades available. The matching lightness level is chosen first. (C) When adjacent teeth have different colours, these should be recorded so that accurate evaluation of the shade shift can be assessed.

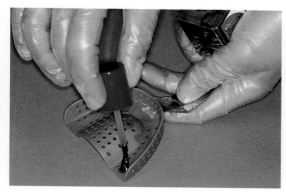

(A)

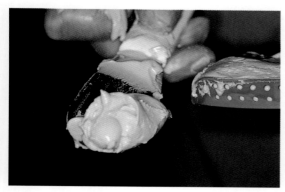

(B)

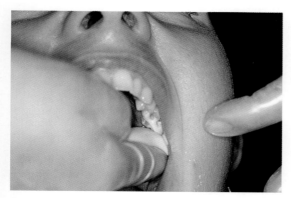

(C)

Figure 5.6

Impression taking: it is essential that an excellent alginate impression be taken in order to make the bleaching tray. (A) The alginate container is shaken gently, to fluff the alginate powder prior to combining it with water. This provides a more consistent mix. Care is taken to dispense the correct amount of powder using the measuring cups provided. Stock trays for alginate can be made of perforated plastic or metal which is more rigid. The metal trays offer less chance of distortion and they are sterilized after use. The plastic trays are disposable. Plastic trays need to have adhesive applied to that the alginate material adheres well to the tray. The perforations are supposed to increase adherence to the tray. Metal trays do not need adhesive as they have in built rim lock devices. (B) Adhesive can be applied to the outside edges of the tray to ensure firm adherence of the borders of the impression. The brush tip is a more precise method of applying the adhesive. Adhesive sprays are also available. The alginate material is then spatulated well when the water is added to the powder. When the mix is ready it is of smooth consistency. The dental assistant provides an amount of alginate on the mixing spatula in order to apply the alginate on to the occlusal surface of the teeth, while the tray which is loaded with the alginate material is brought close to the patient's mouth. (C) Alginate is applied to the incisal surfaces with finger pressure. The alginate material should be placed onto the occlusal surfaces of the molar teeth as well, to prevent air bubbles from building up on the occlusal surface. The tray is placed in the mouth and left in situ for 1 minute to ensure a proper set of the material.

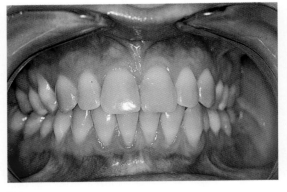

(A)

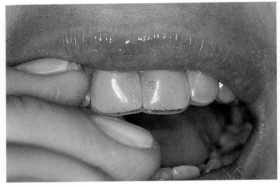

(D)

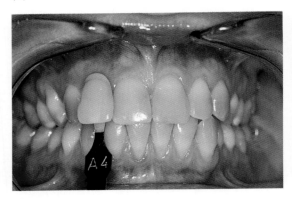

(B)

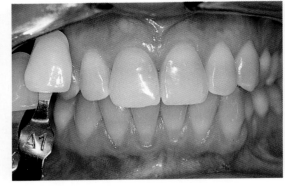

(E)

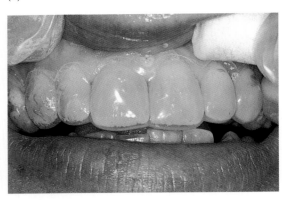

(C)

Figure 5.7

This demonstrates the home bleaching protocol with reference to a patient with mild tetracycline staining. A patient presents to the practice after a 3-week vacation in the sun. She noticed during that time her teeth had discoloured. It is explained to the patient that she has mild tetracycline staining and that the sun caused the teeth to discolour further. Options are discussed for treatment and the patient chooses to have bleaching treatment first. (A) The appearance of the teeth prior to commencing bleaching treatment. (B) The colour of the teeth prior to bleaching showing the porcelain shade tab matching the existing dentition was shade A4. (C) The bleaching tray is tried in to check for correct fit and that there are no over extensions present. It is then loaded with the bleaching material. This is demonstrated to the patient, who is shown how to remove the excess bleaching gel by several methods. A cotton wool roll can be used to remove the excess material. (D) Gentle finger pressure is applied to the tray to improve retention and suction while removing the excess material at the same time. This is demonstrated to the patient by the dentist and the patient copies the action. After the desired amount of tray wearing the tray is removed and the excess material (if any) is brushed off.

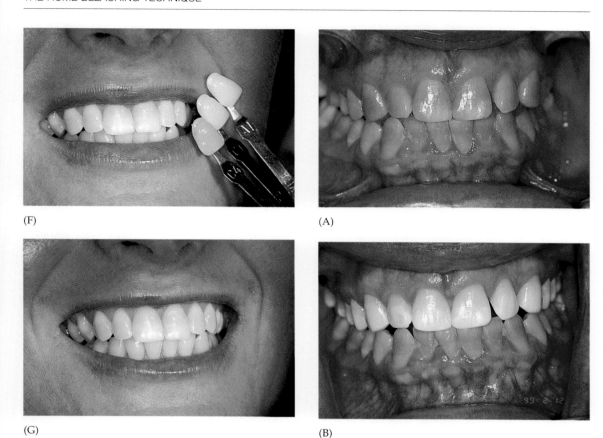

(F)

(A)

(G)

(B)

Figure 5.7 continued

The tray is rinsed under running water to ensure that all the residual bleaching material is removed from the tray. (E) The patient's smile and result after 2 weeks bleaching on the upper teeth. There have been several shade shifts. The porcelain shade tabs are placed next to the teeth in order that a comparison can be made between the original shade and the bleached shade. Note also the comparison between the bleached upper teeth which have lightened and whitened and the yellow lower teeth which had not yet been bleached. This demonstrates the purpose of bleaching the upper teeth first in order to have a colour comparison. (F) The patient's smile after a further 3 weeks of bleaching treatment. The lower teeth had whitened successfully. The range of colour change is shown. (G) The appearance of the teeth after bleaching.

Figure 5.8

(A) Tetyracycline staining. (B) Results after 6 months of home bleaching (by courtesy of Dr Van Haywood).

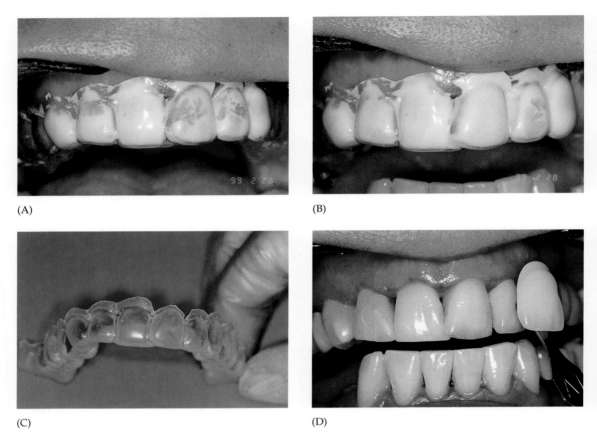

(A)   (B)

(C)   (D)

Figure 5.9

(A) Insufficient material is placed into the tray. There are many air voids present. The tray is over-extended and should be cut back. (B) More material has been added to the tray. This is a more suitable amount, and fills the tray well. (C) There is an excess of at least 2 mm to be cut back from the tray edge. The edge is rough and should be re-polished using a rubber wheel or flame smoothed. (D) This patient still experienced gingival irritation where the trays were rubbing on both upper and lower teeth. As the patient only had 10 teeth present, bleaching treatment was done simultaneously, using the upper and lower bleaching trays.

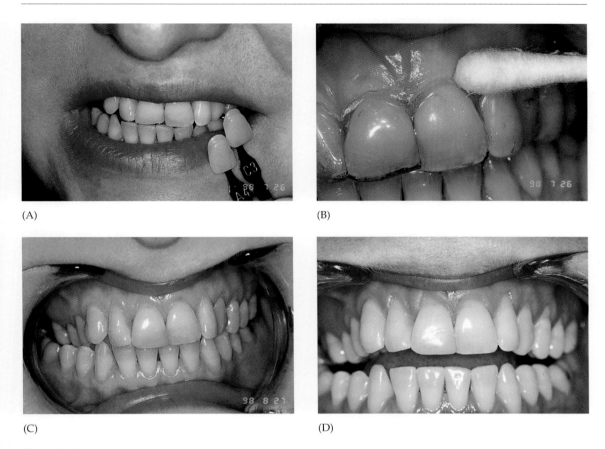

(A)

(B)

(C)

(D)

Figure 5.10

This patient had yellow teeth that were discoloured from a combination of coffee drinking, inherent yellow colour and smoking. Bleaching treatment was undertaken, although the patient had gingival recession and translucent teeth and was therefore not an ideal case. (A) The pre-operative appearance of the teeth. As the patient had some gingival recession on the upper anterior teeth, she was warned that she might experience some thermal sensitivity. If this happened she was to refrain from using the bleach for a few days and instead supplement her home care regime with twice-daily fluoride mouthwash. However, as the patient was going to live abroad and wanted to complete the treatment as soon as possible, both arches were bleached at the same time. There was a natural discrepancy in shade between the upper and lower teeth. The anterior teeth had different lengths and were aligned at different angles. (B) The bleaching tray was tried to check for correct fit. The tray was cut away from the recession areas to reduce the chance of sensitivity. A small amount of the bleaching material was placed into the tray to demonstrate to the patient how much material to apply. The excess material can be removed with a cotton bud. In addition to the bleaching kit, cotton buds and cotton wool rolls are provided to remove the excess material. (C) The result after 3 weeks. The patient had already achieved a colour change of two shades. However, as expected the upper right central incisor had become sensitive. A class 4 restoration was placed to cover over the exposed incisal edge. This stopped the sensitivity on this tooth. It is not ideal to place restorations during the bleaching procedure, as the enamel bond strength is weaker. It is preferable to wait at least a week after bleaching before placing new composite restorations. (D) The final result after cosmetic contouring of the upper and lower teeth, and bonding to the upper right central and lateral incisor.

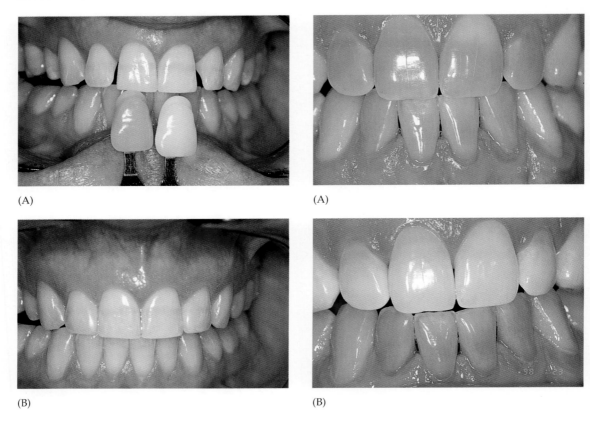

(A)   (A)

(B)   (B)

Figure 5.11

(A) This figure shows the patient during bleaching treatment. The upper teeth have been bleached and the lower teeth will be bleached soon. (B) This patient went on to have further aesthetic dentistry by closing the diastemas between the central and lateral teeth with composite resin bonding. This treatment was undertaken several months after completing home bleaching treatment. (Dentistry by Dr Lambert Fick.)

Figure 5.12

(A) Tetracycline stained teeth prior to treatment. (B) The appearance of the upper teeth after four months of dentist-supervised home bleaching treatment. The grey colour of the upper teeth has been removed and replaced with white. (Courtesy of Dr Van Haywood.)

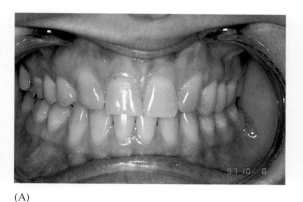

(A)

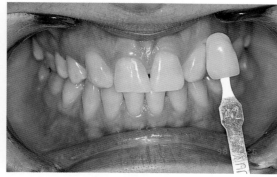

(B)

Figure 5.13

(A) This patient had mild tetracycline staining and missing upper lateral incisors. The appearance of the teeth prior to bleaching treatment. (B) The shade change measured by the shade tab after 3 months.

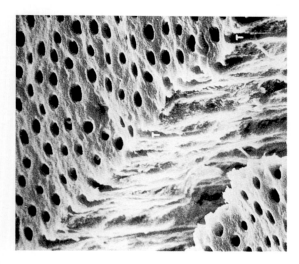

Figure 5.14

The structure of dentine, as revealed on a scanning electron micrograph. (Courtesy of Dr Ilan Rotstein)

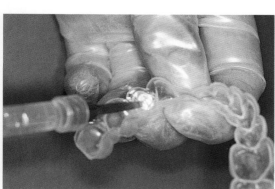

Figure 5.15

Treatment of sensitivity. Desensitizing toothpaste can be used 2 weeks prior to bleaching, applied into the bleaching tray or directly on to the sensitive cervical parts of the teeth. Neutral sodium fluoride gel can be used for desensitizing. It can similarly be applied directly with a brush on to the teeth or it can be placed into the bleaching tray and the tray seated in the mouth. The tray can be worn overnight. The fluoride works by blocking the tubules. This restricts the ingress of fluids according to the hydrodynamic theory of pain. Proprietary agents containing potassium nitrate can be applied directly into the tray. The potassium nitrate reduces sensitivity via chemical interference that prevents the pulpal sensory nerve from repolarizing after initial depolarization, or it aids the release of nitric acid.

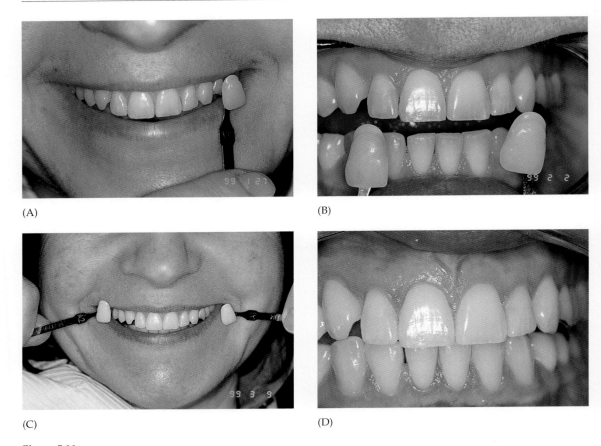

(A)

(B)

(C)

(D)

Figure 5.16

(A) This patient had yellow staining on her teeth due to tea and coffee drinking and had noticed that her teeth had recently become more yellow. The shade is Vita Shade A3,5. (B) Intraoral view of the patient verifying the shade to be Vita Shade A3,5. (C) Smile of the patient showing the shade shift to between Vita Shade A1 and A2. (D) Intraoral view of the final result.

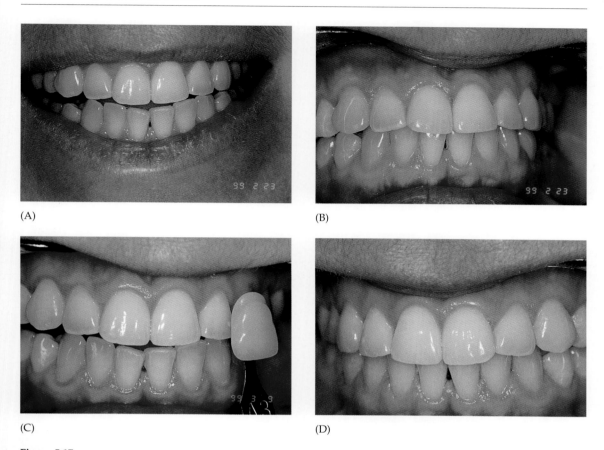

Figure 5.17

(A) Prior to treatment, the patient's teeth are naturally yellow in colour and the canines are darker than the other anterior incisors. (B) Intraoral view prior to treatment. (C) After 3 weeks of bleaching treatment on the upper teeth, the teeth have lightened. The lower teeth are used as a comparison and the difference in the colour of the upper and lower teeth can be noted. (D) Intraoral view of the teeth after bleaching is completed on the upper and lower teeth.

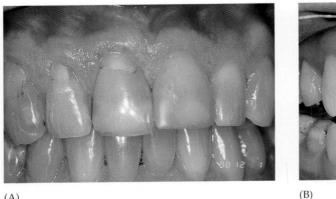

(A)

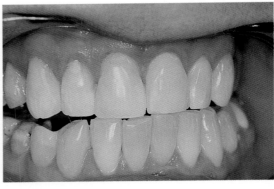

(B)

Figure 5.18

(A) The patient has age-yellow staining with multiple composite restorations on the anterior teeth and gingival inflammation. This case is not ideal, but it demonstrates how bleaching treatment can improve the patient's smile in a very simple way. The patient may need further restorative dentistry once the gingival condition has resolved, but bleaching can enhance the patient's confidence and willingness to continue with further restorative and aesthetic dentistry. Intraoral view of the teeth showing leaking composite restorations and many large anterior composite restorations. The gingiva is inflamed and hypertrophic. (B) The appearance of the teeth after 2 weeks of bleaching treatment. Note the improvement of the gingival condition. The lower teeth are used as a colour comparison. Note the upper teeth are much lighter.

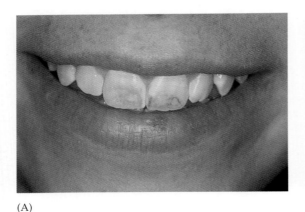

(A)

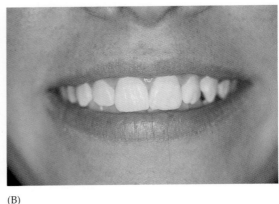

(B)

Figure 5.19

(A) Smile of the patient prior to bleaching showing the brown discoloration on the central incisors. (B) Smile of the patient after 4 weeks of home bleaching. The brown discoloration is permanently removed and the colour of the teeth has whitened. (Courtesy of Dr Martin Kelleher.)

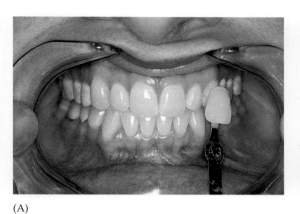

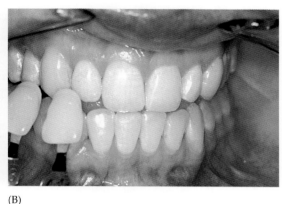

(A)

(B)

Figure 5.20

(A) Portrait of the patient prior to bleaching. She has a wide aesthetic smile. She noticed that the teeth had become a little stained from coffee drinking. She had very mild fluorosis staining on the teeth. The appearance of the teeth prior to bleaching was at Vita Shade A3. (B) The appearance of the teeth after 3 weeks of treatment. The yellow staining was removed from the teeth and the teeth returned to a paler colour. The teeth went from Vita Shade A3 to A1.

6 HOME BLEACHING TRAYS: HOW TO MAKE THEM

INTRODUCTION

The appropriate design and construction of the bleaching trays for home bleaching is essential to successful bleaching treatment and patient compliance. Excess tray material can cause impingement of the soft tissues and irritation of the gingivae. Uncomfortable bleaching trays can lead to the patient failing to comply with the home bleaching regime and discontinuing treatment. This chapter will discuss different tray design features and fabrication options and demonstrate the step-by-step procedures of how to make the bleaching trays.

PROPERTIES OF THE IDEAL BLEACHING TRAY

- It should be strong enough to avoid damage by the patient during wear.
- It should not distort during use.
- It should be made from a material that is bioinert (Greenwall 1999).
- It should not cause irritation to the soft tissues, gingivae, mucosa, tongue or teeth.
- It should not impinge too far on to the papillae.
- It should be thin enough to be well tolerated in the mouth.
- It should be smooth and well polished so that there are no rough edges.
- It should fit comfortably and not feel too tight in places.
- It should not extend into deep undercuts.
- It should be correctly trimmed with freedom of movement for the frenum attachments if the 'full vestibule' design used.
- It should have good retention.

- It should be easy to clean and rinse.
- It should not distort during storage.

There are several designs that can be used depending on the nature and location of the discoloration and the specific case (Haywood 1991). For example if the front teeth are particularly dark and discoloured while the colour of the rest of the teeth is satisfactory a tray can be designed to lighten the central incisors only. Conversely, windows can be cut into the trays to exclude certain teeth (see Figures 6.14 and 6.27).

TRAY DESIGN FEATURES

There are several types of trays which can be used for at-home bleaching.

- Full vestibule upper or lower trays.
- Trays with reservoirs.
- Trays with no reservoirs.
- Trays with a foam liner. Haywood et al (1993) does not recommend this design as its use does not shorten the bleaching time and may impinge on the occlusion.
- Trays with/without windows.
- Tray with scalloping or anatomical cut out. The tray follows the tooth–gingiva interface.
- Non scalloped: straight-line trays.
- Tray with shortened borders.

TRAYS WITH RESERVOIRS

A **reservoir** is a void or space which has been created in the bleaching tray. The *Oxford*

Table 6.1 Tray design options

Design	Indication	Comments
Full vestibule	This type of tray is not commonly used.	Would provide excellent retention but the impingement on the gingivae would cause irritation.
Scalloped/reservoir	Where minimal tissue contact is desired. For highly viscous materials which supply retention. For the maxillary arch to conserve material use.	Saliva ingress is a problem unless insoluble material is used (thick and sticky). Special trimming scissors facilitate fabrication.
Non-scalloped/non-reservoir	This design will provide maximum retention of the bleaching tray. It will provide for maximum retention of the material at the cervical area of the tooth. It is useful for fluid and honey-like bleaching materials. It is indicated for the mandibular arch where the occlusion contacts the buccal/facial of the tooth.	It allows tissue contact which may cause gingival irritation. It cannot extend into undercuts. It should not terminate on soft tissue peak such as rugae or impinge on frenum movement or the canine eminance.
Facial/buccal scalloped reservoir	This type of design is used where taste is a problem to the patient. It can also be used where there has been a problem with tongue irritation from the edges on the tray.	It avoids spill over the material onto the tongue from the lingual side. It provides a smooth edge for tongue contact.
Scalloped reservoired buccal and lingual surfaces, no occlusal surface	This type of tray can be used for TMD patients who cannot tolerate fine changes to the occlusal surfaces.	Using a vicous bleaching gel will allow excellent bleaching of the teeth. There should be no difference in bleaching rates with the occlusal surfaces removed.
Scalloped non-reservoir	This type of tray is used for fluid or paste materials, (e.g. Colgate Platinum; see Figure 6.29) when tissue avoidance is desired, but allowing for maximum retention of the tray.	There is no apparent difference in the bleaching rate with or without reservoirs. As there is no apparent difference between bleaching rates, Miller (2000) has recommended that the reservoirs are not necessary anymore.
Non-scalloped reservoir	This design is used when seating a tray with viscous material where a better seal is desired.	The mandibular arch is best with the non-scalloped design for retention of the material and tissue comfort.

(Modified from Haywood 1997.)

Handy Dictionary definition (1988) of a reservoir is a receptacle for fluid. The reservoir in the tray acts as a receptacle for the bleaching material. The viscous bleaching material is better retained if a reservoir has been created in the bleaching tray. It is normally used to hold extra bleaching material near the surface of the tooth. It is made by placing or flowing a light cured resin/composite on to the buccal surfaces of the teeth on the plaster model. The reservoir can also be called a **spacer**.

Function of the reservoir

It has been determined that the reservoir or spacer performs many important functions.

Advantages

1 It retains and contains the bleaching material better, particularly the more viscous bleaching materials such as Opalescence (Ultradent Products, Optident, UK) and prevents it from leaking around the gingivae.
2 It allows the bleaching material to stay in contact with the tooth for longer.
3 It may help to keep the bleaching material active for longer (Matis et al 1999).
4 It allows gel in areas with a higher concentration of carbamide peroxide to be transferred to areas with a lower concentration (Matis et al 1999).
5 It holds more bleaching material (Miller 1999).
6 It prevents wash out of the bleach.
7 The reservoir aids in seating highly viscous materials (Oliver and Haywood 1999).
8 It prevents the occurrence of pinching pressure.

Disadvantages

1 It causes the tray to become less retentive (Haywood 1995).
2 More bleaching material is required to fill the tray.
3 It makes the tray more bulbous and slightly thicker.
4 There may be the potential for occlusal interference on the mandibular arch.
5 It requires additional time and products to be made.

Reservoirs are normally placed on the buccal/facial surfaces of the tooth. There is no apparent difference in bleaching rate with or without reservoirs (Haywood 1997). Reservoirs can be used depending on:

- the viscosity of the bleach used. Some materials, e.g. Opalescence, are very viscous. The material is retained in place better if there is a reservoir that allows for easier seating. If the bleaching agent has a thin viscosity, a reservoir is not needed (Haywood 1995).
- tooth anatomy. If a tooth is more bulbous than the rest it may not be necessary to place a reservoir. Teeth with less aesthetic

demands (e.g. second molar teeth) do not require placement of reservoirs.
- tooth darkness. The darker the tooth the thicker the reservoir should be (see Figure 6.24).
- a dark cervical margin. These cases should have the tray designed 1 mm over the gingivae and could have a reservoir as more bleach is required to go into the dark cervical margin.

Where should the reservoir be placed?

The reservoir should be placed on the buccal surfaces of the model of the teeth at least 1 mm away from the gingivae. This will seal the tray at the gingivae. The block-out resin can be placed to the incisal edge.

SCALLOPED TRAYS

Scalloped trays allow for minimal soft tissue contact. They cause minimal gingival irritation and use a minimal amount of bleaching material. The tray follows the tooth–gingiva interface. The tray should be cut back 1 mm so that the gingivae are not impinged on those patients that have a high lip line. Scalloping prevents soft tissue contact and reduces gingival irritation. However, saliva may ingress at the neck of the tooth and may remove material from the tray. Furthermore, the tongue or lip can become irritated from the scalloped edges of the tray. Additional time is required to make this type of tray.

NON-SCALLOPED STRAIGHT-LINE TRAYS

These trays are cut out 2 mm over the labial incisors. Touati et al (1999) recommend using this type of tray. They state that this design is easier to use, is simpler to carry out, is less traumatic to the rest of the mouth, and provides a better border seal than the anatomical tray design. This design has the interproximal spaces filled in and a central thin reservoir in the middle of each tooth.

TRAYS WITH SHORTENED BORDERS

Although this tray design is not ideal, it can be made in certain circumstances such as a patient with excessive gingival recession, or pre-existing sensitivity, or a patient who gags easily. Capillary action will transmit the bleach to the cervical part of the tooth. This is not often recommended because the trays could theoretically act as an orthodontic retainer, or anterior bite splint if the tray is worn for a long period. Intrusion and uncontrolled orthodontic movement of the teeth could result from prolonged wearing of a shortened bleaching tray. It is usually better to have full occlusal coverage of all the teeth.

TRAYS WITH WINDOWS

This depends on the location of the discoloration and can allow for a single or group of teeth to be bleached. Windows can be used to exclude certain teeth from the bleaching process. This is usually when some of the teeth have a light colour and the others are darker. Windows can be cut around the light teeth (see Figure 6.14). Windows can be used also to bleach single dark teeth where the teeth surrounding the dark tooth are cut back so that they are not bleached. Windows can also be used when further restorative dentistry may be contemplated after bleaching treatment.

THICKNESS OF THE TRAY

There are many varying thicknesses of plastic used for the trays and it depends on the patient. If the patient has a bruxing habit, it is advisable to use a thicker tray material as the patient may wear through a thin tray in a matter of days (see Figure 6.23). If the patient gags easily it would be advisable to use a very thin tray that is scalloped well so that it is easily tolerated. It is possible to make trays with no occlusal coverage for those patients who have

temporomandibular joint dysfunction (TMD) syndrome. In this case the tray material would cover the labial and lingual surfaces and be cut away from the occlusal surfaces. The standard thickness is the 'Sof-Tray' size 0.035 inch made by Ultradent Products Inc., Utah, USA (supplied by Optident Company).

MAKING THE TRAY

EQUIPMENT NEEDED

1   Cast of the teeth.
2   Block-out resin and applicator.
3   Curing light box or light-cure hand-held machine.
4   Cold mould seal (Figure 6.3) and applicator.
5   Sheet material, e.g. plastic sheets ready cut to the appropriate shape (Sof-Tray, Ultradent, USA; Figure 6.4).
6   Heat/vacuum tray-forming machine.
7   Pair of scissors for trimming the gross excess.
8   Scalpel handle (Bard Parker) and blade (No. 12) with access to a flame.
9   A polishing trimmer, cotton wheel (Figure 6.8).
10 Straight/laboratory slow handpiece.
11 Stone, spatula and mixing machine (if available) (Greenwall 1999).

STEP-BY-STEP GUIDE

1. Take a good alginate impression

Spatulate the alginate well. Alginator machines can be used to reduce the occurrence of air bubbles in the alginate mix. (See Chapter 5 on home bleaching for impression taking in further detail.) Alginate can be wiped on the occlusal surface with a finger to avoid air entrapment (Haywood and Powe 1998). Load the tray and seat it gently. Leave the alginate to set for 1 minute. Once the alginate has set, remove from the mouth. Ensure that there are no air bubbles on the occlusal, facial or lingual surfaces of the impression. Disinfect the impression and rinse the disinfectant to ensure that the impression is not distorted (Figure 6.20). Wrap the models in a damp paper towel and send to the laboratory.

2. Cast a model

Pour stone into the impression and ensure that there is no air entrapment in the stone. Suggestions for stone include Microstone (Whipmix, Louisville KY 40217), Kaffir D stone, Gnathastone (Panadent UK, London), a fast setting stone Snapstone (Whipmix) which can set in 8 minutes. Follow the manufacturer's instructions on the setting times carefully. The cast should be free from bubbles, voids or excess plaster. Any minor voids can be blocked out. Any excess plaster bubbles should be removed from the occlusal and cervical areas (see Figure 6.1).

3. Trim the model

The model should be carefully trimmed so that the base of the model is flat and parallel to the occlusal plane. The cast can be trimmed further around the base into a horseshoe shape so that it is easier to remove the heated plastic from the cast. However, do not over-trim the model as this could make it too weak and thin (Miller 1999) and it may fracture. It is best to allow the model to dry for 24 hours to allow the stone to set fully and to stop further expansion of the stone. This will prevent distortion of the tray. However, the fast-setting stone models can be trimmed after 10 minutes.

4. Place the block-out resin

Using the block-out composite material, gently place it in the middle of each tooth. (See Figures 6.1 and 6.2.) Start in the midline and work your way back. The block-out kit comes with an applicator, which has a brush tip on the end to enable ease of placement.

5. Cure the resin

Once the desired amount of block-out resin has been added around the teeth, it can be placed in a light box (the one used in our laboratory is the Triad 2000 light box from Dentsply/York Division). We set the machine to 4 minutes to ensure that an all-round full cure is achieved. Place the cast in the centre of the stand to ensure an even cure.

6. Apply separator/cold mould seal

Once the curing is complete place a thin layer of cold mould seal over the model (Figure 6.3). This will facilitate ease of removal of the plastic press down from the model at a later stage. Remove the excess seal by air drying with compressed air.

7. Choose the tray sheet material

There are several types of plastic which can be used to make the trays. Some manufacturers supply the tray material inside the bleaching kits. The most common tray material is ethyl vinyl acetate (Eva). The Eva material is a flexible material of the type used for sports guards but it is much thinner (Newman and Bottone 1995). The size 0.035 inch is the most common thickness used, but there are thinner ones at 0.02 inch and thicker ones for patients with a bruxing habit at size 0.05 inch. For the purpose of demonstration we have used the 'Sof-Tray' size 0.035 inch made by Ultradent Products, Inc., Utah, USA (supplied by Optident Company). The sheets come in squares with a protective backing.

Some press-down machines only take round sheets, not square ones. These can be cut down by using a specific template and scalpel. It is also possible to buy round sheets pre-cut. The machine should be preheated for 10 minutes prior to starting the procedure. It is essential to remove the protective backing prior to placing the plastic sheet in the machine (see Figure 6.4). Ensure that the sheet is placed into the correct location and in the centre of the holder. It is kept in place with three lugs.

8. Cast the plastic in the vacuum tray-forming machine

Place the cast with the teeth face-up in the centre of the machine making sure that the plastic sheet is directly above it. The machine used was a Drufomat-TE (Dreve-Dentamid GmbH, Unna, Germany supplied by Panadent Ltd, London, UK). Wait until the plastic has melted, is hanging down and just touching the cast before pulling the machine down over the cast (Figure 6.4). The machine should be pulled down slowly to avoid generating any creases of the plastic. Sufficient time should be allowed for the vacuum to be properly adapted to the cast. The resultant effect will be the heated plastic sheet vacuum-suctioned over the cast. To avoid tray distortion, the plastic should cool down sufficiently before the trays are trimmed. Remove the plastic sheet from the case; the gross excess can be removed using a small pair of scissors.

9. Trim the tray

Continue trimming the tray with scissors until about 1 cm above the gingival margin (see Figures 6.6 and 6.7.) Put the bleaching tray back on to the model and with a heated scalpel carefully trim the palatal margins close to the clinical crown margin of the teeth (Figure 6.17). Remove the excess flash as you go along. The buccal/facial parts of the tray can be scalloped first (Figure 6.6). Once the buccal part has been completed, start trimming the palatal margins by using the same technique, i.e. with the heated scalpel. This time, scallop the edge 1–2 mm above the clinical crown margin. However, if the patient has particularly sensitive teeth prior to starting the bleaching procedure, the tray should be cut back to 1 mm below the clinical crown height. This design of tray is good for those patients who have particularly dark cervical margins.

10. Polishing the tray

Remove the tray from the model again and start polishing and finishing the edges with a soft cotton wheel so that there are no rough parts (Figure 6.8). To ensure that the frenum attachments have freedom of movement, the tray may need to be further relieved in certain areas. Place the tray back on the model for the final polishing as at this stage it can easily distort. Some techniques advise flame polishing of the edges if it distorts.

THE FINISHED TRAY

The finished tray is shown in Figure 6.9. Once the trays are completed they are returned to the dentist and put back on to the plaster models. These trays are useful to demonstrate how to wear the trays on the model with the blue resin acting as a good contrasting background. The dentist will check the tray for correct fit and make any necessary adjustments.

BIBLIOGRAPHY

Haywood VB. (1991) Overview and status of mouth-guard bleaching. *J Esthet Dent* **3**(2):157–61.

Haywood VB. (1995) In: RE Goldstein, Garber DA, editors. *Complete dental bleaching*. Quintessence: Chicago. 71–100.

Haywood VB. (1997) Nightguard Vital Bleaching: current concepts and research. *J Am Dent Assoc Suppl* **128**:19S–25S.

Haywood VB, Powe A. (1998) Using double poured alginate impressions to fabricate bleaching trays. *Operative Dentistry* **23**:128–31.

Haywood VB, Leonard RH, Nelson CF. (1993) Efficacy of foam liner in 10% carbamide peroxide bleaching technique. *Quintessence Int*, **24**:663–6.

Greenwall LH. (1999) How to make home bleaching trays. *Independent Dentistry* **4**(7):71–5.

Matis BA, Gaiao U, Blackman D, Schultz FA. (1999) In-vivo degradation of bleaching gel used in whitening teeth. *J Am Dent Assoc* **130**(2):227–35.

Miller MB. (editor) (1999) *Reality: The information source for esthetic dentistry*. Reality Publishing: Houston, TX.

Miller MB. (editor) (2000) *Reality: The information source for esthetic dentistry*, Vol 14. Reality Publishing Company: Houston.

Newman SM, Bottone PM. (1995) Tray forming technique for dentist supervised home bleaching. *Quintessence Int* **26**(7):447–53.

Oliver TL, Haywood VB. (1999) Efficacy of Nightguard Vital Bleaching technique. Beyond the borders a shortened tray. *J Esthet Dent* **11**(2):95–101.

Oxford Handy Dictionary (1988), 6th edn. Oxford University Press and Chancellor Press: London.

Touati B, Miara P, Nathanson D. (1999) *Esthetic dentistry and ceramic restorations*. Martin Dunitz: London.

MAKING A SCALLOPED RESERVOIRED BLEACHING TRAY

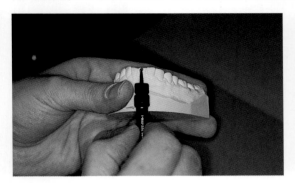

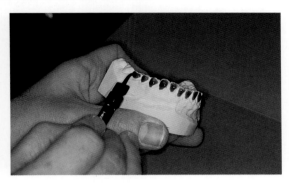

Figure 6.1

Check that the model is free from surface blebs or air bubbles that can interfere with the exact fit of the tray at the cervical edges and thus the correct seating of the tray. Place the block-out composite resin on to the first tooth to create a reservoir. The resin is positioned in the centre of the tooth, avoiding the incisal edges and gingival crevices. Ensure that it is applied evenly.

Figure 6.2

Start from the midline, place the resin all along the buccal surfaces of the tooth. This takes a matter of seconds. Teeth that have lower aesthetic concerns need not have reservoirs placed such as lower second and third molars.

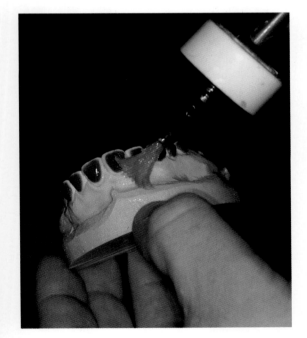

Figure 6.3

The light box is set for 4 minutes to fully cure all the resin. Place the cast in the centre of the tray table. The tray table rotates around the light source for 4 minutes to ensure an even cure. Once the blue resin has set, it is firm and has a slightly oily feel to it. It is advisable to place a thin layer of cold mould seal separating medium over the teeth and the model. This will facilitate easy removal of the tray material from the model after it has been vacuum formed. Apply the cold mould seal to the buccal and lingual surfaces of the model. Blow the excess off the cold mould seal using the compressed air hose.

124 BLEACHING TECHNIQUES IN RESTORATIVE DENTISTRY

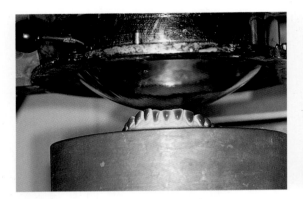

Figure 6.4

The sheets come in varying sizes, shapes and thicknesses. The 0.035 inch thickness is the standard size which are boxed in 25 sheets. As the machine only takes round sheets, these are cut into the correct shape using a template and scalpel. It is essential to remove the backing from round plastic sheet, since otherwise it will not melt properly. Ensure that the plastic sheet is placed into the holder correctly. The machine has three holding lugs to keep the plastic in place. Place the model on the base section of the vacuum tray-forming machine. Ensure that the plastic sheet is properly placed over the model. Raise the model to the heating element at the correct height. When the plastic has sufficiently melted it will hang over and just touch the model. At this stage it is ready for starting the press-down procedure.

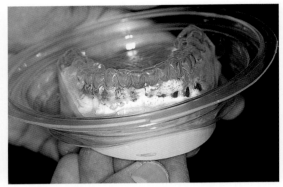

Figure 6.5

The plastic sheet is now more easily removed from the press. The application of the cold mould seal underneath the plastic leaves a white residue.

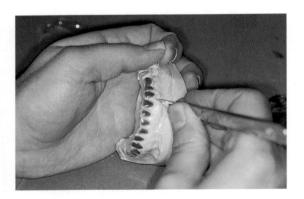

Figure 6.6

Scalloping the tray on the buccal/facial surface of the model using a heated scalpel blade for better accuracy. The tray can be trimmed to 1 mm above the gingival margin or just above the neck of the tooth. The excess flash is easily removed at the same time.

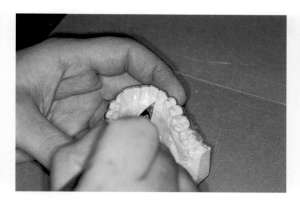

Figure 6.7

The palatal lingual portion is then scalloped in the same manner. Using a scalpel heated with a flame, trim off the excess of plastic around the palatal cervical margin of the teeth. Remove the flash which should come away easily.

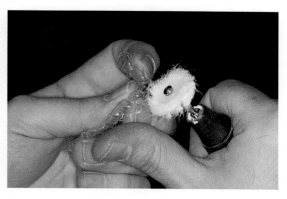

Figure 6.8

The edges of the tray should be carefully polished gently with a special soft cotton wheel. The thin trays can be carefully polished into the scalloped areas, by gently bending the tray. The polishing discs used to polish the scalloped margin.

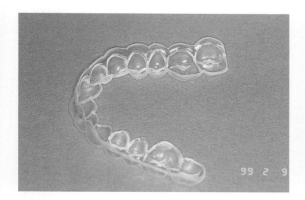

Figure 6.9

A finished upper tray.

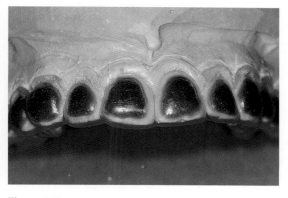

Figure 6.10

Place the finished tray back on to the cast after and during polishing to ensure that the tray does not distort. The trays are returned from the laboratory to the dentist. The model shows the areas where the scalpel was used to trim the tray.

VARIOUS TRAY DESIGNS

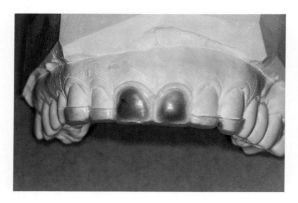

Figure 6.11

A shortened bleaching tray with a shortened dental arch. Even though the tray is shortened, it can still assist with tooth lightening (Oliver and Haywood 1999). Shortened bleaching trays are only recommended for very specific cases and should not be used routinely.

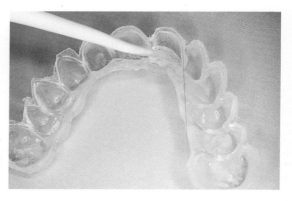

Figure 6.12

A design for a bleaching material that has a honey-like consistency. This has a non-scalloped design on the palatal part and a scalloped design on the buccal/facial part. The scalloping on the facial portion is very rough and needs to be polished more as it can cause gingival irritation.

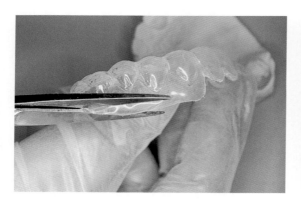

Figure 6.13

Modifications necessitated by change to a different bleaching material. The tray has had to be modified from a full vestibule non-scalloped design to scalloped design.

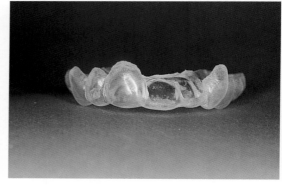

Figure 6.14

Shows a different light cure block-out resin. This patient has very dark canine teeth, so more block-out resin was placed on the canines. The upper left central and lateral are a good colour and do not need to be lightened. The tray has been cut out from this area so that these teeth are not lightened. The palatal portion is covered to avoid any changes to the occlusion.

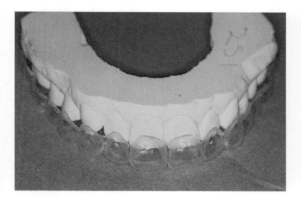

Figure 6.15

This tray has a scalloped, non-reservoir design, for a bleaching material that has a toothpaste-like consistency.

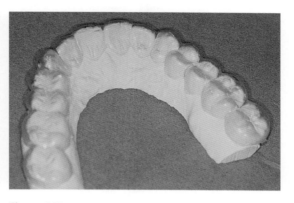

Figure 6.16

The plaster cast has been cut back into a horseshoe design to facilitate the scalloping process.

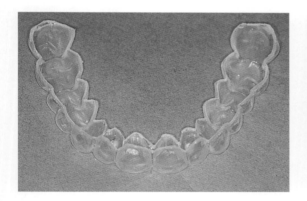

Figure 6.17

The scalloped non-reservoir tray.

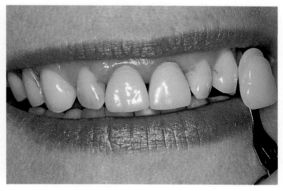

Figure 6.18

This patient, who needs extensive restorative dentistry, is not happy with the colour of her remaining four anterior natural teeth. She required a full mouth rehabilitation, which included long-term provisional restorations, the opening of the occlusal vertical dimension, a sinus lift procedure and implants were to be placed in the edentulous upper posterior section. This figure shows the colour of the teeth before bleaching treatment and before extensive restorative dentistry was undertaken (see Chapter 12).

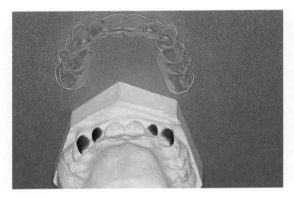

(A)

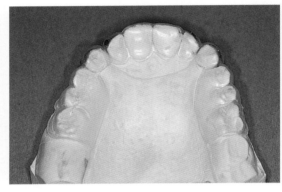

(B)

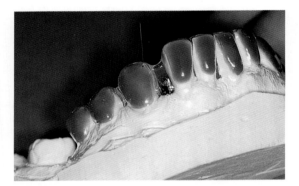

(C)

Figure 6.19

(A) As the patient was wearing a partial chrome denture a tray was designed to fit over the denture. This figure shows the block-out resin which was placed on the lateral incisors and the canines only. The tray was extended on to the denture teeth for extra retention. Some authors advise making two trays for denture wearers. One to use with the dentures in place and one to use when the dentures are not being worn. (B) The bleaching tray on the model, showing the anterior palatal scalloping. (C) A bleaching tray design showing a model with spacing of the teeth. When this occurs the plastic continues into the space between the teeth.

PROBLEM-SOLVING AND TROUBLESHOOTING TO ENSURE SUCCESS

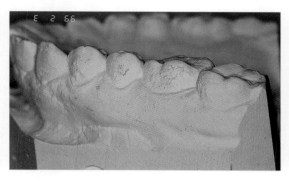

Figure 6.20

Shows that the excess disinfectant has not been washed off the impression prior to pouring the impression. This has left a residue behind on the buccal surface. A new impression should be taken as it is possible that distortion of the cast has resulted. Do not attempt to make a bleaching tray on such a model.

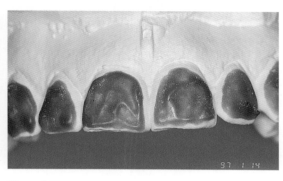

Figure 6.21

The block-out material has not been evenly placed onto the model. This can result in an uneven reservoir formation, which may be uncomfortable for the patient to tolerate on the labial mucosa. In this case wax was used as block-out material and melted unevenly when placed into the vacuum machine. Block-out resins are better to use because they do not melt under the heat of the machine.

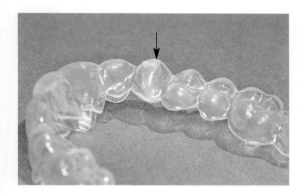

Figure 6.22

After 2 weeks of night time wear, this patient has worn roughened areas on her tray due to bruxing habits. Note the roughened canine (arrow). The trays should be inspected at recall sessions. The roughened tray could irritate the tongue and should be polished in this area. Even if the tray has not completely worn through, it may be better to re-design and remake it using a thicker tray material.

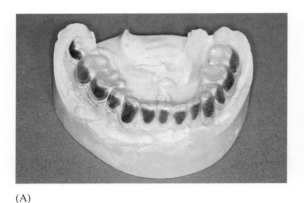
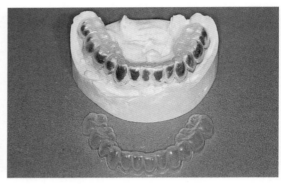

(A)   (B)

Figure 6.23

Trays should always cover all occlusal portion of the teeth in an arch to prevent temporomandibular joint problems. (A) This tray was made without including the last tooth of the arch. The patient reported that in the morning her 'bite' felt strange as she could feel the back tooth only in contact. (B) The tray was remade using a thicker material and included occlusal coverage on all the teeth.

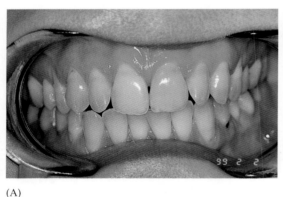
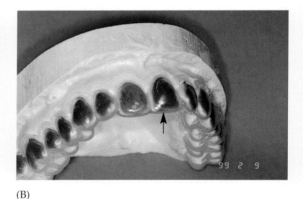

(A)   (B)

Figure 6.24

(A) Two central incisors having different colours. (B) Extra reservoir space can be placed on the darker tooth (arrow). This will allow for extra material to be retained for longer and help to lighten the teeth to the same colour as the other one. The scalloped reservoired bleaching tray is shown over the plaster model of the teeth.

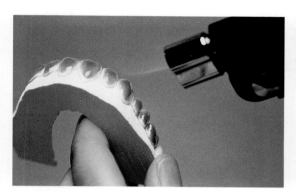

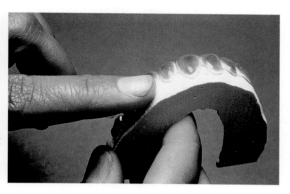

Figure 6.25

Sometimes after scalloping the edges of the tray with a pair of scissors, there can be distortion at the cervical area. If this should occur, the tray can be reheated on the model.

Figure 6.26

The reheated plastic tray is pressed back into place using gentle finger pressure. This will help to achieve close fitting margins at the cervical area.

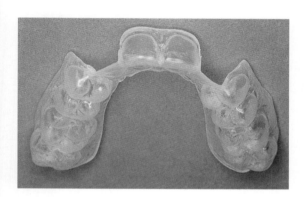

Figure 6.27

This patient had veneers that were lighter than her existing teeth. A tray was designed to exclude these teeth from the bleaching procedure. Reservoirs were placed on all teeth except the lateral incisors. The tray design is shown with the lateral teeth cut from the arch. In this case a non-scalloped design was used to give the tray extra strength.

POWER BLEACHING AND IN-OFFICE TECHNIQUES

George A Freedman, Gerald McLaughlin
and Linda Greenwall

INTRODUCTION

Clinical techniques for destaining teeth can be classified into two complementary modalities: in-office bleaching covered in this chapter and at-home bleaching covered in Chapter 5. Each of these techniques has certain advantages. Both can, and should be used by dentists in combating dental discoloration.

Some dentists and patients prefer in-office or power bleaching. A high concentration of hydrogen peroxide is administered to the teeth with an activating or promoting method (e.g. heat, light or laser) to expedite the whitening effect (Barghi 1998). Many variations of the technique are available but insufficient research has been carried out to verify if it is more effective than at-home bleaching, which has the advantage of requiring less total chair time and a lower patient fee. The whitening materials that are used for at-home bleaching are often of a lower concentration and therefore use of rubber dam is not involved.

In-office bleaching is useful in the removal of stains throughout the arch (for example, age or tetracycline staining), or for lightening a single tooth in an arch (such as post-endodontically), or perhaps even treating specific areas of a single tooth (such as in some types of fluorosis). The dentist is in complete control of the process throughout treatment. This provides the advantage of being able to continue treatment or to terminate the decolouring process at any time. In-office bleaching is usually so rapid that visible results are observed even after a single visit. As patients become visually motivated at the first appointment, they tend to be more compliant for the second and third appointments that are often required to complete the in-office process. Many patients prefer bleaching by the dental professional because it requires less active participation on their part.

In order to best serve their patients, dentists should ideally be familiar with both at-home and in-office treatment modalities. It is not uncommon to combine both techniques for a customized whitening treatment of a single patient. In this way, the patient sees immediate results and is encouraged to continue the treatment both at home and in the office. By the combination of these two techniques, the whitening process is continued in-between the office bleaching sessions, and thus the final result is achieved more rapidly than if either technique were to be used alone. In either case, a colour indicator signals the completion of the oxidation process. Users will find that in a single application, it is not uncommon to note a one- to two-shade value change (see Chapter 5).

TERMINOLOGY

There are many names associated with in-office bleaching.

- Chairside bleaching
- Power bleaching
- Laser bleaching (the term is often used loosely for any light source)

- Dentist administered/applied bleaching (Barghi 1998)
- Assisted bleaching (Miller 1999)/dentist supervised bleaching (Barghi 1998)

WHAT MATERIALS ARE AVAILABLE FOR POWER BLEACHING?

- 35% hydrogen peroxide liquid, liquid/powder products or a gel (thick, containing a stabilizer, or thin, red coloured gel) called a 'power gel' or 'laser bleaching gel'.
- 35% carbamide peroxide.
- Various concentrations or combinations of the above materials.
- Dual-activated bleaching system (Toh 1993). This material (containing 35% hydrogen peroxide gel) is both light and chemically activated.

BENEFITS OF POWER BLEACHING GELS

Manufacturers claim the use of a gel for in-office bleaching decreases the incidence of tooth sensitivity by reducing the tooth desiccation commonly observed with the liquid and the liquid/powder products. The gel contains 10–20% water which rehydrates the tooth as bleaching continues. The consistency of the gel allows it to remain in intimate contact with the tooth (Tam 1992). The presence of water in the gel reduces the shelf-life and some of these products need mandatory refrigeration (Barghi 1998). The gels minimize the possibility of soft tissue contact as they remain in the area where they are placed. It appears that the viscous nature of the gels may promote better penetration of the oxidizing ions through the enamel by acting as a blanket to prevent the escape of oxygen ions. Gels can be freshly mixed just before the treatment commences. The shelf-life of hydrogen peroxide is very short (approximately 6 months). It is important to check the shelf-life of the hydrogen peroxide liquid prior to combining it with the powder to form a gel. This can affect the bleaching efficacy of the gels. A fresh solution should be mixed for each patient.

EQUIPMENT NEEDED

1. *The power bleach materials.* The bleaching gel materials are now more effective because they are less likely to release heat. Many require less time to be activated and to penetrate the teeth. Some contain a stabilizer which makes them more effective while they remain on the teeth.
2. *Tissue protector.* Although the standard rubber dam (Figure 7.8) with mucosal protector can be used, many light-activated liquid resins are available to protect the gingivae, which have gained popularity (e.g. Paint-on-Dam by Den-Mat Corporation and Opaldam, by Ultradent, USA).
3. *Energizing/activating source.* This can be by heat or light. The light source activates/catalyses the bleaching material. There are many different lights available:

- Traditional bleaching light. The traditional light used heat and light to activate the 35% hydrogen peroxide while the patient sat under the rubber dam for about an hour. The great heat generated from this source may cause dehydration. It is now considered obsolete.
- Regular halogen curing light.
- Plasma arc light.
- Argon and CO_2 lasers.
- Xenon power arclight.

Note that the use of resin-curing lights with bleaches does not provide enhancement of the bleaching outcome (Christensen 2000).

4. *Heat source.* It appears that a heat source may not be necessary to enhance the bleaching effect: the teeth are not bleached significantly lighter and the oxygen release is not significantly higher (Christensen 2000). Some bleaches are heated in hot water first or heated over a flame before application on to the tooth. The use of the radiosurgery unit spoon-shaped electrode has been advocated for accelerated bleaching procedures (Sherman 1997). The curing lights and plasma arc lights produce only a relatively small amount of heat, however. The plasma arc light has a clear glass bleaching probe which can be attached to the light. It emits more heat and thus should be held a short distance away from the teeth.

Plasma arc lights generate their energy from a high frequency electrical field, using a wider frequency than a laser. Plasma arc lights have been claimed to speed up the bleaching reaction using the power gels (Croser 1999 and Apollo 95E manufacturer's instructions); however, there is little published research on the use of bleaching and plasma arc lights (Christensen 1999).

5. *Protective clothing and eyewear.*

6. *Mechanical timer.* It can be tedious to hold the light in position; a timer helps to make the procedure more accurate. Some lights have inbuilt timers.

INDICATIONS

These are similar to home bleaching (see Chapter 5), but may be especially suited to tenacious stains.

- Developmental or acquired stains
- Stains in enamel and dentine
- For removing yellow–brown stains
- Age-yellowed smiles
- For blending white colour changes
- Mild to moderate tetracycline stains

ADVANTAGES OF POWER BLEACHING

Patients may prefer power bleaching to home bleaching because they do not have the time to devote to home bleaching, or have an inability to tolerate wearing the trays and gag easily or may not be manually dextrous enough to use the trays. They may also have existing sensitivity, or an inability to tolerate the taste (Haywood 1998). On the positive side, the procedure takes less time than the overall time for home bleaching and the results are almost immediate which enhances the perceived value of the bleaching programme. It removes yellow–brown stains and does not damage the enamel. The patients may thus be motivated to continue home bleaching after seeing the results and to comply with the recommended protocol. A

scanning electron microscope study showed that there were no surface morphological effects and no etching was produced by heated 35% carbamide peroxide gel or 35% hydrogen peroxide gel (Klutz et al 1999).

DISADVANTAGES OF POWER BLEACHING

Unfortunately, there are several disadvantages to power bleaching. It takes more surgery time; thus it can be more expensive. It may also be unpredictable as it is not known how much the teeth will respond to the bleaching.

First, longer and more frequent appointments are needed, as one session is normally not enough to get sufficient colour change. Rosensteil et al (1991), studying the darkening effect following use of 30% hydrogen peroxide to bleach teeth in vivo, reported that 50% of the immediate lightening effect remained after only 1 week, and only 14% remained after 6–9 months. These results indicate that although hydrogen peroxide alone is an efficient bleaching agent, significant darkening occurs with time following one bleaching treatment. Therefore more appointments are needed and the lightening should be followed by the home bleaching treatment.

Second, the teeth are dehydrated during treatment which can lead to further problems or false evaluation of actual shade change. Rehydration of desiccated bleached teeth depicts slightly darker coloration and is mistakenly interpreted by patients as rebound discoloration (Barghi 1998).

Third, there are serious safety considerations. The bleach is normally a stronger, caustic concentration and so is more dangerous. Tissue burns can result on the patient's lips, cheeks and gingivae. Protection of the patient's face, soft tissues, eyes, skin and lips is mandatory (see Figure 7.4D). The dental assistants can also be subject to tissue burn as they prepare to clear up the material after use (Figure 7.3A). Meticulous procedures are therefore required for preparing and disposing of the bleaching materials, as well as for protecting the mouth and mucous membranes. It should be noted that 35% hydrogen peroxide is unstable, has a very short shelf-life and should be stored at cool temperatures (Tam 1992).

Additionally, the cost of re-treatment is the same cost as that of the initial treatment, whereas that for home bleaching is much less. Regression of the colour may occur much quicker (Haywood 1996). The teeth may be more sensitive using this technique alone (Bowles and Thompson 1986, Bowles and Ungwuneri 1987).

Finally, there is not much research by way of clinical controlled studies to support the technique as being more effective than home bleaching.

SIDE EFFECTS OF STRONGER CONCENTRATIONS

As we have seen, the stronger concentrations of 35% hydrogen peroxide can cause soft tissue damage, gingival ulceration (Figure 7.3C,D) and skin burns (Figure 7.3A). Normally these burns appear as a white lesion in the area, followed by a red rim. The patient may notice that the gums are burning or tingling during the bleaching treatment and should be questioned during the procedure to check that this is not happening. If patients should get a burn, it should be rinsed with copious amounts of water to neutralize the effects on the soft tissue. Gingival burns or 'blanching' can unfortunately be common. These disappear after a few minutes, heal quickly and do not cause any permanent damage. If these do occur the patient should be told, shown and reassured.

Some stronger concentrations of carbamide peroxide (e.g. 35%) can also cause soft tissue and gingival burning. It is advisable to use soft tissue protection with rubber dam or light-activated soft tissue protector, in the case of liquid resin.

HOW DOES POWER BLEACHING WORK?

The techniques work by lightening the enamel to give the appearance of whiteness (McEvoy

1998). The exact mechanism of lightening remains unknown (Swift 1988). One theory is that the large coloured organic molecules responsible for the stain are reduced to smaller, less noticeable molecules by a process of oxidation. The hydrogen peroxide acts as both an oxygenator and an oxidant. The stain removing process is selective and there are fewer side effects (McEvoy 1998).

Another theory is that the peroxide penetrates into the enamel and dentine and oxidizes tooth discolorations. The passage of the nascent oxygen into the tooth structure occurs first in the enamel and then in the dentine (Haywood 1996, Klutz et al 1999). (See also Chapter 1.).

GENERAL PROCEDURE

The patient is assessed clinically and radiographically. A proposed treatment plan is discussed. Consent forms are completed and signed. Pre-operative photographs of the teeth are taken.

The teeth are isolated with a protective mucous membrane seal and the gingivae are protected. A rubber dam is placed (Figure 7.8). The teeth are ligated with floss to protect the material from creeping under the dam. The teeth are cleaned with pumice prophylaxis paste. It was thought that etching of the teeth enhanced the colour change during bleaching, but it has been shown to be of no benefit (Hall 1991).

The bleaching material is now applied to the teeth. The light is applied close to the teeth. If the plasma arc light is used, this is applied 6–7 mm away from the gel. A composite curing light can be used in addition or on its own. This is held at the same distance from the bleaching material. Strict adherence to the manufacturer's instructions should be observed, particularly in relation to the appropriate timing that the materials remain on the teeth. The plasma arc light emits 3-s bursts of light applied on to each tooth in turn (Radz 1999). This is generally continued for a period of three, 3-min intervals (depending on the instructions) or 10–15 min, and the bleach is removed from the teeth via the high volume aspirator (Figure 7.4c). This can also be done with a damp gauze to avoid splutter or cotton wool. The teeth are then washed, rinsed and the bleach is reapplied for a further 10 min. The process is repeated for 45 min to 1 h. The teeth are polished with diamond polishing paste or aluminium oxide discs of varying degrees of abrasiveness to achieve an enamel lustre.

The dam is then removed. The mucosal protectant is also removed and the mouth is rinsed. The shade of the teeth is now assessed. The patient is shown the result by use of a hand mirror or the intraoral camera. Post-operative photographs can be taken.

Although the use of heat or light has been thought to further accelerate the bleaching process, they are not necessary to activate the oxidation process (Goldstein 1997, Christensen 2000). Local anaesthetics are not administered during power bleaching treatment in order that the dentist can monitor any patient discomfort and avoid tissue tingling or burns. During the first 24 hours after treatment, the patient may require local analgesics to eliminate any post-treatment discomfort. The second and third appointments are scheduled 3–6 weeks later to allow the pulp to settle. The patient then returns in 6 weeks for a further session. This process can be repeated in 6-week increments until the desired shade is achieved (Garber 1997).

ASSISTED BLEACH TECHNIQUE OR WAITING ROOM BLEACH TECHNIQUE

This bleaching technique can be used for both vital and non-vital teeth. (For a description of non-vital bleaching see Chapter 9.) This bleaching technique was invented by Den-Mat when the Quick-Start product was introduced to be used to initiate the bleaching procedure and for the patient to continue bleaching at home. The Reality reference source book coined the phrase Assisted Bleaching (Miller 2000).

The 35% carbamide peroxide (which breaks down to 10% hydrogen peroxide) is marketed as a power bleaching agent. The teeth are

polished with prophylaxis paste. Cheek and lip retractors are placed. The 35% carbamide peroxide can also be heated gently, by holding the syringe under hot running water for 2–3 minutes, prior to use, but this is not mandatory. The heating of the syringe accelerates the activity of the material before it is loaded into the mouth guard (Klutz et al 1999). The dentist applies the 35% carbamide peroxide into a custom-made bleaching tray (see Figure 7.6). After the excess material is removed, the patient returns to the waiting room for a period of about 30 minutes with the bleaching tray in the mouth. The patient can remain in the operatory during this time. After 30 minutes, the bleach is suctioned off the teeth before rinsing. Each tooth is then rinsed keeping the high volume evacuator on the tooth that is being rinsed (Miller 2000).

This 35% carbamide peroxide technique has also been advocated for at-home use in certain selected cases (Broome 1999), but pending laboratory and clinical trials this technique should be used cautiously and under close supervision. No changes in surface morphology were noted by scanning electron microscopic analysis (Klutz et al 1999).

There are no published studies on this technique to show that it is better or more effective than the 10% carbamide peroxide home bleaching technique. However, an in-vitro study to test laser bleaching with 10% or 20% carbamide peroxide showed that the latter produced most perceivable colour change after 2 weeks when measured with a colorimeter (Jones et al 1999). The 20% carbamide peroxide is used in home bleaching syringes. It can also cause a little soft tissue irritation (see Figure 7.7).

COMPRESSIVE BLEACHING TECHNIQUE

Miara (2000) suggests that the power bleaching technique could be made more effective by compressing the bleaching material on the tooth. He recommends using 35% hydrogen peroxide in a bleaching tray, sealing the tray's edges with light-cured resin to prevent damage to the soft tissues. The benefit of the technique is that it influences the penetration of oxygen ions into the tooth enamel, which improves the tooth shade significantly. However, further research on this promising technique is essential.

THE IN-OFFICE DUAL-ACTIVATED TECHNIQUE

The Hi-Lite in-office bleaching system is formulated for both light and chemical activation. It includes ferrous sulphate, which serves as a chemical activator that completes the bleaching process in 7–9 minutes. In addition, the formulation includes manganese sulphate, which is light activated and can accelerate the bleaching process to as little as 2–4 minutes. This technique uses hydrogen peroxide in a strong concentration of 19–35%. A feature of the Hi-Lite material (Shofu) is that it has blue-green indicator dye which starts off as blue and as it becomes deactivated changes to white. This helps the dentist to minimize the amount of time the bleach is kept on the teeth and maximize the results.

The procedure may be summarized as follows:

- The teeth are isolated with the rubber dam in the standard manner.
- The Hi-Lite material is placed on the teeth
- The material is left on for 6–10 minutes and then removed.
- The process can be repeated again (as many as six times per visit if necessary, depending on the type and severity of the stain: Goldstein 1997).
- The teeth are cleaned with prophylaxis paste.

In a study by Toh (1993) on 23 university students using this technique, teeth were observed to be a half to two shades lighter after each treatment session. It required one to three treatment sessions to achieve the desired results except for severe tetracycline stained teeth. Different concentrations of 35% and 19% hydrogen peroxide were tested. They found that there was no visible difference in the results achieved by the different concentrations. However, it took 3 to 5 minutes

longer for the 19% hydrogen peroxide to effect a similar change in colour.

PATIENT EVALUATION

A thorough medical and dental history must be elicited before initiating any therapy. In addition to the conventional health history, information should be taken regarding the possible causes of the patient's present dental coloration, as well as the patient's hopes and expectations for dental appearance at the termination of treatment.

As 'before-and-after' photographs are essential to the documentation of the bleaching (or any other aesthetic) treatment, they should be taken prior to any whitening procedure. This set of photographs or slides should include at least one image with a standard shade guide tab in the field for colour reference.

If some other method of colour assay is available, such as a full spectrum colorimeter, then it may be used in place of the standard method of comparison with shade tabs. A colorimeter is currently being developed by Dr François Duret.

Notations are made in the patient's chart describing the shade and condition of the teeth prior to any treatment. Generally, it is best to involve the patient in the determination of their 'before' shade.

The dentist then carefully inspects all teeth that will come into contact with the whitening materials. Of particular interest at this stage is the discovery of any endodontically compromised tooth, or the presence of teeth with major cracks, or decay or leakage under existing fillings. Transillumination can be of great assistance in detecting some of these problems (see Figure 7.9).

Any necessary endodontic treatments should be completed prior to the initiation of the whitening process. It is generally best to restore decayed teeth after the whitening process is complete in order to take advantage of the colour change that has been achieved. The dentist should also make a note of any cervical abrasion, exposed root structure, or severely diminished enamel thickness for reasons of future reference (Figure 7.10).

The patient must be informed that all other existing tooth-coloured restorations will remain chromatically unchanged, even though the teeth themselves are expected to whiten. In fact, the degree of whitening can often be gauged by the contrast that has developed between the existing composite fillings and the surrounding tooth structure (Figure 7.11).

Naturally, the dentist must inform the patient prior to the whitening process that all visible anterior fillings or crowns (that match to the darkened teeth) will likely need replacement at the end of the whitening procedure.

Following the establishment of these baseline conditions, a thorough prophylaxis of the teeth is performed. This will facilitate the next several steps (Figure 7.12).

A complete examination follows. At this point, it is important, although not critical, to ascertain the type of discoloration exhibited by the teeth. This analysis will help in predicting the degree of lightening to be expected, along with the treatment time that will be required.

Careful discussion utilizing good listening skills (on the part of the dentist/hygienist) should be employed to gauge the patient's level of expectation from the procedure. Once the type and severity of the discoloration have been diagnosed, the patient's expectations can be aligned with realistically predicted results.

Treatment planning can be made more meaningful by showing the patient photographs of results which have been achieved in similar situations with other patients. It is important, however, to make the patient aware that every tooth is different, and the photographic examples cannot constitute a guarantee of similar results in their particular case.

Patients should be fully informed about the course of the treatment. They are naturally interested in any potential discomfort, whether they will be able to talk during the procedure, and how long the procedure will take. Prior to initiating any sort of treatment, all of these aspects should be discussed and financial arrangements made.

If the prophylaxis has somewhat destained the teeth, then another baseline photograph may be taken. Once again, some method of colour assay should be performed, whether it be simply matching the teeth to a shade guide, or a more precise measurement of shade by machine.

BLEACHING PROCEDURE

After the photographs, the active bleaching procedure can begin. First, the gingiva is isolated with a rubber dam (Figure 7.13) and protected by a continuous coating of either Mucoprotectant (Bright Smile, Birmingham, Alabama), Orabase or Vaseline (Figure 7.14).

This rubber dam should be tight-fitting, and may be ligated with waxed floss for additional protection.

Protective eyewear for both the patient and the dental staff is used to diminish the risk of dental materials irritating the eyes (Figure 7.15).

Another prophylaxis is performed on the isolated teeth to clean off any film or debris that may have contaminated the enamel or dentin surface. This prophylaxis is performed using flour of pumice without any oils, glycerine or fluoride.

The Hi-Lite powder should be tumbled in its container to assure a more homogeneous mix. One level scoop of the uncompacted powder is dispensed on to a mixing pad for every three labial surfaces to be bleached. One drop of liquid per level scoop is placed alongside the powder. This will provide sufficient liquid to create a medium viscosity gel. The final proportions of powder to liquid are not critical. It is more important to create a comfortable working consistency.

The liquid should be incorporated into the powder to create a uniform gel. A good consistency is one that is fluid enough to carry to the tooth easily and to spread smoothly on the surfaces of the tooth, while still being viscous enough to remain where it is placed (Figure 7.16).

During the mixing phase, it is desirable to minimise the exposure of the gel to any bright source of illumination such as the operatory light, as such light may create premature oxidation of the bleaching material.

Immediately upon mixing, the gel is applied to the entire surface of the teeth to be bleached. This application forms a substantial layer of 1–2 mm in thickness (Figure 7.17).

In the case of teeth that are particularly dark, it may be necessary to apply the gel to the lingual surfaces as well.

As soon as the liquid comes into contact with the powder, the oxidation process is initiated. It is significantly accelerated, however, when exposed to a bright light. The operatory light provides some acceleration, but a composite curing light with a minimum output of 300 mW/cm^2 is preferable (Figure 7.18). Heat lamps or conventional bleaching lights are contraindicated because of the heat output created by these sources.

A maximal bleaching power is realised by leaving the mixed gel on the tooth for approximately 2 minutes prior to light activation.

As the paste oxidizes, it turns from a blue-green to a cream colour (Figure 7.19).

After the oxidation is complete and the bleaching material is a chalky white, the spent material can be wiped away using a damp cotton gauze (Figure 7.20).

The application of Hi-Lite may be repeated, up to six times per treatment session, depending upon the severity and type of the stain being treated provided the patient does not experience any sensitivity.

At the end of the session, all the bleaching material is rinsed off the teeth using a continuous flow of water (preferably heated to body temperature) for 60 seconds before removing the rubber dam.

The patient is then allowed to rinse, and instructed to avoid any activities that might stain the teeth in the first 24 hours after the session.

Where post-bleaching bonding is required, it is best to complete the bleaching first and to then schedule the bonding for a subsequent visit. There are two reasons for this. First, research indicates that the potential exists for decreased composite bond strength to recently bleached enamel and dentine (Torneck et al 1990a, 1990b, Cullen et al 1993, Garcia-Godoy et al 1993, Toko and Hisamatsu 1993). The decrease in potential composite bond strength is, however, short lived. Testing has shown that the potential bond strengths return to pre-bleach levels within a week (Bishara et al 1993, Dishman et al 1994).

The second reason is the slight fall-back of colour that occurs after bleaching has been completed. As accurate colour matching of restorations is very important, the dentist should wait a minimum of 1 week prior to placing fillings in a tooth or taking a shade for a crown. Otherwise a composite which has

been selected to match a tooth immediately after a bleaching session will probably be found to be too white after the colour equilibration has occurred.

CASE REPORT

This is a typical example of results using the dual-activated bleaching materials (Figure 7.21). This case was completed by Dr Fred Hanosh and Dr G. Scott Hanosh. The patient was a 23-year-old woman. Prior to beginning treatment, a proper history was elicited, pre-treatment photographs were taken, the diagnosis and treatment plan were discussed and agreed upon.

At the first treatment visit, the teeth were cleaned with flour of pumice.

The gingiva was coated with Orabase, and then further isolated through the use of a rubber dam. Because the teeth were significantly darker along the gingival third of her teeth, they were selectively etched in those areas. This was accomplished using a 37% orthophosphoric acid gel for 15 seconds. The teeth were then rinsed with water for 30 seconds and dried.

Three drops of Hi-Lite liquid were mixed with one spoonful of powder. At this point the mixture was a green colour.

The paste was then applied over the entire surface to be bleached in a layer approximately 2 mm thick.

The paste was irradiated with a standard composite curing light for approximately three minutes.

By the end of that time, the paste changed from a green to a light yellow/off-white colour, indicating that the oxidation had finished.

The teeth were rinsed off using copious amounts of water for approximately one minute, and a new batch of paste was mixed and applied. The process was repeated for three cycles during the first visit.

The teeth were then polished using a Ceramiste point and cup. There was a contrast between the treated maxillary anterior teeth and the non-treated mandibular dentition. The gingival third of teeth numbered 6 and 8 were then spot-treated for additional whitening in these difficult areas.

POWER BLEACHING TECHNIQUES USING HEAT

Research has been undertaken to assess the effect of heat and hydrogen peroxide on the pulp (Zach and Cohen 1965, Cohen 1979, Robertson and Melfi 1980, Seale and Wilson 1985). It appears that heat may cause the liquid in the dentinal tubules to expand which results in an outward flow of the odontoblast processes and a decrease in pulpal circulation, pulp inflammation and irregular dentine formation. This could explain why some patients experience sensitivity after power bleaching. Thus heat can damage the odontoblasts in the dentine and possibly result in irreversible pulpal damage. These heat activation studies show that an increase in the intrapulpal temperature would cause inflammatory changes to the pulpal tissues. No irreversible damage was evident in the above study. Hydrogen peroxide by itself has been shown to inhibit pulpal enzyme activity. A small amount penetrates the pulp.

Using a heated instrument. The rubber dam is placed on the teeth as above and the mucosa protected. Gauze soaked in 35% hydrogen peroxide liquid is placed on the teeth. A heating instrument can be placed on to the teeth to enhance the effect of the bleach. Depending on the individual's tolerance level, it is applied for a period of 1–3 minutes. This technique has been superseded by the introduction of the power bleaching gels.

Using a bleaching light. Gauze soaked in 35% hydrogen peroxide is placed on the teeth and left for a period of 30 minutes with the light set approximately 30 cm from the teeth. This procedure may be repeated at one or two week intervals (Tam 1992) for three to five appointments. Typically, the teeth were sensitive for a few days after treatments due to the heating effect of the light (Radz 1999). This technique has also been superseded by the bleaching gels used with halogen lights, but is included here for completeness.

Using heated bleaching gels (Rembrandt Products). This chairside technique employs the use of 35% carbamide peroxide gel, heated to 80°C and applied directly on to the tooth.

Procedure

1. Isolate the treatment area using a paint-on protective coating to the labial gingivae, 4 mm of cover around the papillae and to the palatal gingivae 2–3 mm. Extend the protection to the area between the canine and first premolar.
2. Heat up the bleach by using one of two methods: immerse the bleaching material in a water bath at 80°C; or boil the bleach in a crucible over a flame or with hot air. The bleach should be heated until it starts bubbling.
3. Place the heated bleach on to the isolated teeth for 2 minutes.
4. Remove the material using a gauze cotton square; do not use the water spray as this will chill the teeth and the bleach will not be as effective.
5. Apply 3–4 times for 2–3 minutes each for a period of about 20 minutes.
6. Rinse the teeth, remove the protection, review the new shade of the teeth.
7. The teeth will dessicate while the protective coat is on the gingivae and the teeth will appear more dessicated, or lighter. This effect will diminish after the procedure is completed and the mouth is rehydrated.
8. Patients can continue to do the at-home bleaching procedure using 10% carbamide peroxide at home for 1 hour per day for 7 days.
9. Review the patient after 1 week. The lower teeth can be 'hot bleached' the following week. As the mandibular teeth are thinner, the technique works more quickly.
10. Review after 1 week. A further hot bleach session can be undertaken.

THE LASER BLEACHING TECHNIQUE

Laser-assisted bleaching has been introduced as a bleaching technique, in an attempt to accelerate the bleaching process. Laser bleaching officially started in 1996 with the approval of Ion Laser Technology's argon and carbon dioxide lasers by the FDA. The public are fascinated by lasers and patients are keen to try laser bleaching (Christensen 1997) which is promoted as being superior to other bleaching techniques. However, this is the technique for which there is the least amount of clinical research. Long-term effects using laser-assisted bleaching are not yet established (ADA Council on Scientific Affairs 1998). There is little data to prove that lasers are more effective than the traditional bleaching methods (Garber 1997). Most of the reports are anecdotal and empirical.

An in-vitro study by Jones et al (1999) showed that one session of laser bleaching did not demonstrate any perceivable colour change and recommended that additional or longer applications may be required. In their study, exposure to 20% carbamide peroxide produced the greatest perceivable colour change. However, this was an in-vitro study and did not take into account the salivary flow wash that takes place and the hydrodynamic pulpal pressure that exists in vivo.

TYPES OF LASERS

There are four lasers that have dental applications. These are the carbon dioxide, argon, neodymium:yttrium–aluminium–garnet (Nd:YAG) and erbium–chromium:yttrium–scandium–gallium–garnet (ErCr:YSGG) lasers. The first two lasers have bleaching uses (Garber 1997). There are two ways to use the lasers for bleaching, individually or in combination.

HOW DO LASERS WORK ON THE BLEACHING PROCESS?

Lasers are used to enhance the activation of the bleaching materials. The lasers provide energy for the hydrogen peroxide to break down into water and oxygen and to release the oxygen into the stained tooth. They catalyse the oxidation reaction. The free radicals of oxygen liberated in the process break apart the double valency bonds into simpler, more stable, less pigmented chains (Garber 1997).

As very little clinical research has been published, most of the available data comes

from the laser manufacturers (ADA Council on Scientific Affairs 1998). The manufacturers claim that the pulp is not affected in laser bleaching as the laser energy heats the bleaching solution more quickly than a conventional heat source. Some manufacturers claim that their own laser is more effective in catalysing the water based bleaching reaction. Others claim that the laser energy is totally absorbed by the bleaching gel resulting in superior whitening.

ADVANTAGES OF LASER BLEACHING

Laser bleaching is faster due to the high concentration of an active ingredient (Christensen 1997). It may act as a jump start for difficult cases by helping to remove difficult stains caused by tetracycline and fluorosis (Christensen 1997).

DISADVANTAGES OF USING LASERS

1 Cost. Purchasing the laser is expensive, although some companies offer a free loan with purchase of the bleaching agent.
2 The procedure is time consuming.
3 Post-operative sensitivity can be high (Christensen 1997).
4 Anecdotal reports indicate moderate-to-severe post-procedural pain following laser-assisted bleaching (ADA Council on Scientific Affairs 1998).

PROCEDURE

Using a rubber dam or light-cured soft tissue protectant isolates the soft tissues and gingivae. The laser bleaching gel is mixed according to the manufacturer's instructions. The gel is placed at a thickness of 1–2 mm on to the buccal surface of the teeth to be bleached (Reyto 1998). The Argon laser light is applied for 30 seconds about 1–2 cm from the buccal surface of each tooth.

The laser light at 488 nm is applied slowly for 30 seconds and moved from right to left over the tooth's surface. After the laser is applied, the gel is left on the tooth for 3 minutes. The gel is then removed from the tooth first by wiping it off and then rinsing off the excess because the 35% hydrogen peroxide gel is very caustic and can cause soft tissue burns. The gel is reapplied in the same manner five more times to equal about a 1 hour session of bleaching.

An alternative technique involves using both the argon and carbon dioxide laser. The argon laser is used as described previously and then the carbon dioxide laser is employed with another peroxide-based solution to promote penetration of the bleaching agent into the tooth to provide bleaching below the surface. (ADA Council on Scientific Affairs 1998). Treatment time for this system ranges from 1–3 hours.

TETRACYCLINE STAINING

Tetracycline staining is one of the most difficult aesthetic problems faced by dentists today. Typically, stains that are extrinsic in origin can be more readily removed through use of bleaching materials that are applied externally. Tetracycline discoloration presents a dual problem: it is not only intrinsic, but tends to increase in darkness over time. Clinically, the patients who are most likely to be concerned with the aesthetic drawbacks created by this type of staining are younger individuals.

One approach to solving this problem of historical significance has been the use of crowns over the stained tooth structure. While this was the only viable solution for many years, it did involve extensive removal of often healthy enamel and dentine. In addition, the potential for aesthetic failure through exposure of the darkened tooth structure at the marginal area, should gingival recession occur, always remained a long-term liability.

With the development of modern tooth whitening techniques, however, a new era in aesthetic treatment of these stains has arrived. Clearly, the most acceptable treatment in this type of situation (Figure 7.22A) has become

the bleaching of the affected teeth. The resulting normalized coloration of the teeth (see the maxillary arch in Figure 7.22B) restores the patient to a more acceptable social and cosmetic appearance. Often bleaching alone is sufficient to bring the patient to optimal aesthetic balance. If necessary, the bleaching can be followed by bonding procedures 2 weeks later.

The patient's smile is evaluated to determine which teeth show during the largest smile. Generally, it is safest to whiten up to and including the second bicuspids. A rubber dam is applied to the arch being treated. The dam is passed through tight interdental contacts with dental tape floss, a braided and waxed material that will not tear the dam. It is necessary to protect the peridental tissues from the bleaching materials as hydrogen peroxide based tooth whiteners can irritate gingival tissues significantly (see Figure 7.23).

All the teeth to be whitened are exposed through the rubber dam in a manner that exposes as much tooth surface as possible.

It is preferable to provide dental bleaching without anaesthesia. This allows the patient to monitor the procedure for dental sensitivity as it is being performed. For this reason, it is preferable not to use rubber dam clamps, which may dig into the gingiva or the potentially sensitive cemento-enamel junction. Instead of the traditional metal clamps, a small piece of rubber dam can function just as effectively in retaining the entire apparatus. The small piece is stretched until thin, passed between the teeth, and then allowed to spring back to its full thickness. The tightness of the interdental space will prevent the dam from slipping off the teeth.

If the rubber dam is not applied completely and evenly, there may be a small amount of seepage through to the soft tissues. Therefore, it is prudent to protect the gingiva and the mucosa with a mucoprotectant gel that will neutralize any hydrogen peroxide that oozes through the dam (Figure 7.23).

The appropriate amounts of Hi-Lite powder and liquid are dispensed on to a mixing pad. They are then mixed with a plastic spatula. Immediately upon mixing, the material will turn a bright green. This indicates that the material is in the process of releasing oxygen and ready to be placed on to the tooth surface.

It is important that the Hi-Lite bleaching agent be mixed to the consistency of a fairly viscous slurry prior to its application to the dentition. This will prevent it from spreading easily to unintended areas. In cases where only specific areas of the teeth are to be selectively bleached, a higher viscosity of the mix will allow precise application and treatment control.

The mixed Hi-Lite is picked up with a brush and applied directly to the surfaces of the teeth to be bleached.

The bleaching agent is usually first applied by brush to the area in the gingival half of the tooth that is most stained by the tetracycline (Figure 7.24A). By increasing the bleaching time (or the number of applications) to areas of the teeth which are originally darker, the overall shade of the tooth can not only be lightened, but made more homogeneous, as well. Once the Hi-Lite has been applied to all the areas of tetracycline banding in the exposed teeth, the material is allowed to sit on the dentition for approximately two minutes. This first stage of whitening is the 'passive' phase.

Once the green colour of the Hi-Lite begins to fade, the bleaching activity is reactivated by shining the curing light (Demetron) on each tooth in turn, for 60 seconds (Figure 7.24B). As the bleaching activity is continued through light activation, the originally green gel will turn a chalky white (Figure 7.24C).

Naturally, because of the time involved in treatment, the patient may experience excessive saliva pooling behind the rubber dam. This can be easily solved by introducing a slow speed suction underneath the dam.

Once the bleaching gel has turned white, it is wiped off the teeth with a wet gauze. Wiping, rather than spraying, prevents the powder from being blown to inappropriate places such as eyes and noses.

At this stage, the teeth should have visibly whitened (Figure 7.24D). The dentist must then decide whether to continue the whitening process, or if the decoloration is adequate. Generally, the Hi-Lite system is repeated 3–5 times at the same appointment for optimal whitening results. When all the bleaching procedures have been completed, the teeth are washed with a gentle stream of water, preferably lukewarm (Figure 7.24E). The use of heated water will prevent the thermal sensitivity that is often observed with cold tap water.

If there is any surface roughness of the teeth, they may be polished with the polishing points and cups. Any remaining interproximal surface stain may be eliminated with polishing disks. The teeth are rinsed again, to show the full decoloration achieved.

The rubber dam is removed from the teeth, and the colour of the upper teeth is compared to the stain of the lower dentition. Notice that the decoloration extends as far back as the teeth that were exposed through the rubber dam (Figure 7.24F).

Ultimately, the final evaluation for the success of tooth whitening is made by the patient looking at his or her own smile. In the vast majority of cases, tetracycline stains can be diminished or eliminated through the use of dental bleaching. When bleaching is combined with porcelain veneers, very striking results may be observed.

THE SINGLE DISCOLOURED TOOTH

The dental practitioner often encounters a tooth that is far darker than its neighbours. This can be quite unsightly if it occurs in the anterior areas of the mouth. The discoloration may be due to any one of several factors, including trauma, disease, discoloration from dental materials, or idiopathic pulpal recession.

In the case of trauma, the precipitating incident may have been a recent occurrence but it may even have been an event in the distant past that has been forgotten, except for its effect on the tooth. Various diseases and materials have been implicated in pulpal necrosis and dentinal discoloration. Idiopathic pulpal recession is sometimes the most difficult situation for the dentist to deal with, and for the patient to accept, in that there is no evident reason or cause for the condition.

Typically the affected teeth are not only dark, but continue to darken with time, despite the best efforts of the dentist. Even if the whitening process can be successfully completed, the ongoing discoloration of these teeth will tend to cause a chromatic relapse. Therefore, it is important in selecting these cases that the patient accepts that long-term continuous maintenance will be required to keep these teeth at their optimal aesthetic levels. This implies regular recall bleaching visits, as often as required by the chromatic shift.

Bleaching the traumatically injured tooth should therefore be considered a provisional process; the treatment may only be effective for a limited period. The dentist and the patient should not consider the temporary nature of the benefits as a failure; to the contrary, the longer that one can stave off a more invasive procedure, the more successful the treatment has been.

While these cases pose some specific challenges, they can also be very rewarding for both the patient and the dentist. Here is an example of just such a treatment. The right lateral in Figure 7.25A was severely discolored with respect to the other teeth in the arch. The patient vaguely remembered a moderate trauma approximately ten years previously. The tooth had darkened slightly following the impact, and had then stabilized. Seven years following the original trauma, the colour of the tooth began to deteriorate yet again. Radiographic examination did not indicate an abscess. Vitality tests showed the tooth to be vital.

The tooth was isolated with a rubber dam and ligated with floss. Five consecutive applications of Hi-Lite were administered over an hour. The tooth had whitened considerably, but would continue to whiten for some time as the oxygen diffused through the enamel and dentine. When the patient returned 10 days later, the lateral was significantly lighter in shade.

After two more sessions with Hi-Lite bleaching, the tooth's coloration was almost equivalent to the other teeth in the arch (Figure 7.25B). The patient was very satisfied with the aesthetic result and decided to undertake a series of other cosmetic dental procedures.

It was made very clear that the decoloration could only be maintained through regular touch-ups (every 6 months for this patient),

and that a time might come when bleaching was no longer adequate, and veneering or full coverage ceramics would have to be considered.

A NOTE OF CAUTION

The ADA Council on Scientific Affairs (1998) does not recommend laser-assisted bleaching. This is due to the continuing concerns and unknowns about laser interactions with hard tissue and the lack of controlled clinical studies. The Council encourages manufacturers and other interested parties to conduct appropriate studies on this technique so that the profession and the public can benefit from technological improvements that are safe and effective in clinical dentistry.

CONCLUSION

There are still several unanswered questions about power bleaching, particularly about the heat source (as to whether the heat should be applied to the tooth gradually or at sudden, very high temperatures – and, indeed, whether it is justified in terms of results). There are few controlled studies compared with the vast clinical research that is emerging on home bleaching. Reports from manufacturers claim that the pulp is not damaged by these high temperatures because the process is likened to drinking a hot cup of coffee. The use of the light source to activate the bleach has not been proved to be more effective than the home bleaching technique. Laser-assisted bleaching still poses a number of unanswered questions. In all, further research on power bleaching is necessary to justify its popular use.

REFERENCES

ADA Council on Scientific Affairs. (1998) Laser-assisted bleaching: an update. *J Am Dent Assoc* **129**:1484–7.

Appollo 95E: curing was never so easy and comfortable. Manufacturer's Instructions 1999.

Barghi NB. (1998) Making a clinical decision for vital tooth bleaching: at-home or in-office? *Compend Contin Educ Dent* Aug; **19**(8):831–8.

Bishara SE, Sulieman AH, Olson M. (1993) Effect of enamel bleaching on the bonding strength of orthodontic brackets. *Am J Orthod Dentofacial Orthop* Nov; **104**(5):444–7.

Bowles WH, Thompson LR. (1986) Vital bleaching: the effect of heat and hydrogen peroxide on pulpal enzymes. *J Endodont* **12**:108–12.

Bowles WH, Ungwuneri Z. (1987) Pulp chamber penetration by hydrogen peroxide following vital bleaching procedures. *J Endodont* **13**:375–7.

Broome JC. (1999) At-home use of 35% carbamide peroxide bleaching gel: a case report. *Compend Contin Educ Dent* **19**(8):824–9.

Christensen G. (1997) Tooth bleaching, start-of-art. *CRA Newsletter* **21/4**.

Christensen G. (1999) New resin curing lights, high intensity vs. multimode intensity. Status Report 2. *CRA Newsletter* **23/5**: 6.

Christensen G. (2000) Why resin curing lights do not increase tooth lightening. Status Report. *CRA Newsletter* **24/6**: 3.

Cohen SC. (1979) Human pulpal responses to bleaching procedures in teeth. *J Endodont* **5**:134–8.

Croser D. (1999) The Light Fantastic. *Dental Practice* **37**.

Cullen DR, Nelson JA, Sandrick JL. (1993) Peroxide bleaches: effect on tensile strength of composite resins. *J Prosthet Dent* Mar; **69**(3):247–9.

Dishman MV, Covey DA, Baughan LW. (1994) The effects of peroxide bleaching on composite to enamel bond strength. *Dent Mater* Jan; **10**(1):33–6.

Garber DA. (1997) Dentist-monitored bleaching: a discussion of combination and laser bleaching. *J Am Dent Assoc Suppl* **128**:26S–30S.

Garcia-Godoy F, Dodge WW, Donohue M, O'Quinn JA. (1993) Composite resin bond strength after enamel bleaching. *Oper Dent* Jul–Aug; **18**(4):144–7.

Goldstein RE. (1997) In-Office bleaching: where we came from, where we are today. *J Am Dent Assoc Suppl*. **128**:11S–15S.

Hall DA. (1991) Should etching be performed as part of a vital bleaching technique. *Quintessence Int* **22**:679–86.

Haywood VB. (1996) Achieving, maintaining and recovering successful tooth bleaching. *J Esthet Dent* **8**(1):31–8.

Haywood VB. (1998) Quick tips: Nightguard Vital Bleaching and in-office bleaching. *Contemp Esthet Restor Prac* July/August:78–81.

Jones AH, Diaz-Arnold AM, Vargas MA, Cobb DS. (1999) Colorimetric assessment of laser and home bleaching techniques. *J Esthet Dent* **11**(2):87–94.

Klutz J, Kaim J, Scherer W, Gupta H. (1999) Two in-office bleaching systems: a scanning electron microscope study. *Compend Contin Educ Dent* **20**(10):965–9.

McEvoy S. (1998) Combining chemical agents and techniques to remove intrinsic stains from vital teeth. *Gen Dent*. March/April:168–72.

Miara P. (2000) An innovative chairside bleaching protocol for treating stained dentition: initial results. *Pract Perio Aesth Dent* **12/7**:669–78.

Miller M. (editor) (1999) *Reality: the information source for esthetic dentistry*. Vol. 13. Reality Publishing Company: Houston, Texas.

Miller M. (editor) (2000) *Reality: the information source for esthetic dentistry*. Vol. 14. Reality Publishing Company: Houston, Texas.

Radz GM. (1999) In-office bleaching system for quick esthetic change. Chairside with RW Nash. *Compend Contin Educ Dent* **20**(10):986–90.

Reyto R. (1998) Laser tooth whitening. *Dent Clin North Am* **21**(4):755–62.

Robertson WD, Melfi RC. (1980) Pulpal response to vital bleaching. *J Endodont* **5**:134–8.

Rosensteil SF, Gegauff AG, Johnston WM. (1991) Duration of tooth colour change after bleaching. *J Am Dent Assoc* **123**:54–9.

Seale NS, Wilson CFG. (1985) Pulpal response to bleaching in dogs. *Pediatr Dent* **7**:209–14.

Sherman JA. (1997) *Oral radiosurgery*, 2nd edn. Martin Dunitz: London.

Swift EJ. (1988) A method for bleaching discoloured vital teeth. *Quintessence Int* **19**(9): 607–9.

Tam L. (1992) Vital tooth bleaching: review and current status. *J Can Dent Assoc* **58**(8):654–63.

Toh CG. (1993) Clinical evaluation of a dual-activated bleaching system. *Asian J Aesthet Dent* **1**(2):65–70.

Toko T, Hisamitsu H. (1993) Shear bond strength of composite resin to unbleached and bleached human dentine. *Asian J Aesthet Dent* Jan; **1**(1):33–6.

Torneck CC, Titley KC, Smith DC. (1990a) Adhesion of light-cured composite resin to bleached and unbleached bovine dentin. *Endodont Dent Traumatol* Jun; **6**(3):97–103.

Torneck CD, Titley KC, Smith DC, Adibfar A. (1990b) The influence of time of hydrogen peroxide exposure on the adhesion of composite resin to bleached bovine enamel. *J Endodont* Mar; **16**(3):123–8.

Zach L, Cohen G. (1965) Pulp response to externally applied heat. *Oral Surg* **19**:515–30.

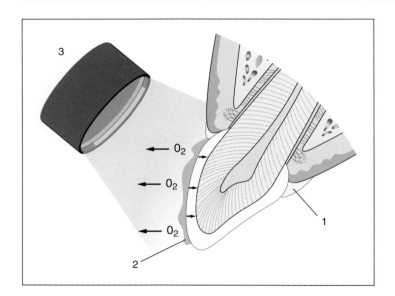

Figure 7.1

The conventional power bleaching technique: 1, light-cured resin, to seal gingival margin; 2, high-concentration gel; 3, light source.

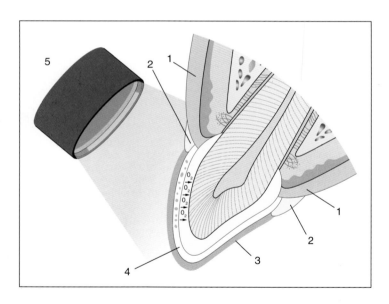

Figure 7.2

The compressive bleaching technique (Miara 2000): 1, gingival protection; 2, light-cured resin, to seal tray; 3, polyethylene tray; 4, high-concentration gel; 5, light-source.

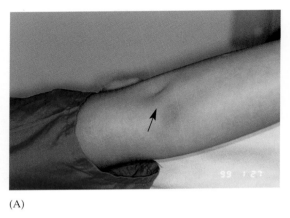

(A)

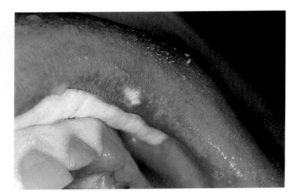

(B)

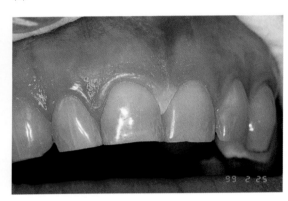

(D)

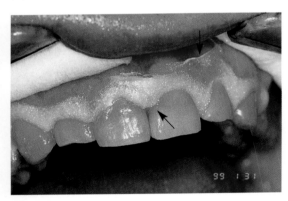

(C)

(E)

Figure 7.3

Side effects of stronger concentrations of bleaching gels. (A) Damage to dental assistant's arm incurred clearing-up after a bleaching treatment. (B) Chemical burn on the patient's upper lip from 35% hydrogen peroxide during power bleaching. The material used was quite runny and thus it was difficult to control. This white area occurred under the plastic cheek retractor. (C) Gingival ulceration from power bleach gel on the mandibular gingiva. (D) Bleaching on the papilla. This disappears within about 10 minutes. Patients should rinse the mouth with copious amounts of water. (E) This chemical burn can be avoided by attention to detail and meticulous care when applying the bleaching gel and the tissue protectant resin. In this case the resin had been applied in a sloppy manner. The resin should extend into the inter-papillary areas and there should be a thicker layer for extra protection (see arrows pointing to the errors).

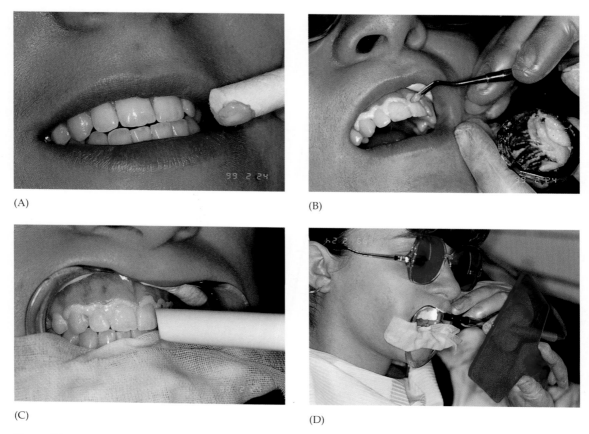

(A)

(B)

(C)

(D)

Figure 7.4

The general procedure applied to a patient with yellow discoloration of the teeth from tea drinking. (A) Lip protector is placed on the lips of the patient. (B) Light-cured protectant resin is placed around the gingival margins. The bleaching gel is placed on to the tooth by using a flat plastic instrument. The lower lip and mucosa are protected by using a damp gauze over the lip. The cheeks are protected with a lip retractor and cotton wool rolls. (C) After a 10 minute period, the material is suctioned away first to prevent the material splashing on to the gingival area. The teeth are rinsed thoroughly and the teeth reassessed. More light-cured protectant is added if necessary and then more gel is applied to the teeth. (D) This figure demonstrates the protection that is needed for the patient. This includes protective glasses, cheek retractor, cotton rolls, damp gauze and light shield to protect from the glare of the light for the dentist and assistant. The dentist and assistant should wear protective gloves and eye wear.

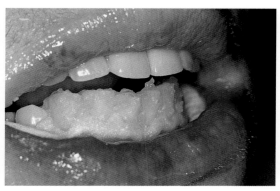

(E)

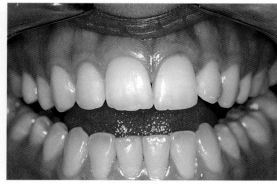

(F)

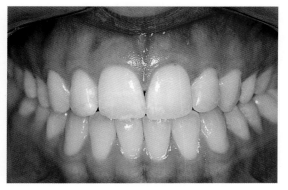

(G)

Figure 7.4 continued

(E) The technique demonstrated on the lower teeth. In this figure the gel has been applied for nearly 10 minutes. After this time the gel appears as peaks and crystal formation. It can then be aspirated away, rinsed and reapplied. (F) The patient continued bleaching treatment at home. This is the result of home bleaching for 2 weeks on the upper teeth. (G) Six weeks after bleaching treatment was completed, an aesthetic bonded restoration was placed on the upper left lateral incisor tooth to bring this tooth into better proportion and to make it longer.

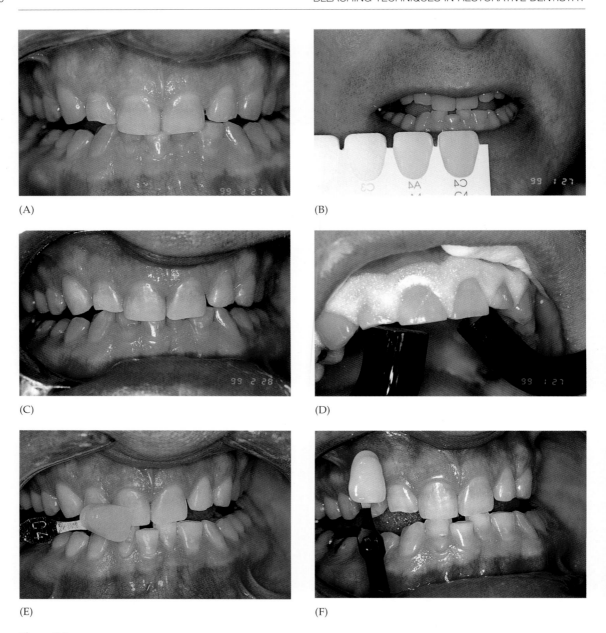

(A)   (B)   (C)   (D)   (E)   (F)

Figure 7.5

Minocycline staining. This patient took minocycline antibiotics for acne as a teenager for 3 years. It was only after that period that he noted that his teeth had discoloured. He was unaware that whitening treatment was available. Treatment involved two sessions of power bleaching and this was followed by home bleaching for a period of 4 months. The shade of the teeth went from Shade C4 to Shade C1. (A) Appearance of the teeth prior to bleaching treatment. (B) Assessing the shade using the customized shade guide from the Opalescence Bleaching Kit for the patient to verify shade changes at home. Existing shade was shade C4. (C) Appearance of the teeth after one power bleaching session. (D) The protective resin was placed on to the teeth. The mucosa was also isolated with cotton wool rolls and a plastic cheek retractor. The power arc light and the halogen light are used simultaneously to activate the bleaching gel. (E) After 2 months of bleaching, the teeth had gone to Shade C2. (F) Appearance of the teeth after 4 months of bleaching.

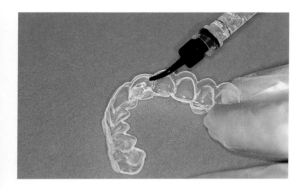

Figure 7.6

The assisted bleach technique. The first-generation materials were packaged in tubs. Later editions were packaged in syringes to conform with regulations in some countries that the bleaching materials were medical devices. A small nozzle helps application using a syringe. The syringe can be heated in hot water to make it more effective. When it is warmed, it is also more runny, and so more difficult to retain on the tooth and it is then better to apply the material in the tray.

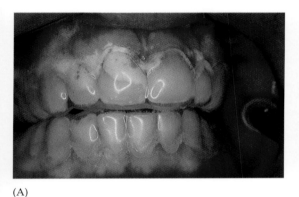

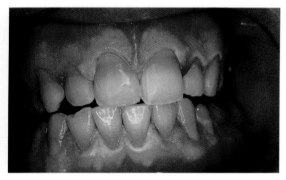

(A)   (B)

Figure 7.7

(A) The dangers of inappropriate application of the assisted bleach technique. Errors encountered with first generation assisted bleaching materials. (i) The material is not properly loaded in the tray. (ii) The tray is not retaining the material well and it is dispersing on to the mucosa. (iii) The material is very runny. (iv) The excess material has not been removed sufficiently. (v) The excess material is resting on the gingiva and soft tissues. (B) The result of poor technique shows numerous tissue burns on the marginal gingivae.

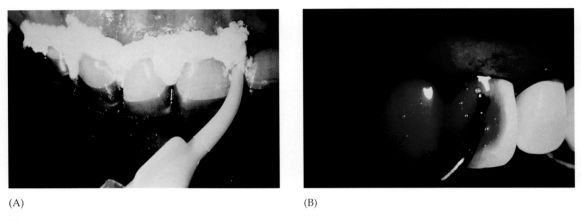

(A)   (B)

Figure 7.8

The Opalescence Xtra technique (slides courtesy of Ultradent). This material contains 35% hydrogen peroxide in a pre-mixed syringe. It also contains carotene, a red pigment which converts the blue wavelength of the blue halogen light to heat energy. It is not necessary to use a light source for this technique. (A) Rubber dam is an excellent barrier to use for power bleaching teeth. Oraseal protective material is placed underneath the rubber dam on the gingival margins, embrasures and mucosae. (B) A rubber dam instrument is used in combination with an air to invert the margins of the rubber dam, in order to seal the area better. Rubber dam clamps are applied to the molar teeth to keep the dam sturdy. Prior to bleaching, the dam should be checked for tears or leakage. The Opalescence Xtra is then applied on to the tooth with a brush tip over the labial surface. The material is also applied on a quarter of the lingual incisal surface. A light-reflective resin can also be used to protect the gingival area. High-volume suction should be used to remove the material after the appropriate time.

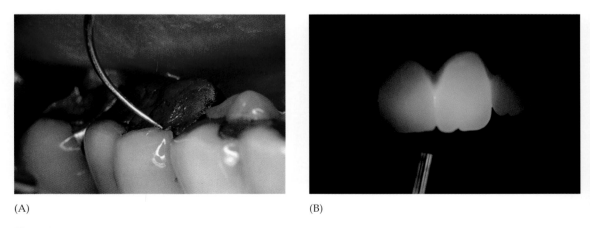

(A)   (B)

Figure 7.9

(A) Teeth should be examined carefully for any existing compromise or defect. (B) Transillumination helps with the detection of cracks or decay.

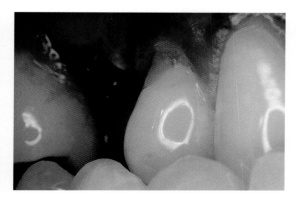

Figure 7.10

Decay in any tooth should also be noted in advance of treatment.

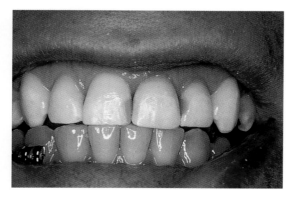

Figure 7.11

A contrast will develop between existing composite fillings and the surrounding tooth structure.

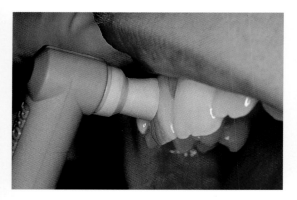

Figure 7.12

Prophylaxis of the tooth is performed as a preliminary to examination.

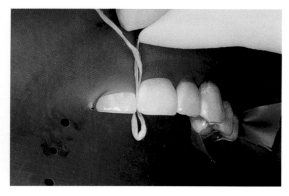

Figure 7.13

The gingiva is isolated with a rubber dam.

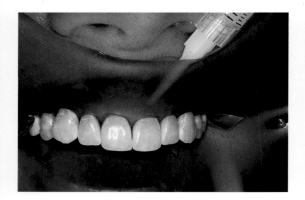

Figure 7.14

The gingiva is protected with a continuous coating.

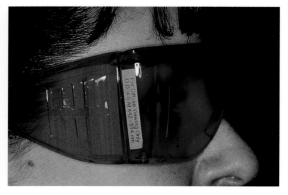

Figure 7.15

Protective eyewear is mandatory for patient, dentist and dental assistant.

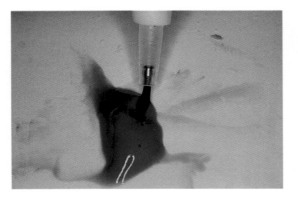

Figure 7.16

Good consistency in the mixed gel.

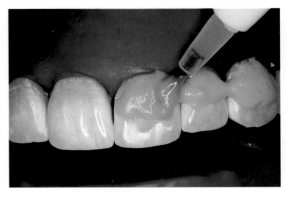

Figure 7.17

Application of the gel.

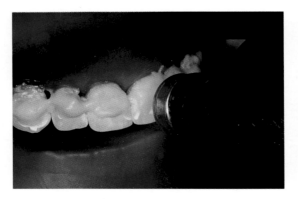

Figure 7.18

Operation of a composite curing light may accelerate the oxidation process.

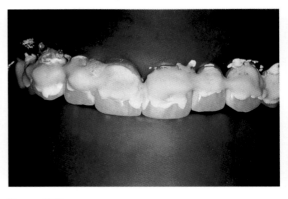

Figure 7.19

The oxidizing paste changes to a cream colour.

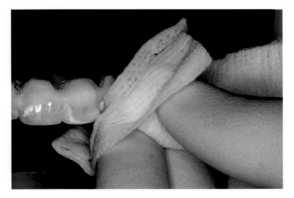

Figure 7.20

Removal of the spent bleaching material.

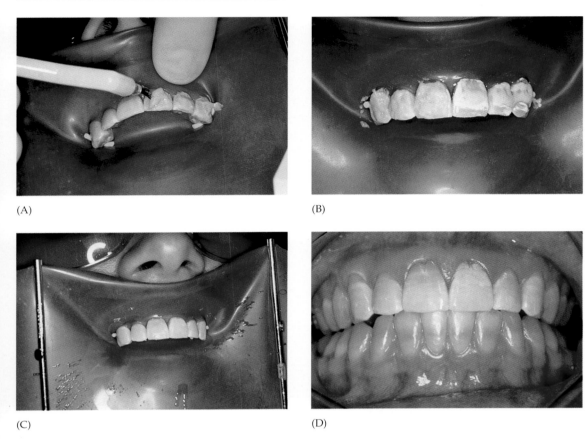

(A)

(B)

(C)

(D)

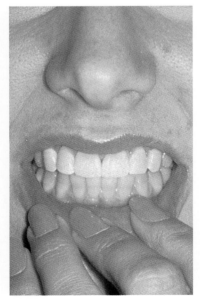

(E)

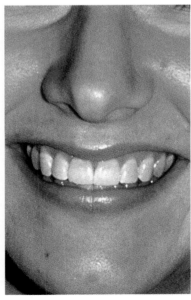

(F)

Figure 7.21

(A) The darker portions of the patient's teeth are selectively etched with an acid gel for 15 seconds. (B) The oxidizing paste, green in colour at this stage, is applied over the entire surface to be bleached in a layer approximately 2 mm thick. (C) A composite curing light was then used to irradiate the paste for approximately 3 minutes. (D) When the paste was a light yellow/off-white colour, oxidation had finished. (E) The results after the first bleaching session: there is a contrast between the treated maxillary anterior teeth and the non-treated mandibular dentition. (F) The final appearance of the teeth after additional spot-treatment.

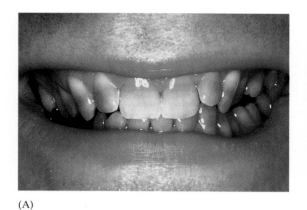

(A)

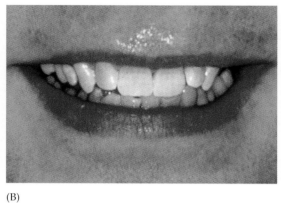

(B)

Figure 7.22

(A) Tetracycline staining. (B) A successful aesthetic result.

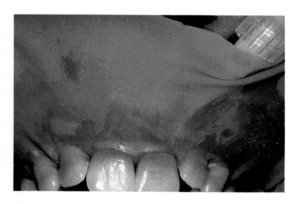

Figure 7.23

A mucoprotectant gel will neutralize any hydrogen peroxide that oozes through the dam.

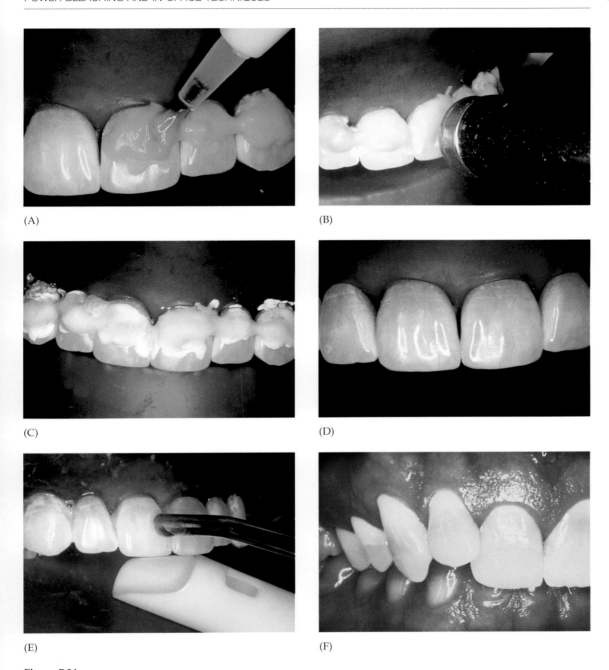

(A)

(B)

(C)

(D)

(E)

(F)

Figure 7.24

(A) Application of the bleaching agent to the gingival half of the tooth most stained. (B) Once the original colour of the agent begins to fade, the curing light is shone on each tooth in turn for 60 seconds. (C) The bleaching agent turns a chalky white under light activation. (D) Once the spent gel has been wiped from the teeth, they are visibly whitened. (E) The teeth may finally be washed with a gentle stream of warm water. (F) Decoloration matches the area exposed through the dam.

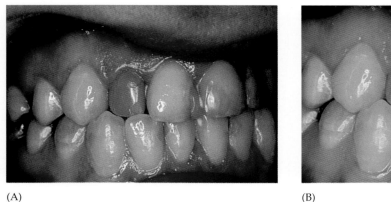
(A)

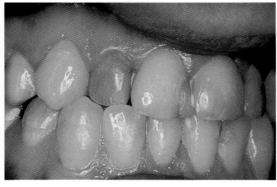
(B)

Figure 7.25

(A) The patient's right lateral was severely decoloured in comparison to the other teeth in the arch, following a moderate trauma 10 years previously. (B) 10 days after five consecutive applications of bleaching agent, the lateral was significantly lighter in shade. After two further sessions the tooth coloration (shown here) was almost equivalent to that of the other teeth in the arch.

8 INTRACORONAL BLEACHING OF NON-VITAL TEETH

Ilan Rotstein

INTRODUCTION

Intracoronal bleaching of non-vital teeth involves the use of chemical agents within the coronal portion of an endodontically treated tooth to remove tooth discoloration (American Association of Endodontists 1998). It may be successfully carried out at various times (see Figure 8.1), even many years after root canal therapy and discoloration. The successful outcome depends mainly on the aetiology, correct diagnosis and proper selection of bleaching technique (Rotstein 1998).

The methods most commonly employed to bleach endodontically treated teeth are the walking bleach and the thermo/photo bleaching techniques.

WALKING BLEACH PROCEDURE

The walking bleach technique (Figure 8.2) should be attempted first in all cases requiring intracoronal bleaching. Walking bleach is preferred as it requires less chairtime and is safer and more comfortable for the patient (Spasser 1961, Nutting and Poe 1963, Holmstrup et al 1988).

The technique involves the following steps (Figure 8.3):

1 Familiarize the patient with the possible causes of discoloration, the procedure to be followed, the expected outcome and the possibility of future rediscoloration.
2 Take radiographs to assess the status of periapical tissues and quality of endodontic obturation. Endodontic failure or questionable obturation should always be retreated prior to bleaching.
3 Assess the quality and shade of any restoration present and replace it if defective. Tooth discoloration frequently is the result of leaking or discolored restorations. In such cases cleaning the pulp chamber and replacing the defective restorations usually suffice.
4 Evaluate tooth colour with a shade guide and take clinical photographs at the beginning of and throughout the procedure. These provide a point of reference for future comparison.
5 Isolate the tooth with rubber dam. The dam must fit tightly at the cervical margin of the tooth to prevent possible leakage of the bleaching agent on to the gingival tissue. Interproximal wedges and ligatures may also be used for better isolation. If hydrogen peroxide is used, protective cream, such as Orabase or Vaseline, must be applied to the surrounding gingival tissues prior to dam placement.

Table 8.1 Indications and contraindications for intracoronal bleaching of non-vital teeth

Indications
Discolorations of pulp chamber origin
Dentine discolorations
Discolorations not amenable to extracoronal bleaching

Contraindications
Superficial enamel discolorations
Defective enamel formation
Severe dentine loss
Presence of caries
Discoloured composites

6 Remove all restorative material from the access cavity, expose the dentine and refine the access. Verify that the pulp horns as well as other areas containing pulp tissue are properly exposed and clean. Tissue remaining in the pulp chamber disintegrates gradually and may cause discoloration. Pulp horns must always be included in the access cavity to ensure removal of all pulpal remnants.

7 Remove all materials to a level just below the labial gingival margin. Orange solvent, chloroform or xylene on a cotton pellet may be used to dissolve sealer remnants. Etching of dentine with phosphoric acid is unnecessary and may not improve bleaching prognosis (Casey et al 1989).

8 Apply a sufficiently thick layer, at least 2 mm, of protective white cement barrier, such as polycarboxylate cement, zinc phosphate cement, glass ionomer, intermediate restorative material or cavit, on the endodontic obturation. The coronal height of the barrier should protect the dentine tubules and conform to the external epithelial attachment (Steiner and West 1994) (see Figure 8.1F).

9 Prepare the walking bleach paste by mixing sodium perborate and an inert liquid, such as water, saline or anaesthetic solution, to a thick consistency of wet sand. With a plastic instrument, pack the pulp chamber with the paste. Remove excess liquid by tamping with a cotton pellet. This also compresses and pushes the paste into all areas of the pulp chamber.

10 Remove excess bleaching paste from undercuts in the pulp horn and gingival area and apply a thick, well-sealed temporary filling directly against the paste and into the undercuts. Carefully pack the temporary filling, at least 3 mm thick, to ensure a good seal.

11 Remove the rubber dam. Inform the patient that the bleaching agent works slowly and that significant lightening may not be evident for several days.

12 Recall the patient approximately 2 weeks later and if necessary repeat the procedure several times. Repeat treatments are similar to the first one.

13 As an optional procedure, if initial bleaching is not satisfactory, strengthen the walking bleach paste by mixing the sodium perborate with gradually increasing concentrations of hydrogen peroxide (3–30%) instead of water. Although a sodium perborate and 30% hydrogen peroxide mixture bleaches faster, in most cases, long-term results are similar to those with sodium perborate and water, and therefore should not be used routinely (Holmstrup et al 1988, Rotstein et al 1991d, 1993) (see Figure 8.8). The more potent oxidizers may permeate into the tubules and cause damage to the cervical periodontium (Rotstein et al 1991b, 1991c).

SODIUM PERBORATE BLEACHING MATERIAL

This oxidizing agent is available in a powdered form or as various commercial preparations. When fresh, it contains about 95% perborate, releasing about 9.9% available oxygen. Sodium perborate is stable when dry but, in the presence of acid, warm air or water, decomposes to form sodium metaborate, hydrogen peroxide and nascent oxygen. It acts synergistically with hydrogen peroxide; a stronger concentration of hydrogen peroxide in combination with sodium perborate potentiates the effect of the sodium perborate. If initial bleaching is not satisfactory, hydrogen peroxide can be mixed into the perborate in an increased concentration.

Various types of sodium perborate preparations are available: monohydrate, trihydrate, and tetrahydrate. They differ in oxygen content which determines their bleaching efficiency (Weiger et al 1994). Commonly used sodium perborate preparations are alkaline and their pH depends on the amount of hydrogen peroxide released and the residual sodium metaborate (Rotstein et al 1991d).

Sodium perborate is more easily controlled and safer than concentrated hydrogen peroxide solutions. Therefore, it should be the material of choice in most intracoronal bleaching procedures.

THERMO/PHOTO BLEACHING PROCEDURE

The techniques involve placement of the oxidizing chemical, generally 30–35% hydrogen peroxide, in the pulp chamber followed by either heat application by electric heating devices, light application by specially designed lamps, or both (Figure 8.6). Generally, the techniques involve the following steps:

1 Familiarize the patient with the probable causes of discoloration, the procedure to be followed, expected outcome, and the possibility of future rediscoloration.
2 Take radiographs to assess the status of periapical tissues and quality of endodontic obturation. Endodontic failure or questionable obturation should be re-treated prior to bleaching.
3 Evaluate tooth colour with a shade guide and take clinical photographs before and throughout the procedure. Assess the quality and shade of any restoration present and replace if defective.
4 Apply a protective cream to the surrounding gingival tissues and isolate the teeth with rubber dam and waxed dental floss ligatures. If a heat lamp is used, avoid placing rubber dam metal clamps as they are subjected to heating and may be painful to the patient.
5 Do not use anaesthesia.
6 Position protective sunglasses over the patient's and operator's eyes.
7 Apply a sufficiently thick layer, at least 2 mm, of protective white cement barrier, such as polycarboxylate cement, zinc phosphate cement, glass-ionomer, intermediate restorative material (IRM) or cavit, on the endodontic obturation. The coronal height of the barrier should protect the dentine tubules and conform to the external epithelial attachment (Steiner and West 1994).
8 Soak a small amount of 30–35% hydrogen peroxide solution on a small cotton pellet or a piece of gauze and place in the pulp chamber. A bleaching gel containing hydrogen peroxide may be used instead of the aqueous solution.
9 Apply heat with a heating device or a light source. The temperature should be less than the patient can comfortably tolerate, usually between 50 and 60°C. Re-wet the cotton pellet and pulp chamber with hydrogen peroxide as necessary. If the tooth becomes too sensitive, discontinue the bleaching procedure immediately. Preferably, bleaching should be limited to separate 5-min periods rather than being performed during a long continuous period (Rotstein et al 1991b).
10 Remove the heat or light source and allow the teeth to cool down for at least 5 min. Then wash with warm water for 1 min and remove the rubber dam.
11 Dry the tooth and place walking bleach paste in the pulp chamber.
12 Recall the patient approximately 2 weeks later and evaluate the effectiveness of bleaching. Take clinical photographs with the same shade guide used in the pre-operative photographs for comparison purposes. If necessary, repeat the bleaching procedure.

INTENTIONAL ENDODONTICS AND INTRACORONAL BLEACHING

The technique involves standard endodontic therapy followed by an intracoronal bleaching. It was mainly advocated for treating intrinsic tetracycline discolorations. Such discolorations and other similar stains are incorporated into tooth structure during tooth formation, mostly into the dentine, and therefore very difficult to treat from the external enamel surface. Intracoronal bleaching of tetracycline discoloured teeth has been shown to be predictable, and to improve tooth shade without significant clinical complications (Abou-Rass 1982).

The procedure should be carefully explained to the patient, including the possible complications and sequelae. A treatment consent form is strongly recommended. Sacrificing pulp vitality should be considered in terms of the overall psychological and social needs of the individual patient as well as the possible complications of other treatment options. Preferably, only intact teeth without coronal defects, caries or restorations should be treated. This prevents the need for any additional restoration, thereby reducing the possibility of coronal fractures and failures.

COMPLICATIONS AND ADVERSE EFFECTS

EXTERNAL ROOT RESORPTION

Clinical reports (Harrington and Natkin 1979, Lado et al 1983, Montgomery 1984, Shearer 1984, Cvek and Lindvall 1985, Goon et al 1986, Latcham 1986, Friedman et al 1988, Gimlin and Schindler 1990, Al-Nazhan 1991, Heithersay et al 1994) and histologic studies (Madison and Walton 1990, Rotstein et al 1991a, Heller et al 1992) have shown that intracoronal bleaching may induce external root resorption. This is probably caused by the oxidizing agent, particularly 30–35% hydrogen peroxide. The mechanism of bleaching induced damage to the periodontium or cementum has not been fully elucidated. Presumably, the irritating chemical diffuses via unprotected dentinal tubules and cementum defects (Rotstein et al 1991c, Koulaouzidou et al 1996) and causes necrosis of the cementum, inflammation of the periodontal ligament and finally root resorption. The process may be enhanced if heat is applied (Rotstein et al 1991b) or in the presence of bacteria (Cvek and Lindvall 1985, Heling et al 1995). Previous traumatic injury (see Figures 8.7A–C) and age may act as predisposing factors (Harrington and Natkin 1979).

CHEMICAL BURNS

Hydrogen peroxide (30–35%) is caustic and causes chemical burns and sloughing of the gingiva. When using such solutions, the soft tissues should always be protected.

DAMAGE TO RESTORATIONS

Bleaching with hydrogen peroxide may affect bonding of composite resins to dental hard tissues (Titley et al 1993). Scanning electron microscopy observations suggest a possible interaction between composite resin and residual peroxide causing inhibition of polymerization and increase in resin porosity (Titley et al 1991). This presents a clinical problem when immediate aesthetic restoration of the bleached tooth is required. It is therefore recommended that residual hydrogen peroxide is totally eliminated from the pulp chamber prior to composite placement. This may be done by injecting catalase prior to bonding (Rotstein 1993). Catalase removes the residual oxygen from the dentine. A glass ionomer restoration can be placed immediately and the rest cut back 2 weeks later for the composite restoration.

It has been suggested that immersion of peroxide-treated dental tissues in water at 37°C for 7 days prevents the reduction in bond strength (Torneck et al 1991). Another study (Rotstein 1993) suggested that 3 minutes of catalase treatment effectively removed all the residual hydrogen peroxide from the pulp chamber.

SUGGESTIONS FOR SAFER NON-VITAL BLEACHING

- *Isolate tooth effectively*. Intracoronal bleaching should always be carried out with rubber dam isolation. Interproximal wedges and ligatures may also be used for better protection.
- *Protect oral mucosa*. Protective cream, such as Orabase or Vaseline, must be applied to the surrounding oral mucosa to prevent chemical burns by caustic oxidisers. Animal studies suggest that catalase

Table 8.2 Suggestions for safer intracoronal non-vital bleaching

Isolate tooth effectively
Protect oral mucosa
Verify adequate endodontic obturation
Use protective barriers
Avoid acid etching
Avoid strong oxidizers
Avoid heat
Recall periodically

applied to oral tissues prior to hydrogen peroxide treatment totally prevents the associated tissue damage (Rotstein et al 1993).

- *Verify adequate endodontic obturation*. The quality of root canal obturation should always be assessed clinically and radiographically prior to bleaching. Adequate obturation ensures a better overall prognosis of the treated tooth. It also provides an additional barrier against damage by oxidizers to the periodontal ligament and periapical tissues.

- *Use protective barriers*. This is essential to prevent leakage of bleaching agents which may infiltrate between the gutta-percha and root canal walls, reaching the periodontal ligament via dentinal tubules, lateral canals or the root apex. In none of the clinical reports of post-bleaching root resorption was a protective barrier used. Various materials can be used for this purpose. Barrier thickness and its relationship to the cemento-enamel junction are most important (Rotstein et al 1992, Steiner and West 1994). The ideal barrier should protect the dentinal tubules and conform to the external epithelial attachment.

- *Avoid acid etching*. It has been suggested that acid etching of dentine in the chamber to remove the smear layer and open the tubules, would allow better penetration of oxidizer. This procedure has not proven beneficial (Casey et al 1989). The use of caustic chemicals in the pulp chamber is undesirable, as periodontal ligament irritation may result.

- *Avoid strong oxidizers*. Procedures and techniques applying strong oxidizers should be avoided if they are not essential for bleaching. Solutions of 30–35% hydrogen peroxide, either alone or in combination with other agents, should not be used routinely for intracoronal bleaching.

- *Avoid heat*. Excessive heat may damage the cementum and periodontal ligament as well as dentine and enamel, especially when combined with strong oxidizers (Madison and Walton 1990, Rotstein et al 1991a). Although no direct correlation was found between heat applications alone and external cervical root resorption, it should be limited during bleaching procedures.

- *Recall patients periodically*. Bleached teeth should be frequently examined both clinically and radiographically. Root resorption may occasionally be detected as early as 6 months after bleaching. Early detection improves the prognosis as corrective therapy may still be applied.

REFERENCES

Abou-Rass M. (1982) The elimination of tetracycline discoloration by intentional endodontics and internal bleaching. *J Endodont* **8**: 101.

Al-Nazhan S (1991) External root resorption after bleaching: a case report. *Oral Surg* **72**:607.

American Association of Endodontists. (1998) *Glossary of Contemporary Terminology for Endodontics*, 6th edn. AAE: Chicago: p. 7.

Casey LJ, Schindler WG, Murata SM, Burgess JO. (1989) The use of dentinal etching with endodontic bleaching procedures. *J Endodont* **15**:535.

Cvek M, Lindvall AM. (1985) External root resorption following bleaching of pulpless teeth with hydrogen peroxide. *Endodont Dent Traumatol* **1**:56.

Friedman S, Rotstein I, Libfeld H, Stabholz A, Heling I. (1988) Incidence of external root resorption and esthetic results in 58 bleached pulpless teeth. *Endodont Dent Traumatol* **4**:23.

Gimlin DR, Schindler WG. (1990) The management of postbleaching cervical resorption. *J Endodont* **16**:292.

Goon WWY, Cohen S, Borer RF. (1986) External cervical root resorption following bleaching. *J Endodont* **12**:414.

Harrington GW, Natkin E. (1979) External resorption associated with bleaching of pulpless teeth. *J Endodont* **5**:344.

Heithersay GS, Dahlstrom SW, Marin PD. (1994) Incidence of invasive cervical resorption in bleached root-filled teeth. *Austral Dent J* **39**:82.

Heling I, Parson A, Rotstein I. (1995) Effect of bleaching agents on dentin permeability to *Streptococcus faecalis*. *J Endodont* **21**:540.

Heller D, Skriber J, Lin LM. (1992) Effect of intracoronal bleaching on external cervical root resorption. *J Endodont* **18**:145.

Holmstrup G, Palm AM, Lambjerg-Hansen H. (1988) Bleaching of discoloured root-filled teeth. *Endodont Dent Traumatol* **4**:197.

Koulaouzidou E, Lambrianidis T, Beltes P, Lyroudia K, Papadopoulos C. (1996) Role of cementoenamel junction on the radicular penetration of 30% hydrogen peroxide during intracoronal bleaching in vitro. *Endodont Dent Traumatol* **12**:146.

Lado EA, Stanley HR, Weisman MI. (1983) Cervical resorption in bleached teeth. *Oral Surg* **55**:78.

Latcham NL. (1986) Postbleaching cervical resorption. *J Endodont* **12**:262.

Madison S, Walton RE. (1990) Cervical root resorption following bleaching of endodontically treated teeth. *J Endodont* **16**:570.

Montgomery S. (1984) External cervical resorption after bleaching a pulpless tooth. *Oral Surg* **57**:203.

Nutting EB, Poe GS. (1963) A new combination for bleaching teeth. *J South Calif Dent Assoc* **31**:289.

Rotstein I. (1993) Role of catalase in the elimination of residual hydrogen peroxide following tooth bleaching. *J Endodont* **19**:567.

Rotstein I. (1998) Bleaching nonvital and vital discolored teeth. In: Cohen S, Burns RC. *Pathways of the pulp*, 7th edn. Mosby: St Louis; 674.

Rotstein I, Friedman S, Mor C, Katznelson J, Sommer M, Bab I. (1991a) Histological characterization of bleaching-induced external root resorption in dogs. *J Endodont* **17**:436.

Rotstein I, Torek Y, Lewinstein I. (1991b) Effect of bleaching time and temperature on the radicular penetration of hydrogen peroxide. *Endodont Dent Traumatol* **7**:196.

Rotstein I, Torek Y, Misgav R. (1991c) Effect of cementum defects on radicular penetration of 30% H$_2$O$_2$ during intracoronal bleaching. *J. Endodont* **17**:230.

Rotstein I, Zalkind M, Mor C, Tarabeah A, Friedman S. (1991d) In vitro efficacy of sodium perborate preparations used for intracoronal bleaching of discolored non-vital teeth. *Endodont Dent Traumatol* **7**:177.

Rotstein I, Zyskind D, Lewinstein I, Bamberger N. (1992) Effect of different protective base materials on hydrogen peroxide leakage during intracoronal bleaching in vitro. *J Endodont* **18**:114.

Rotstein I, Mor C, Friedman S. (1993) Prognosis of intracoronal bleaching with sodium perborate preparations in vitro: 1 year study. *J Endodont* **19**:10.

Rotstein I, Wesselink PR, Bab I. (1993) Catalase protection against hydrogen peroxide-induced injury in rat oral mucosa. *Oral Surg* **75**:744.

Shearer GJ. (1984) External resorption associated with bleaching of a non-vital tooth. *Austral Endodont Newslett* **10**:16.

Spasser HF (1961) A simple bleaching technique using sodium perborate. *NY State Dent J* **27**:332.

Steiner DR, West JD. (1994) A method to determine the location and shape of an intracoronal bleach barrier. *J Endodont* **20**:304.

Titley KC, Torneck CD, Smith DC, Chernecky R, Adibfar A. (1991) Scanning electron microscopy observations on the penetration and structure of resin tags in bleached and unbleached bovine enamel. *J Endodont* **17**:71.

Titley KC, Torneck CD, Ruse ND, Krmec D. (1993) Adhesion of a resin composite to bleached and unbleached human enamel. *J Endodont* **19**:112.

Torneck CD, Titley KC, Smith DC, Adibfar A. (1991) Effect of water leaching on the adhesion of composite resin to bleached and unbleached bovine enamel. *J Endodont* **17**:156.

Weiger R, Kuhn A, Löst C. (1994) In vitro comparison of various types of sodium perborate used for intracoronal bleaching. *J Endodont* **20**:338.

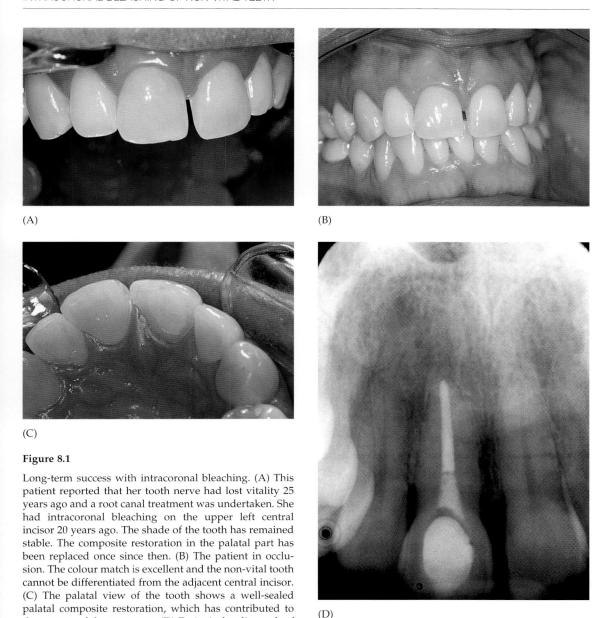

(A)

(B)

(C)

(D)

Figure 8.1

Long-term success with intracoronal bleaching. (A) This patient reported that her tooth nerve had lost vitality 25 years ago and a root canal treatment was undertaken. She had intracoronal bleaching on the upper left central incisor 20 years ago. The shade of the tooth has remained stable. The composite restoration in the palatal part has been replaced once since then. (B) The patient in occlusion. The colour match is excellent and the non-vital tooth cannot be differentiated from the adjacent central incisor. (C) The palatal view of the tooth shows a well-sealed palatal composite restoration, which has contributed to the success of the treatment. (D) Periapical radiograph of the tooth that was bleached. The barrier is placed at the cemento-enamel junction. A well condensed root canal is in place.

continued on the next page

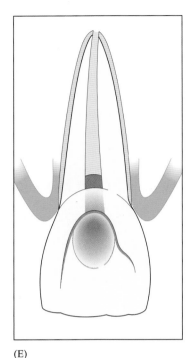

(E)

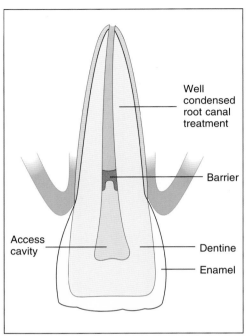

Well condensed root canal treatment

Barrier

Access cavity

Dentine

Enamel

(F)

Figure 8.1 continued

(E) All existing restorative material is removed. Root filling is removed to 2 mm apical to cemento-enamel junction. A small quantity of glass ionomer mixed to a putty is packed to form a 1.5–2.00 mm 'assurance' sealing plug. (F) The design of the barrier – it should have the appearance of a bobsleigh from the facial view and a ski slope from the proximal view.

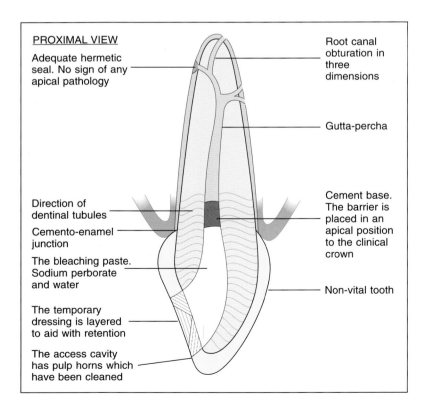

PROXIMAL VIEW

Adequate hermetic seal. No sign of any apical pathology

Direction of dentinal tubules

Cemento-enamel junction

The bleaching paste. Sodium perborate and water

The temporary dressing is layered to aid with retention

The access cavity has pulp horns which have been cleaned

Root canal obturation in three dimensions

Gutta-percha

Cement base. The barrier is placed in an apical position to the clinical crown

Non-vital tooth

Figure 8.2

The walking bleach technique.

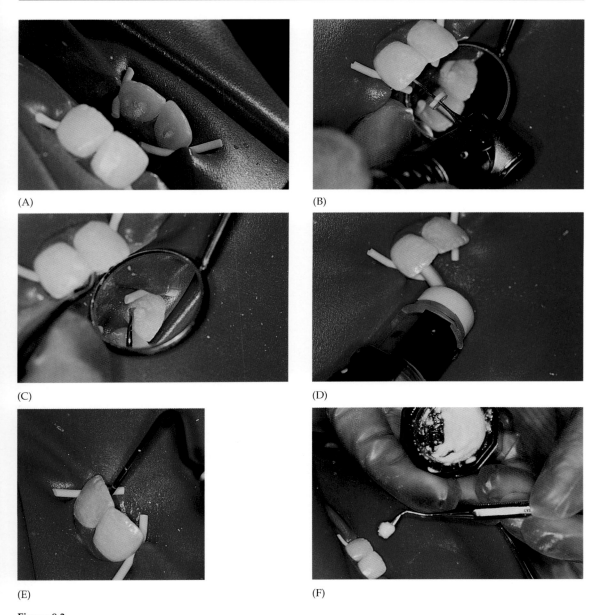

(A)

(B)

(C)

(D)

(E)

(F)

Figure 8.3

Preparation for intracoronal bleaching technique (A) The rubber dam is placed on the teeth and they are well isolated. Care is taken that the dam fits tightly at the cervical margin. Rubber 'wedges' are used to keep the dam in place. The coronal access cavity and restoration are removed. The gutta-percha is situated just underneath the restoration. All restorative material is removed from the access cavity. The dentine should be exposed and the access cavity refined. (B) The gutta-percha can be removed in several ways: by using a heated instrument (electric or manual) directly on to the gutta-percha, or by using Gates–Glidden burs measured to the exact barrier depth (about 3 mm below the cemento-enamel junction). This figure shows the Gates–Glidden bur being inserted. A rubber stopper is placed on to the bur to reach the correct length. Orange solvent, chloroform or xylene can be used to dissolve the sealer remnants. (C) The pulp remnants can be removed with an excavator shown here or with an ultrasonic cleaning device. It has been suggested that a small calcium hydroxide layer be placed directly over the gutta-percha, before the barrier is placed, but this is empirical. (D) Encapsulated chemically cured glass ionomer material is used for the barrier placement in this case. *continued on next page*

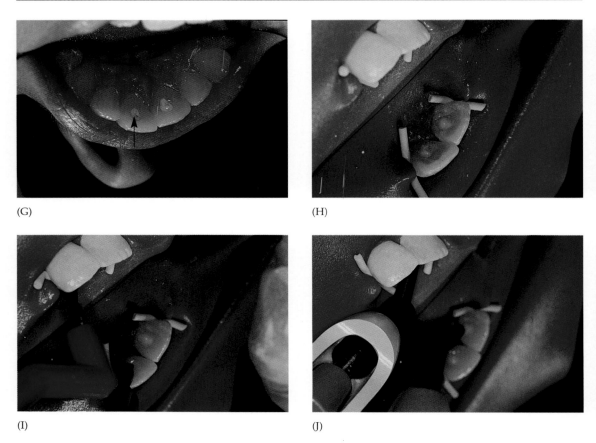

(G)   (H)

(I)   (J)

Figure 8.3 continued

(E) The material is placed at the correct depth snugly, using a flat plastic or an endodontic plugger. Once the material is set and the excess scraped away, the intracoronal material can be mixed using a commercial form of the sodium perborate bleaching material. (F) It is best to mix a stiff mix, which is easier to place within the canal; it should be the consistency of wet sand. The bleaching material is placed into the access cavity with a flat plastic instrument and the material is packed in tightly. Excess liquid is removed by tamping with a cotton wool pellet. This also compresses the paste into all areas of the pulp chamber. Excess bleaching material is removed from the pulp horn and gingival area. A temporary dressing is placed over this to seal the access cavity. This can be sealed with a bonding agent to prevent oxygen escaping. (G) When the patient returns after 2 weeks, there are small defects in the restoration where the oxygen has escaped despite placing bonding agent over the palatal surface. (H) The rubber dam is applied on to the teeth again and the temporary dressing removed. The bleaching material can be changed or if satisfactory lightening has occurred, the bleaching material is removed. The pulp chamber is rinsed out with water or sodium hypochlorite and a restoration can be placed into the coronal access cavity. Glass-ionomer can be used as a base over the barrier or composite material can be placed into the tooth. A segmental build-up technique should be employed. Here glass-ionomer is used as a base; the material is then cut back and the enamel and cavosurface margin is etched. (I) A bonding agent is then applied with a fine brush. (J) Composite material is packed into the tooth using a segmental build-up.

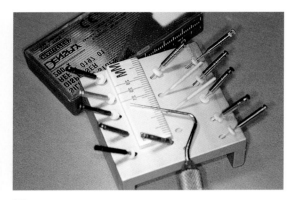

(A)

(B)

Figure 8.4

Armamentarium used in the walking bleach procedure. (A) A holder placing all instruments together for efficient use: Gates–Glidden burs in ascending order. The endodontic plugger (with the green handle) is also shown. Each size has a stripe near the end for easy identification. The end tip has a safe cutting edge which will not destroy excess dentine. (B) Parapost burs can be used, just for the initial removal of the gutta-percha.

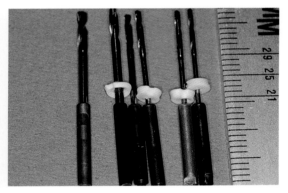

(A)   (B)

Figure 8.5

This patient had been involved in a traumatic impact through a sports accident. The upper right central incisor tooth had become non-vital and a root canal treatment was undertaken. A few months later the tooth became discoloured. The non-vital tooth was bleached intracoronally. After sealing the access cavity, walking bleach treatment was undertaken. This was followed by home bleaching treatment with a tray. (A) Portrait of the patient a few months after the endodontic treatment. (B) Portrait of the patient prior to commencing intracoronal bleaching. It appears as though the tooth has darkened further.

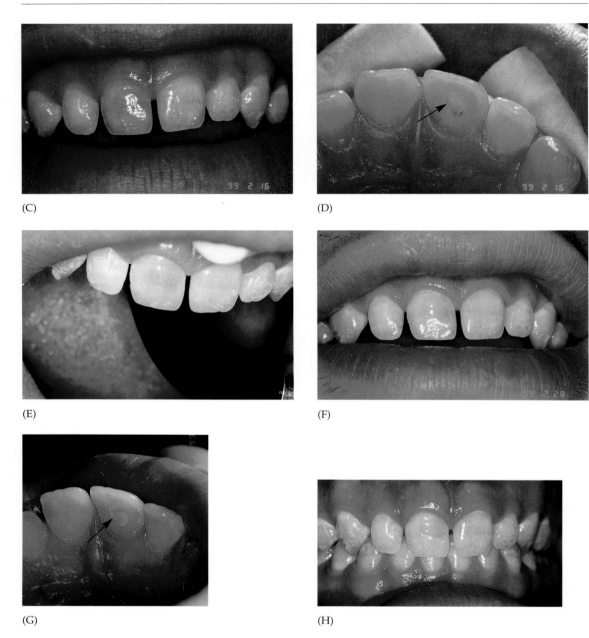

(C) The appearance of the tooth prior to commencing intracoronal bleaching. (D) The composite restoration at the back of the tooth was removed. The access cavity cleaned and a small pulp remnant was noticed. Further gutta-percha was removed to a level just below the labial gingival margin. Cotton wool isolation was used. (It would have been better to place a rubber dam for better isolation.) (E) The light-cured glass-ionomer cement was mixed and placed into the tooth to form a barrier and protection for the gutta-percha from the sodium perborate. The barrier was light-cured. The bleaching mixture was placed into the tooth and packed down. The provisional restoration was placed over this and sealed well. (F) The appearance of the tooth after 12 days of intracoronal bleaching. (G) The palatal mirror view of the provisional restoration after 12 days of bleaching. (H) The bleaching tray was tried in for the patient, who was instructed in the use of the home bleaching materials. The appearance of the tooth is shown after 10 days of home bleaching.

continued on next page

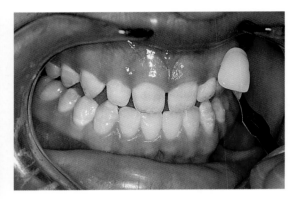

(I)

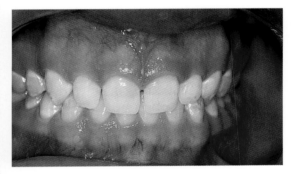

(J)

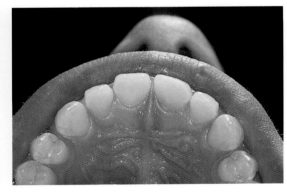

(K)

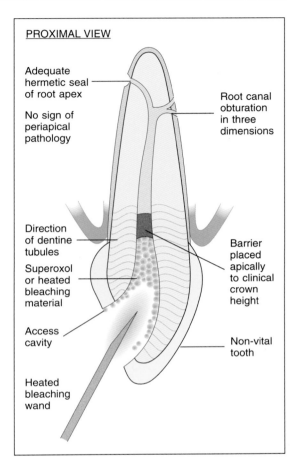

PROXIMAL VIEW

Adequate hermetic seal of root apex

No sign of periapical pathology

Root canal obturation in three dimensions

Direction of dentine tubules

Superoxol or heated bleaching material

Access cavity

Heated bleaching wand

Barrier placed apically to clinical crown height

Non-vital tooth

Figure 8.6

The thermocatalytic bleaching technique.

Figure 8.5 continued

(I) After a further 2 weeks of bleaching. The final shade of the tooth was an A1 shade. (J) The teeth in occlusion at 3-months' follow-up show no further regression of the shade. (K) Access cavity with a well-sealed composite restoration.

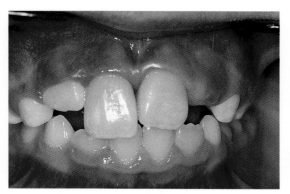

(A)

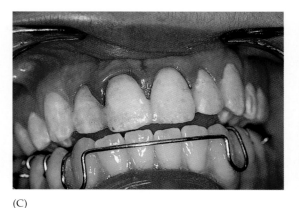

(C)

Figure 8.7

Contraindications to bleaching. (A) This young patient fell on to her two front teeth. The trauma caused the tooth to become devitalized. As the roots were still immature and apexogenesis had not occurred, the roots have remained short and are not yet fully closed. With such a severe traumatic impact, and short roots, it is probably best not to attempt intracoronal bleaching. (B) Shows a periapical radiograph of the root treated teeth. (C) This patient tripped and fell on to a hard surface. The upper right central incisor was avulsed completely and the upper left incisor pushed forwards out of occlusion. The teeth are shown immediately after the right central was reinserted and the left central was repositioned. The teeth were splinted lightly with composite material. As the patient had completed orthodontic treatment recently she was still wearing a retainer. The upper retainer acted as a splint for several weeks. Because of the unpredictable prognosis of these teeth, it is probably best not to attempt intracoronal bleaching.

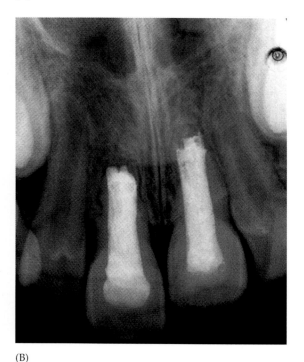

(B)

9

COMBINING BLEACHING TECHNIQUES

INTRODUCTION

While many stains can be treated successfully with a single agent, some may need to be treated using a combination of approaches. Bleaching treatments can be combined in various ways depending on the nature of the discoloration. When one agent fails to remove a stain completely, or when multiple stains of different origin are present in the same tooth, a combination of bleaching techniques can be used. Power bleaching can be combined with a home bleaching programme (Garber et al 1991). Combinations of bleach in different concentrations can be used. The microabrasion technique can be combined with home or power bleaching. Teeth can even be brightened using pumice and a 10% carbamide peroxide slurry (Baker et al 1992). It is the aim of this chapter to demonstrate how different bleaching techniques can be used in combination by showing various case presentations. A modification of the intracoronal technique will be described.

WHY COMBINE BLEACHING TREATMENTS?

- To make the bleaching programme more effective.
- To motivate patients to continue the bleaching programme at home.
- To treat a specific problem such as a single dark vital tooth or a single non-vital tooth.
- To sequence and stage bleaching treatment in a complex treatment plan.
- To treat difficult stains, such as tetracycline, which may respond better to a combination approach.
- To treat stains of different origins that exist in the same tooth.

THE INSIDE/OUTSIDE BLEACHING TECHNIQUE

This has also been called 'internal/external bleaching' (Settembrini et al 1997) and the 'patient-administered intracoronal bleaching technique' or 'modified walking bleach technique' (Liebenberg 1997). The technique combines the intracoronal bleaching technique with the home bleaching technique. It is used to lighten non-vital teeth in a simple manner. After barrier replacement the access cavity is left open so that the bleaching material, which is normally 10% carbamide peroxide, can be placed into the pulp chamber while the bleaching tray is applied to the tooth to retain the material on the tooth. Bleaching can thus take place internally and externally at the same time (see Figure 9.1). This technique is a modification of the intracoronal bleaching technique (see Chapter 8). At present there are few clinical studies (Carillo et al 1998) and anecdotal case reports published on this combined technique. However, its simplicity and effectiveness warrant description and discussion.

THE PROCEDURE

1. Preparation of the barrier

The non-vital tooth is prepared in the same manner described in Chapter 8 on intracoronal bleaching. It is essential to take a pre-operative X-ray to verify the presence of an acceptable root canal treatment and the absence of apical pathology. The tooth can be isolated with rubber dam in preparation for the meticulous removal of the existing extracoronal restoration; however, utilization of the dental dam is not mandatory as the bleaching material is not caustic (Liebenberg 1997). As in the intracoronal technique, the gutta-percha is removed to 2–3 mm below the cemento-enamel junction (CEJ). The object of the gutta-percha removal is to provide space for the barrier. A protective barrier is placed over the gutta-percha to prevent the bleach escaping into the root canal system at the CEJ. Conventional glass ionomer or a resin modified glass ionomer can be used as a barrier (Settembrini et al 1997). It has been suggested that a calcium hydroxide plug approximately 1 mm in thickness be placed over the exposed gutta-percha. This prophylactic step aims to maintain an alkaline medium because cervical resorption has been associated with a drop in pH at the cervical level (Liebenberg 1997). A periapical radiograph can be taken at this stage to check that the barrier has been well placed, but this is not mandatory.

2. Cleaning the access cavity

The access cavity is cleaned and any remaining pulp horn constituents removed. The access cavity can be etched merely to clean the internal surface. It does not enhance the bleaching effect. A cotton wool pellet is placed into the access cavity to avoid food packing into it.

3. Shade assessment

The pre-operative shade is taken both of the non-vital tooth colour and the surrounding teeth and noted in the patient's records or on the bleaching record sheet (see Chapter 5).

4. Instructions for home bleaching

The bleaching tray is checked for fit and comfort. The patient is instructed not to bite with the anterior tooth during the duration of the treatment (Carillo et al 1998). The patient is sent home with the bleaching instructions and enough bleaching materials. The cotton pellet in

the access cavity is removed with a toothpick before bleaching. The bleaching syringe can be applied directly into the open chamber prior to seating the bleaching tray, or the bleaching material can be applied into the tray with extra material into the space for the tooth with the open chamber. The patient is instructed to remove the excess with a toothbrush or paper tissue. After the bleaching session, the tooth is irrigated with a water syringe and a fresh cotton wool pellet is inserted back into the tooth. After a meal, the tooth is again irrigated with water to ensure the absence of debris and a fresh cotton wool pellet is inserted.

5. Treatment timing

If the patient can change the solution every two hours, five to eight applications may be all that it is necessary to achieve the desired lightening. This may take a matter of days. The more often the solution is changed, the quicker the bleaching will take place. Nightly application will be slower than twice daily application. It has been advised that unless the tooth is severely discoloured, the bleach should be applied during the day so that the lightening can be better controlled.

6. Reassessment of the shade and bleaching results

The patient returns in 3–7 days. The shade changes are assessed. If sufficient lightening has occurred the bleaching procedure may be terminated. The longer the tooth has been discoloured, the longer it can take for the bleaching treatment to remove the discoloration (Carillo et al 1998). Similarly, the darker the tooth, the longer it will take to lighten.

7. Sealing the access cavity

The access cavity is then sealed with a temporary dressing. Placement of the final restoration may need to be delayed for 2 weeks to allow the oxygen to dissipate from the tooth and to allow the bond strength of the enamel/composite to improve (Carillo et al 1998). If it is not possible to wait 2 weeks to place the final restoration, catalase can be placed into the access cavity using a sponge pledget for 3 minutes (Liebenberg 1997). The catalase acts to remove any latent hydrogen peroxide by promoting the decomposition of hydrogen peroxide into water and oxygen (Rotstein 1993).

The access cavity is first irrigated with sodium hypochlorite to flush out any remaining debris. The access cavity can then be cleaned using catalase. The cavosurface margin, the enamel surrounding the access cavity and the pulp chamber dentine are etched for 15 seconds with 37% phosphoric acid according to a chosen adhesive protocol. Dentine bonding agents are then applied. Acetone-containing bonding agents are preferred in this situation as they have been shown to reverse the effects of bleaching on enamel bond strengths. The access cavity is sealed with a composite restoration using incremental build-ups of composite and a flowable composite at the base, over the glass ionomer. A condensable glass ionomer restoration can be placed immediately (Settembrini et al 1997) over the barrier and a shallower composite restoration placed after 2 weeks. The thicker base of glass ionomer can sometimes mask the residual discoloration if the non-vital tooth has not fully bleached to match the adjacent teeth.

8. Review

The tooth should be periodically reviewed and a radiograph taken annually to check for any signs of a cervical inflammatory process.

BENEFITS OF THE INSIDE/OUTSIDE BLEACHING TECHNIQUE

1 More surface area is available both internally and externally for the bleach to penetrate.

2 A lower concentration (10% carbamide peroxide with neutral pH) of the bleach is used.
3 This technique will hopefully eliminate the incidence of cervical resorption that has been reported with the conventional intracoronal bleaching technique (no research yet), as most of the potential factors for resorption are reduced.
4 The need to change the access cavity dressing is eliminated as the access cavity is left open. (Previously, the oxygen that was released during the bleaching process often dislodged the temporary dressing from the tooth. The oxygen can escape normally and there is no build-up of pressure.)
5 Treatment time is reduced to days rather than weeks (Liebenberg 1997) if repeated replenishment is used.
6 The patient can discontinue filling the pulp once the desired colour has been achieved.
7 Using catalase prior to placement of the restoration can eliminate residual oxygen.
8 No heat is required to activate the bleaching material.

RISKS

1 The potential for cervical resorption is reduced but still exists.
2 Non-compliant patients: as the technique is a patient applied technique, it requires the patient to return to have the access cavity filled. Dentists should be careful in their patient selection and education to ensure that the patient returns to have the final restoration placed (Carillo et al 1998).
3 Although some degree of manual dexterity is required by the patient to place the syringe into the access cavity, the patient's desire to achieve a whiter tooth counteracts this problem.
4 The tooth could be over-bleached through over-zealous application of the bleaching material by the patient. However, as a matrix is used to apply and retain the bleaching material, the colour of the other teeth can be lightened evenly to

correct the colour mismatch. It is thus essential to have regular reviews at frequent intervals to assess the colour change taking place.

5 Shade stabilization occurs over a 2-week period (a slight rebound darkening can be expected as with all bleaching procedures 1–2 weeks later the shade can shift by one shade darker).

INDICATIONS

1 Indications can include treatment for adolescents with incomplete gingival maturation.

2 A single dark non-vital tooth where the surrounding teeth are sufficiently light. If this is the case, a window can be cut into the tray at the adjacent teeth to help the patient identify where to place the bleach. An oversized provisional crown form (Wahl 1992) can be used where there is difficulty retaining the bleaching tray (Carillo et al 1998).

OTHER OPTIONS FOR NON-VITAL TEETH

Non-vital teeth can be bleached using the bleaching tray at home using 10% carbamide peroxide in a closed chamber technique. This may take longer than a vital tooth because of the nature of the discoloration and the haemosiderin stained dentine. The benefits of this technique are that rather than removing an existing sound restoration, the bleaching material is applied to the tooth via the bleaching tray (Frazier 1998). This technique may be the treatment of choice when providing a 'top up' treatment or a maintenance bleaching treatment several years after the initial bleaching treatment took place.

The choice of which bleaching agent to use depends on the nature of the discoloration and the severity of the existing discoloration. Previous reports of cervical resorption following internal bleaching noted more problems when heat was applied to the tooth and where the tooth had been previously traumatized prior to revitalization. To avoid cervical resorption, it may be prudent to avoid high concentrations of hydrogen peroxide and heat.

Table 9.1 Treatment options for bleaching non-vital teeth

Intracoronal bleaching. The material is sealed into the access cavity during in-office visits and requires frequent changing of dressings:

❑ Intracoronal bleaching technique (see Chapter 8)
  • Sodium perborate and water sealed into the tooth (Rotstein et al 1991, 1993)
❑ Modified intracoronal bleaching technique using different products sealed into the tooth such as:
  • Various increasing hydrogen peroxide concentrations and sodium perborate in combination[a]
  • Sealing 35% carbamide peroxide into the tooth
  • Sealing 10%, 15% or 20% carbamide peroxide into the tooth (Vachon et al 1998)
❑ Intracoronal bleaching using the thermocatalytic technique or other forms of heat or heating instruments[a]

Open chamber bleaching. Combining intra- and extracoronal bleaching; the material is applied into the pulp chamber directly and retained with a home bleaching matrix.

❑ Inside/outside technique with bleaching tray using:
  • 10% carbamide peroxide (Settembrini et al 1997, Carillo et al 1998, Caughman et al 1999)
  • 5%, 16%, 22% differing concentrations
  • 35% carbamide peroxide – assisted bleaching in tray

Closed chamber bleaching – extracoronal. The bleaching material is placed on the external surfaces of the tooth. Other operations:

❑ Power bleaching using 35% hydrogen peroxide
❑ Nightguard Vital Bleaching using 10%, 15% or 20% applied only to the non-vital tooth in the tray (Frazier 1998)
❑ Assisted bleaching applied to the external surface on its own or via a bleaching tray

[a]Technique *not* recommended; included for completeness only.

COMBINATION OF POWER AND HOME BLEACHING TREATMENTS

This approach is very commonly used to motivate the patients to comply with the home bleaching protocol and continue bleaching at home. Normally one or two power bleach in-office sessions are undertaken (see Figure 9.8). The patient is then given the home bleaching instructions, the tray and enough material to continue the bleaching process at home.

Garber (1997) favours this approach and advises his patients to use the matrix system for only 30–45 minutes at night instead of the longer times proposed for conventional home bleaching. He advises using this alternative days for the first week and thereafter only once per week until the colour remains stable.

BENEFITS OF THE POWER AND HOME BLEACHING COMBINATION

1 It eliminates the tedium of repeated office visits and rubber dam applications; instead only one rubber dam application is used (Garber 1997).
2 The patient can get the best from the different bleaching techniques.
3 The procedure can be adapted to suit the patient's bleaching needs, requirements and lifestyle.
4 It reduces the expense of prolonged office visits.
5 Power bleaching provides a 'jumpstart' and demonstrates some improvement while the tray is being made.

WHICH TECHNIQUE SHOULD BE USED FIRST?

It is essential when planning treatment for patients to discuss that a combination of approaches may be necessary, depending on the severity of the staining. There are few reports in the dental literature that offer suggestions about which agent might be the

Table 9.2 Factors to consider when selecting the sequence of bleaching treatment

Treatment choices are based on the following factors:

- Safety
- Effectiveness
- Permanence
- Efficiency
- Time factor – office time or chairtime
- Patient lifestyle
- Patient preference
- Depth, location and nature of the stain

agent of first choice in cases of superficial enamel discoloration (McEvoy 1998). Safety, effectiveness, permanence and efficiency are all factors to consider when deciding which agent should be used first. Matching agents to stains is only part of the treatment planning, while matching the technique to be used with which agent affects the sequence of care and the final result (McEvoy 1998). However, which technique to use first can often depend on the patient's wishes, time demands and finances.

As the dentist becomes more experienced at using the different techniques, the efficiency and effectiveness of their application can be enhanced. Knowledge of the techniques associated with each agent can help in case selection (see cases in Figures 9.4–9.7 and 9.9) planning treatment and overall success of the bleaching treatment. Approaches may need to be different for different cases.

FLUOROSIS

A combination of bleaching techniques may be necessary to remove the discoloration and improve the appearance of the teeth. Microabrasion and bleaching may also be used in combination. In some cases of fluorosis, the yellow-brown stains may be removed with the microabrasion technique, but it may fail to remove all the white stains. Power bleaching can be undertaken while the rubber dam is still in place. This can be followed by home bleaching for 2–5 weeks. An alternative bleaching regime can use home bleaching techniques first to see what colour change can be improved. After 2–4 weeks, the patient can be reassessed to see if other bleaching techniques are required.

STAINS OF MULTIPLE ORIGINS

Stains that have fluorosis, tetracycline and age-related staining can also have discoloration from a previous endodontic treatment (see Figures 9.5 and 9.9), due to a traumatic incident or discoloration from orthodontic bands. Different teeth in the same mouth can have stains from different causes. Patients who have teeth requiring a combination of different bleaching treatments will need to have treatment carefully planned and charged accordingly for the different techniques used. Success with bleaching these stains of multiple origin is not always predictable and the patient should be told prior to commencing treatment that a combination of different approaches may need to be tried. It is only by undergoing the sequence of bleaching treatments that success may be determined towards the end of the process. (See also Chapter 11.) Alternatives to bleaching such as veneers and crowns should also be discussed with patients prior to commencing the bleaching treatments.

It has also been suggested that for tetracycline stained teeth, veneers are prepared and then bleached after preparation (Sadan and Lemon 1998). However, the bleaching treatment may lighten the shade of the teeth so well that veneers may not be necessary.

Patients have a 'threshold of acceptibility', where although the teeth are severely stained, a moderate improvement may be sufficient to improve the patient's appearance and self esteem (see Figure 9.5).

SUMMARY

Dentists should have a thorough knowledge of the chemical agents used for bleaching and lightening teeth so that they can determine which agents or techniques used in combination are most likely to achieve the desired result. The combination approach to bleaching teeth should incorporate the ability to employ agents and techniques in proper sequence to achieve an excellent aesthetic result. It is best to go from the least invasive, most cost-effective first, unless other circumstances such as time and compliance alter.

BIBLIOGRAPHY

Baker FL, Guillen GE, Frysh H, Rivera Hildago A. (1992) Tooth colour alterations secondary to polishing. *J Dent Res* **71**:540. [Abstract No. 202.]

Carillo A, Trevino MVA, Haywood VB. (1998). Simultaneous bleaching of vital teeth and an open-chamber nonvital tooth with 10% carbamide peroxide. *Quintessence Int* **29**(10): 643–8.

Caughman WF, Frazier KB, Haywood VB. (1999) Carbamide peroxide whitening on nonvital single discoloured teeth: case reports. *Quintessence Int* **30**(3):155–61.

Frazier KB. (1998) Nightguard vital bleaching to lighten a restored, nonvital discoloured tooth. *Compend Contin Educ Dent* Aug; **9**(8): 810–13.

Garber DA, Goldstein R, Goldstein C, Schwartz C. (1991) Dentist monitored bleaching. A combined approach. *Prac Periodont Aesthet Dent* **3**(2):22–6.

Garber DA. (1997) Dentist-monitored bleaching: a discussion of combination and laser bleaching. *J Am Dent Assoc Suppl* **128**(4):26S–30S.

Haywood VB. (1992) Bleaching of vital and nonvital teeth. *Curr Opin Dent* **2**:142–9.

Liebenberg WH. (1997) Intracoronal lightening of discoloured pulpless teeth: a modified walking bleach technique. *Quintessence Int* **28**:771–7.

McEvoy SA. (1998) Combining chemical agents and techniques to remove intrinsic stains from vital teeth. *Gen Dent* March/April: 168–72.

Miller MB. (editor) (2000). *Reality: the information source for esthetic dentistry.* Vol 14. Reality Publishing: Houston, TX.

Rotstein I, Zalkind M, Mor C, et al. (1991) In-vitro efficacy of sodium perborate preparations used for intracoronal bleaching of discoloured nonvital teeth. *Endodont Dent Traumatol* **7**(4): 177–80.

Rotstein I, Mor C, Friedman S. (1993) Prognosis of intracoronal bleaching with sodium perborate preparations in vitro: 1 year study. *J Endodontol* **19**:10–14.

Rotstein I. (1993) Role of catalase in the elimination of residual hydrogen peroxide following tooth bleaching. *J Endodontol* **19**:567–9.

Sadan A, Lemon RR. (1998) Combining treatment modalities for tetracycline-discoloured teeth. *Int J Periodont Restor Dent* **18**(6):564–71.

Settembrini L, Gultz J, Kaim J, Scherer W. (1997) A technique for bleaching nonvital teeth: inside/outside bleaching. *J Am Dent Assoc* **128**: 1283–4.

Vachon C, Vanek P, Friedman S. (1998) Internal bleaching with 10% carbamide peroxide in vitro. *Practical Periodont Aesthet Dent* **10**(9): 1145–54.

Wahl MJ. (1992) At home bleaching of a single tooth. *J Prosthet Dent* **67**(2):281–2.

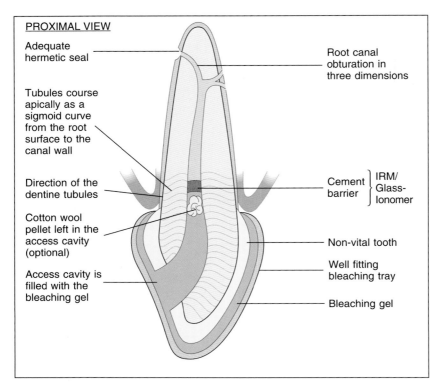

PROXIMAL VIEW

Adequate hermetic seal

Root canal obturation in three dimensions

Tubules course apically as a sigmoid curve from the root surface to the canal wall

Direction of the dentine tubules

Cement barrier } IRM/ Glass-Ionomer

Cotton wool pellet left in the access cavity (optional)

Non-vital tooth

Well fitting bleaching tray

Access cavity is filled with the bleaching gel

Bleaching gel

(A)

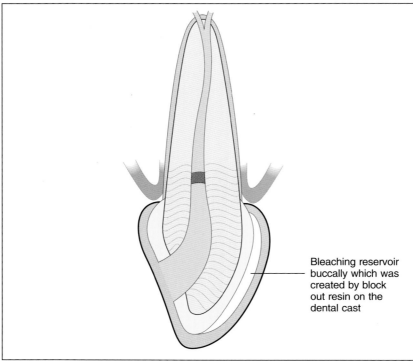

Bleaching reservoir buccally which was created by block out resin on the dental cast

(B)

Figure 9.1

The inside/outside technique. (A) Full tooth in cross section. (B) Sectional close-up of anterior tooth with bleaching tray seated over an open internal access cavity. The glass ionomer forms a base and barrier and seals the gutta-percha from the oral environment during treatment with the carbamide peroxide bleaching material.

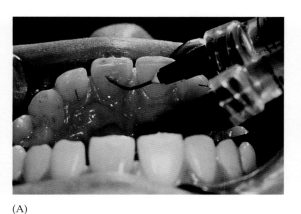

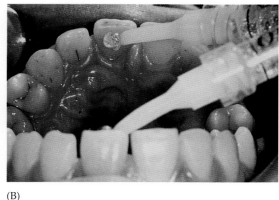

(A)   (B)

Figure 9.2

(A) A non-vital tooth is opened from the access cavity, which is on the lingual side of the tooth. The glass ionomer barrier is placed. A syringe with a fine tip is used to irrigate any debris in the pulp chamber. Water is flushed through in the syringe prior to placing the bleaching material (with permission from the Ultradent Company, Utah, USA). (B) The bleaching material is placed directly into the access cavity using a syringe with a small nozzle which can be bent to enable easier placement of the material.

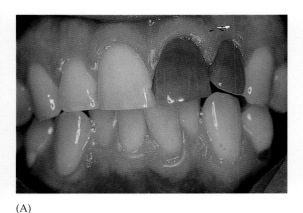

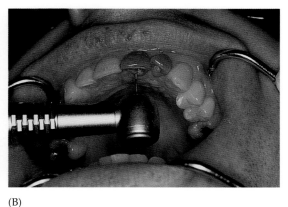

(A)   (B)

Figure 9.3

This patient had two discoloured non-vital teeth adjacent to each other. The palatal restorations were removed and access cavity cleaned out. After barrier placement, the outside/inside technique was used to lighten these teeth. (Courtesy of Dr Martin Kelleher.) (A) This patient had two discoloured non-vital teeth. He delayed previous attempts at treatment, as he did not wish to have the teeth cut down to place crowns on them. (B) A fast handpiece was used to gain palatal access to the coronal restoration. Isolation was achieved by the use of cheek retractors.

continued on the next page

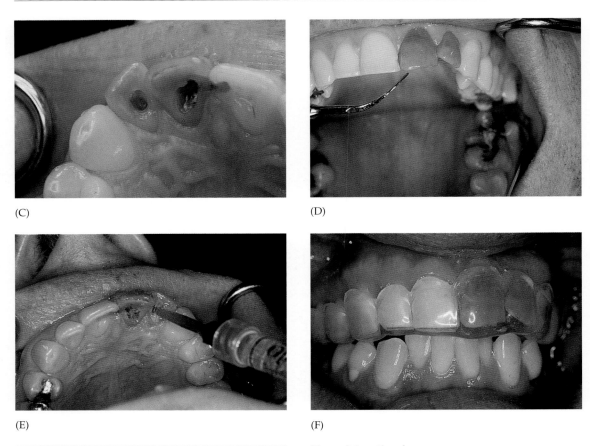

(C)

(D)

(E)

(F)

(G)

Figure 9.3 *continued*

(C) Mirror view. Palatal view: the appearance of the teeth after the restorations had been removed to the level of the gutta-percha. (D) A fine cavitron tip from the ultrasonic cleaning device is used to clean the access cavity and the pulp chamber. Care is taken to ensure that the pulp remnants are removed from the pulp horns because this could contribute to the discoloration of the tooth. If the remnants are not removed, the tooth will not bleach as well and colour regression may occur more quickly. (E) After barrier placement the bleaching material syringe is placed directly into the access cavity. This is demonstrated to the patient. (F) The bleaching tray is fitted over the teeth. The function of the tray is to retain the bleaching material in the palatal part of the teeth and at the same time it allows for bleaching to take place on the labial side of the tooth. (G) The final result.

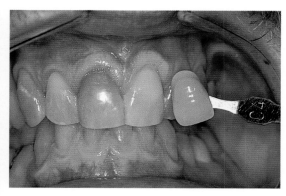

(A)

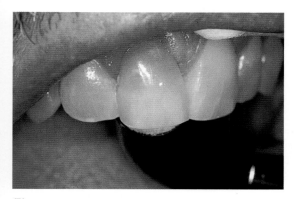

(B)

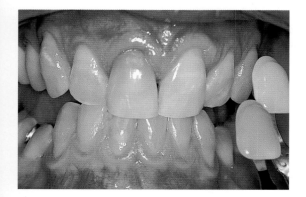

(C)

Figure 9.4

Tetracycline staining and a single non-vital tooth treated with the inside/outside technique and home bleaching. (A) This patient has discoloration from a combination of factors. He has generalized tetracycline staining. The upper right central incisor is non-vital and hence there is further staining from blood pigments and the root canal medication. The lower half of the central incisors is darker as the patient has a short lip; the lip does not cover and protect the entire tooth hence the cervical half of the tooth is lighter. The incisal half has desiccated and is darker. There are also white lines of decalcification near the gingival margins, perhaps caused by an episode of increased sugar intake or poor oral hygiene, or both. The shade of the tooth is taken before bleaching. However, the non-vital tooth is darker than this shade in the main body of the tooth. The canines are approximately this grey shade of C4. (B) The barrier is placed using a light-cured resin modified glass ionomer. The halogen light placed palatally in position for curing. The patient is given the home care instructions with explanations about changing the cotton wool in the access cavity. The severity of the stain is such that it may take several months for the lightening to occur (3–6 months). This is explained to the patient. (C) The appearance of the teeth after 10 days. The access cavity was sealed using a chemically cured glass ionomer restoration. There is whitening from the incisal edge. The patient continues bleaching the teeth using the bleaching tray every evening. The shade change, which has occurred, is from shade C4 to C2.

continued on the next page

Figure 9.4 *continued*

(D) The appearance of the teeth after 1 month. There is now whitening which has occurred on the body of the tooth. (E) The appearance of the teeth after 7 weeks of bleaching. There is further lightening on the lateral teeth. Although the cervical edge is still discoloured slightly, it has lightened considerably. This could have been due to the barrier placement not being placed just below the cemento-enamel junction. As the patient has a very deep bite, care was taken not to place the barrier too deep below the gingival margin. In some areas the shade change was to shade C1. Bleaching treatment was now commenced for the lower incisors. (F) The smile of the patient after 3 months' home bleaching of the upper and lower teeth.

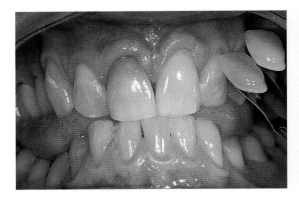

(D)

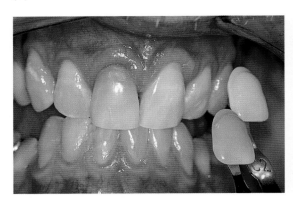

(E)

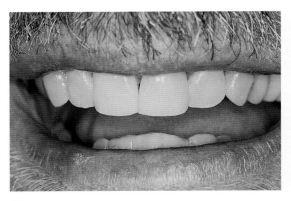

(F)

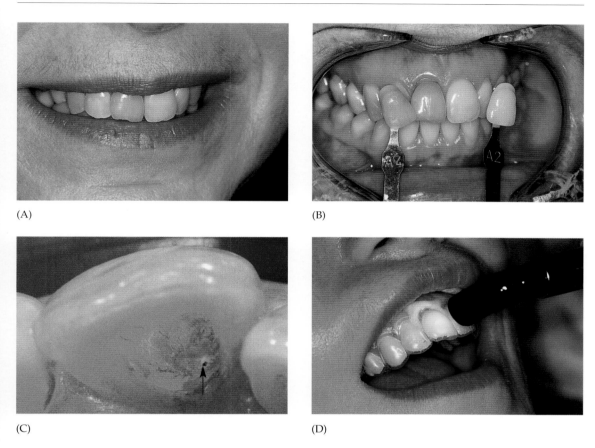

(A)

(B)

(C)

(D)

Figure 9.5

Teeth with multiple stains using assisted bleach followed by the inside/outside technique followed by home bleaching for the upper teeth. (A) Appearance of the teeth before treatment. The canine teeth have an orange-brown intrinsic discoloration. The right central incisor is non-vital. Attempts to bleach via the intracoronal bleaching were attempted 10 years previously with limited success. The patient had resisted suggestions from numerous dentists over the years to place a postcrown on this tooth, as she did not want any invasive treatment. After discussion, she consented to the inside/outside technique and home bleaching. (B) Pre-operative shade assessment using two different shades for contrast demonstrated that the colour of the canine and right central incisor is darker than shade C4. (C) The access cavity was re-entered. It had a large palatal restoration placed 10 years previously. It is difficult to assess whether all the composite material has been removed. The surfaces are gently scratched with a probe to identify which areas still contained the composite material. The residual composite has the grey marks from the probe. The small hole present is the entry to the pulp near the gutta-percha. The remaining composite was removed. Part of the gutta-percha filling was removed (2 mm) at the entry to the canal. A barrier was placed. (D) The assisted bleach technique was used as a chairside procedure. A light-cure tissue protectant is placed on the labial and buccal gingiva. The resin is cured with the tray in place so that the resin will not interfere with the correct seating of the tray.

continued on the next page

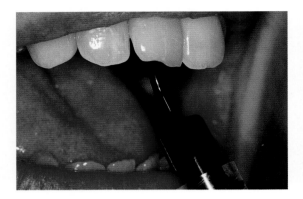

(E)

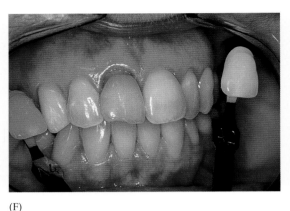

(F)

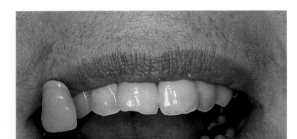

(G)

Figure 9.5 *continued*

(E) The assisted bleach technique utilizes 35% carbamide peroxide, which is heated in hot water for 3 minutes to activate it further. The material is applied to the access cavity via a small tip on the bleaching syringe. The material is left in the tooth for a short time. It is then rinsed out of the tooth and a further application of the assisted bleach material is placed. This is rinsed out and a cotton wool placed in the access cavity. The patient is sent home with instructions on using the inside/outside technique. (F) The results of the inside/outside technique after 1 week. There is less brown discoloration, but not a dramatic improvement. The patient reported that it was difficult to place the bleach into access cavity. The access cavity is sealed over and the home bleaching treatment continues. Note that the brown discoloration has been removed from the canine. (G) After 3 weeks, home bleaching treatment was commenced for the lower teeth. The results after 4 weeks showing the difference using the shade tabs. The lower teeth have whitened. Although the central incisor is considerably lighter than the original shade, there remains residual darkness; however, this is not noticed when the patient smiles. The patient is delighted with the results. Further treatment such as a bonded composite restoration or a porcelain laminate veneer can be undertaken at a later stage.

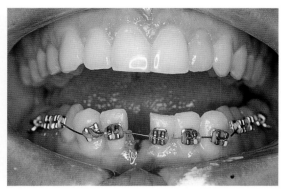

(A)

Figure 9.6

Non-vital tooth, inside/outside staining followed by home bleaching patient with simple restorative needs. (A) This patient's quest for aesthetic dental improvement began 9 years previously when orthodontic treatment was sought to correct lower incisor crowding. The lower right central incisor was extracted to alleviate the crowding and to correct the positioning of the canine teeth. (Courtesy of Dr Neville Bass.)

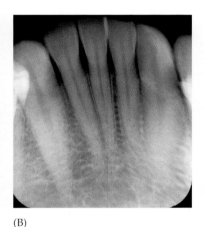

(B)

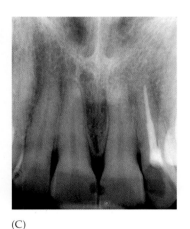

(C)

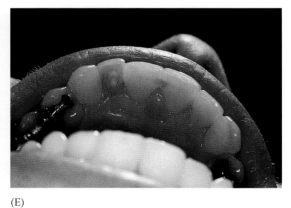

(D)

(E)

(B) Periapical radiograph taken after treatment. (Courtesy Dr Neville Bass.) (C) A periapical radiograph of the upper anterior teeth, showing that the left lateral insecure has had endodontic therapy. The root canal is well sealed and thus this tooth can be used for the inside/outside technique. (D) The appearance of the teeth before treatment. (E) The access cavity is prepared and the glass ionomer barrier is placed. Note the colour of the amalgam restorations.

continued on the next page

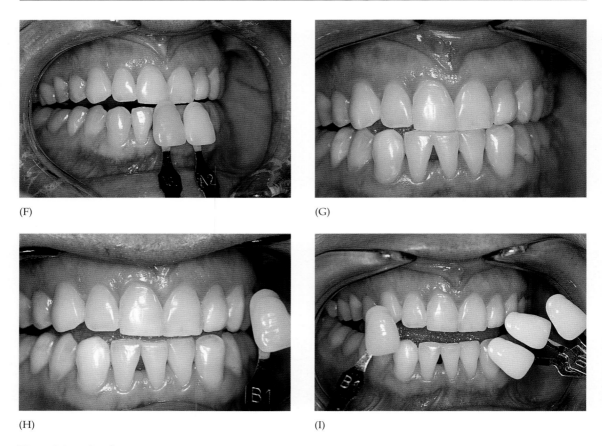

(F)   (G)

(H)   (I)

Figure 9.6 *continued*

(F) Following 1 week of inside/outside bleaching, the access cavity is closed with a glass-ionomer restoration. The patient reported that she had noticed after removing her bleaching tray in the morning that there were areas of black discoloration on the occlusal portions of the tray corresponding to the shapes of the amalgam restorations. Note the colour of the amalgam restorations, which appear lighter. (See Chapter 3 for an explanation of this phenomenon.) (G) The appearance of the teeth after 2 weeks of bleaching treatment on the upper teeth. The patient had been so excited by the tooth lightening results after 1 week, that she insisted on beginning the treatment for the lower teeth at that same time; the result of 1 week's treatment on the lower teeth is shown. The incisal edges are starting to lighten (note the lower right canine tooth). (H) The appearance of the teeth after a further week of bleaching. Note the colour of the lower right canine shows that the body of the tooth has lightened. There has been a shift of 15 shades to shade B1. (I) Some teeth can bleach beyond the value orientated shade guide and the porcelain manufacturers have produced porcelain which matches the shade of bleached teeth. This shade guide was assessed against the shade B1 for the bleached teeth, but was deemed to be too light.

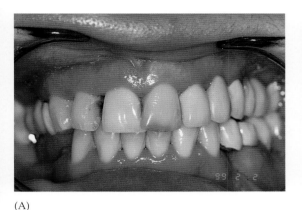

(A)

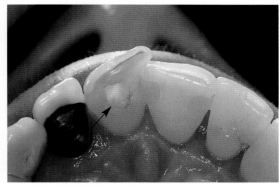

(B)

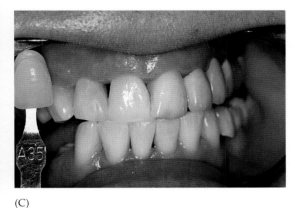

(C)

Figure 9.7

This patient had extensive restorative needs. She was concerned about the single dark non-vital front tooth, which had been discoloured for 10 years. An extensive course of treatment is being planned which includes periodontal therapy, endodontic therapy, and implant fixture placement followed by prosthodontic treatment. The treatment will take about 2 years to complete. However, after an initial course of periodontal treatment, bleaching treatment was started. The excellent bleaching results have motivated the patient to continue with further restorative treatment, which was left untreated for many years. (A) The appearance of the teeth before treatment. A large composite restoration on the lateral tooth was leaking, carious and had an overhanging margin. It was replaced on a temporary basis, so that bleaching could be expedited. There was decay on the distal aspect of the same tooth, but this was very small, so was left until after the bleaching treatment was terminated so that all the restorations could match the new shade of the teeth. (B) A periapical radiograph revealed a well-condensed root canal treatment with a good hermetic seal. The access cavity was re-opened and the composite restoration was removed. This figure shows that there is still composite present on the distal aspect, which should be removed prior to bleaching. (C) The result after 2 weeks of bleaching treatment on the upper and lower teeth. The access cavity was sealed after 1 week and the home bleaching treatment was continued. In this case the upper and lower teeth were bleached together because there were only ten natural teeth, and the existing crown and bridgework acted as a colour control. The treatment plan is to replace all the defective existing restorations, followed by cast posts where needed and provisional crown and bridgework, prior to the definitive treatment, which will commence once the implants have integrated. Following a 1-month period of shade stabilization, the anterior composite restorations will be replaced to match the new bleached shade. The temporary restoration will be replaced with a new shade of composite. This case indicates the importance of bleaching treatment in the course of a complex treatment plan and that it can help to motivate a patient to continue with further restorative treatment.

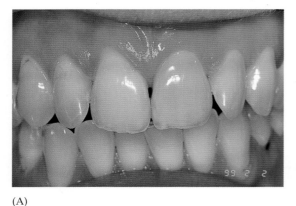

(A)

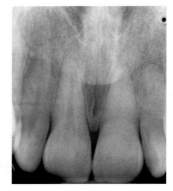

(B)

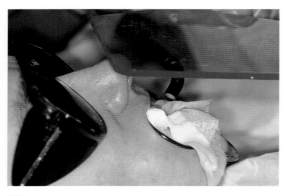

(C)

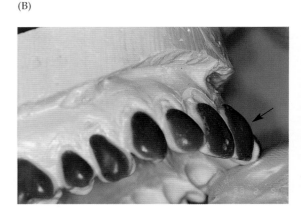

(D)

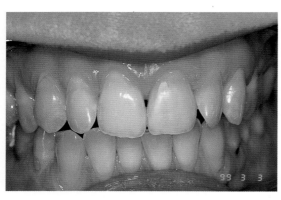

(E)

Figure 9.8

Demonstrates combining power bleaching using in-office techniques with home bleaching and titrating the bleaching treatment to achieve an evenly bleached smile. (A) The appearance of the teeth before treatment showing multi-coloured staining of the teeth. The upper left central incisor had been traumatized 10 years previously and had started to discolour gradually. The tooth responded positively to vitality testing. (B) The periapical radiograph shows that the pulp canal has narrowed and obliterated in some areas. (C) Impressions were taken for home bleaching trays. Power bleaching treatment was undertaken. The patient is well protected: eye cover and isolation with cheek retractors. The lower lip is protected with a damp gauze square to prevent any material dripping onto the lower lip and soft tissues. (D) After the in-office bleaching procedure, the patient is given the upper home bleaching tray in order to continue bleaching treatment at home. As the left central incisor tooth was darker, extra resin was placed in this area. This allowed for a larger reservoir to be held on this tooth which should facilitate bleaching. (E) The appearance of the teeth at the following appointment. Although there had been considerable lightening the upper left incisors were still darker than the right ones.

continued on the next page

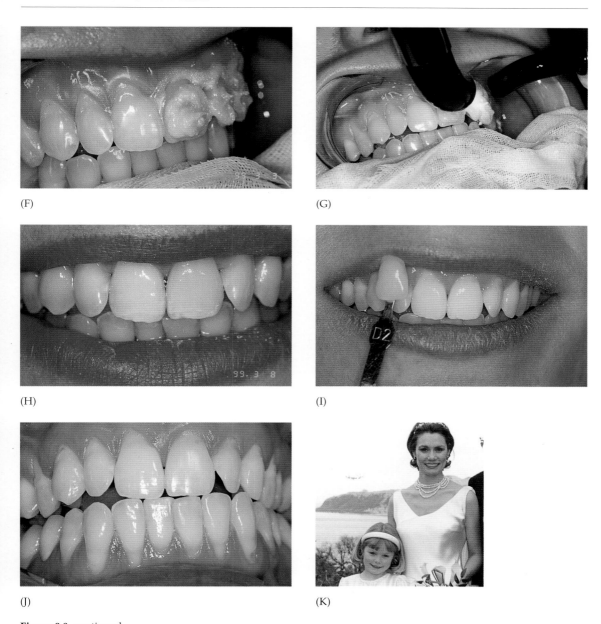

(F)

(G)

(H)

(I)

(J)

(K)

Figure 9.8 continued

(F) A further power bleaching treatment session was undertaken for the three upper left incisors. Light-cure protective resin is placed over the gingival margins of the teeth. The gel is placed on the teeth. (G) Light activation is used to enhance the bleaching action. Two light sources can be used. The light with the wider diameter is a halogen light and the light with the smaller diameter is the plasma arc light used on the bleaching mode. The lower lip is protected with damp gauze. (H) The patient's smile a week later. Note the contrast with the lower teeth, which have not been bleached. (I) The patient's smile 2 weeks later with the shade tab in place. (J) A month after bleaching treatment was completed cosmetic contouring and bonding was carried out on the lower incisors to give the appearance of straight even teeth and to make the teeth appear less crowded. The shapes of the incisal tips were modified and straightened. (K) The final result: wedding photograph of the patient (right) after treatment (with kind permission of the patient).

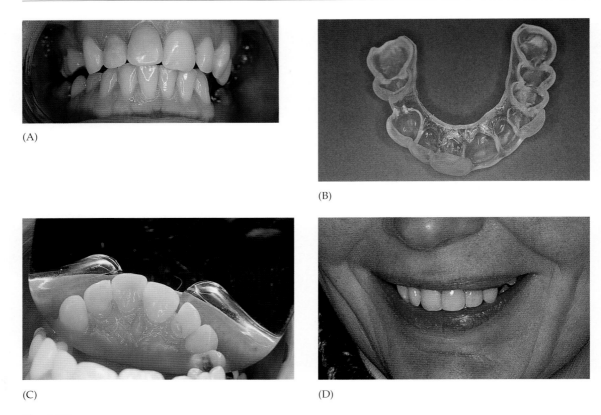

(A)

(B)

(C)

(D)

Figure 9.9

Shows teeth with different staining using a modified bleaching tray for home use. (A) The appearance of the teeth before treatment. The upper right central and lateral incisor were involved in minor trauma several years ago. This caused deposition of secondary dentine in the canal. The teeth when tested were still vital. As the left central and lateral were an acceptable colour, a specially designed bleaching tray was made to exclude the left incisors from the bleaching treatment. (B) The plastic of the special bleaching tray made was slightly thicker so that it could support the teeth that were excluded from the bleaching treatment. (C) The palatal view of the teeth just after removing the rubber dam. The composite restorations still had to be finished and polished. The small excess material on the upper right lateral was removed with a 12-grade tungsten carbide finishing bur. (D) Patient after treatment.

10 BLEACHING AND THE MICROABRASION TECHNIQUE

INTRODUCTION

The small white, brown or mottled lesions that appear on front teeth can be unsightly and patients are often concerned about this type of discoloration (see Figure 10.1). Before the introduction of acid etching, teeth that had these discolorations were cut down to have full coverage restorations. Some enamel discolorations, although intrinsic, are confined to the outermost layers of the enamel. The microabrasion technique can be used in combination with home bleaching or power bleaching to remove these discolorations more effectively. Which procedure is done first depends on the specific case. The microabrasion technique can be used in many different ways, on patients as young as 8–10 years old as well as adolescents and adults.

WHAT IS MICROABRASION?

Enamel microabrasion is a procedure in which a microscopic layer of enamel is simultaneously eroded and abraded with a special compound, leaving a perfectly intact enamel surface behind (Croll 1991a). It is used to treat enamel discolorations which may be the result of hypermineralizations, hypomineralisations or staining. Croll (1991a) called the process 'enamel dysmineralization', which describes the superficial enamel coloration defects resulting from some disturbance of the normal mineralization process. There are advantages in using a combination of chemical and mechanical surface microreduction. In successful cases enamel loss is insignificant and unrecognisable and the patient is left with tooth surfaces that appear normal. When treatment planning and discussing with the patients, this technique can be used either before, after or during the bleaching treatments.

THE DIFFERENCE BETWEEN BLEACHING AND MICROABRASION

Microabrasion improves tooth colour by eliminating the superficial discoloured enamel. Once the discoloration is removed, it is permanent. Microabrasion is preferred when general tooth colour changes are not needed, but a defined isolated surface discoloration is present (Haywood 1995).

Bleaching improves tooth colour by lightening, whitening and brightening the teeth. Unlike microabrasion, bleaching preserves the intact fluoride rich layer of enamel and the tooth shape. The shade of the teeth over many years may darken slightly, but the teeth never return to their original dark colour.

The two techniques can be used in conjunction with each other depending on the specific case (see Figures 10.6 and 10.8). Sometimes after microabrasion, the tooth appears more yellow or darker. Bleaching can thus follow microabrasion to improve tooth colour. The best results and improvements are achieved with a combination of both treatments (Croll 1997).

HYDROCHLORIC ACID

The use of hydrochloric acid to bleach teeth and remove stains from teeth has been advocated for many years (see Chapter 2 on history of bleaching). Hydrochloric acid and pumice are the main ingredients used for the technique. The use of hydrochloric acid depends on the decalcification of enamel, i.e. softening and dissolving the enamel to remove the stain. It should be selectively applied and well controlled (McEvoy 1998). Normally less than 200 μm in total of enamel is removed, but it may be much less. Using the correct concentration, procedure and application can carefully control the degree of enamel loss (Touati et al 1999). The effects of hydrochloric acid are non-selective and superficial. The technique may be enhanced by adding an abrasive (pumice such as advocated by Croll 1986), heat or chemical such as hydrogen peroxide and ether (Touati et al 1999). Which procedure is done first depends on the case.

INDICATIONS

- Developmental intrinsic stains and discolorations (see Figure 10.1) (Croll 1997)
- Superficial surface enamel stains and opacities (see Figure 10.2a)
- Yellow-brown areas (see Figure 10.6A)
- Multicoloured stains (brown, grey or yellow)
- Superficial hypoplastic enamel (Croll 1991 calls this 'enamel dysmineralisation')
- Areas of enamel fluorosis (see Figure 10.5A)
- White patches, white spots (see Figure 10.8A)
- Decalcification lesions from stasis of plaque and from orthodontic bands (see Figure 10.7)
- Some irregular surface textures

CONTRAINDICATIONS

Microabrasion cannot be used for the following conditions:

- Age-related staining

- Tetracycline staining
- Deep enamel hypoplastic lesions (see Figure 10.11A)
- Some concentric areas of hypocalcification that extend to the dentine
- Most amelogenesis imperfecta
- Most dentinogenesis lesions
- Carious lesions underlying regions of decalcification (see Figure 10.11B) (Croll 1997)
- Areas of deep enamel and dentine stains

WHAT IS AVAILABLE?

There are three techniques, which have been suggested for using hydrochloric acid (McEvoy 1998):

1 A cotton pellet soaked in 18% hydrochloric acid and applied to the stain.
2 18% hydrochloric acid mixed with pumice and applied to the stain via a prophy cup.
3 Proprietary kits:

- Prema kit (Premier Dental Products Co, Norristown, PA; Croll 1986) a 10% hydrochloric acid in a preparation of fine grit silicon carbide particles in a water soluble paste that can be applied manually or with a handpiece (see Figure 10.1B).
- The Micro Clean Kit (Cedia Kit, Rue St Honore, Paris, France). This kit contains 5 bottles, which are colour coded. The blue bottle contains 10% hydrogen peroxide gel; the green bottle contains weak hydrochloric acid gel; the red one contains concentrated hydrochloric acid; the mauve one contains a neutralizing gel (which consists of sodium bicarbonate); the orange one contains a fluoride polishing paste (Touati et al 1999).
- Opalustre: this kit packaged in purple syringes, contains hydrochloric acid and silicon carbide microparticles in a water-soluble paste (see Figure 10.8) (Opalustre Kit, Ultradent Products Inc, Utah, USA).

Ideal requirements of proprietary kits

- They should use water-soluble gels for ease of application
- The risk of spillage or splashing should be limited; application procedures should be simple
- Concentration of the gel should be able to be varied for different situations
- The acid should have a low concentration for safety in the mouth
- The abrasive agent should have great hardness to remove enamel easily when combined with the acid
- The abrasive agent should have a small particle size to prevent the enamel from being damaged
- The application method should be slow to prevent splattering of the compound

See further Croll 1989 and Touati et al 1999.

Effect on the enamel/mechanism of action

The rotary application process allows the material to simultaneously abrade and erode the enamel surface and so remove the stain. The enamel surface layer is restructured to form an amorphous prismless layer that clinically appears smooth and lustrous (see Figure 10.8H; Croll 1997). A generalized smoothing effect on the enamel has been documented (Berg and Donly 1991, Donly et al 1992). It consists of an amorphous layer of compacted mineral. This effect has been called the 'enamel glaze' 'abrosion' effect.

Advantages of the technique

- It is easily performed (Rosenthaler and Randal (1998)
- It is a conservative treatment
- It is inexpensive
- Teeth require minimal subsequent maintenance
- It is fast acting (McEvoy 1998)
- It removes yellow-brown, white and multicoloured stains

- It is effective
- Results are permanent

Disadvantages of the technique

- It removes enamel
- Hydrochloric acid compounds are caustic
- It requires protective apparatus for patient, dentist and assistant
- It requires a visit to the dental office
- It cannot be delegated and must be carried out by a dentist

THE PROCEDURE

Clinical evaluation of the teeth

Teeth should be in their usual moist state, and saturated with saliva before and after they are evaluated for the microabrasion technique. There is a camouflaging effect, which is present in the presence of saliva. Although the enamel stain may still be present, the saliva hides it. It is thus not necessary to remove the stain entirely and to evaluate this phenomenon first, before removing more. It is best to be conservative when removing enamel as more applications can be undertaken on another appointment.

Bleaching the teeth often masks the discrepancy between the difference of the dark yellow-brown stains and the natural colour or the white colour and the colour of natural teeth. Patients often ask to have the yellow colour removed and are not aware that the yellow is the natural colour of the tooth, while the white areas are the areas of dysmineralization. When bleaching treatments are undertaken, patients need to be warned that the white areas may appear whiter at first. Once the colour of the teeth changes, the difference becomes hardly noticeable. Microabrasion can be used to remove or reduce in size the remaining white areas after the bleaching process (see Figure 10.9). Again the camouflaging effect should be carefully evaluated and only those white areas which are noticeable should be treated.

EQUIPMENT NEEDED

- Contra-angle slow handpiece: Alternating speed reduction 10:1 or normal rotary slow handpiece. The alternating handpiece prevents splashing.
- The microabrasion material.
- Polishing or prophylaxis paste (see Figure 10.8F).
- Patient protection: gingival protection is normally required in some form such as rubber dam or paint-on dam and lip retractors, protective spectacles.
- Protective coverings: for dentist and assistant.

TREATMENT PLANNING

Case selection is particularly important with this technique. Careful discussion with the patient and their parents (if the patient is under age) as to the consequences, side effects, benefits and further options for treatment such as bleaching, veneers bonding and crowns needs to be discussed. Do not raise the patient's expectations of the expected results. Rather give a slightly pessimistic prognosis, that way the patient is not disappointed with the results. They are pleased when the microabrasion manages to remove the defect in its entirety.

The enamel should be assessed from the incisal edge with the aid of a mouth mirror. This way the labiolingual enamel thickness of the tooth and enamel lesion can be assessed. The depth of the enamel lesion can also be checked (see Figure 10.10).

STEP-BY-STEP GUIDE

1 Clean teeth with rubber cup and prophylaxis paste.
2 Isolate the teeth: rubber dam is the best method, with light-cured resin applied to the gingiva. The rubber dam can be sealed with Copal varnish. Ligatures can be tied around the rubber dam. It is not always necessary to use clamps. 'Wedjits' (Hygienic Corporation, USA) interdental rubber strips can be used to hold down the dam (see Figure 10.7B).
3 Protect the lips with a vaseline barrier.
4 Protect the soft tissues.
5 Microreduce the lesion to begin the treatment, by using a fine grit diamond or tungsten carbide bur (Croll 1997). This decreases overall treatment time.
6 Apply the microabrasion compound to the areas in 60 second intervals with appropriate rinsing. Check manufacturer's instructions on specific timings. A timer can be used to ensure correct amount of time for application of the compound and bristle cup.
7 The applicator head has special fluting to capture as much material as possible and compress the compound on to the tooth and to keep it in contact with the tooth (see Figure 10.1B).
8 Apply the material for short periods of time only. Cautionary note: Damage to soft tissue can occur if the material is left for too long. This may be in the form of blanching or whitening of the gingiva or soft tissues or may result in small ulceration of the mucosa.
9 Wipe off first to prevent splashing and wash the teeth.
10 Check periodically from the labiolingual aspect that minimal enamel reduction is taking place.
11 Repeat the procedure.
12 Polish the teeth using a fine grit fluoridated prophylaxis paste (see Figure 10.8E).
13 Rinse the teeth.
14 Re-evaluate the teeth when wet as some white areas disappear when wet (see Figure 10.8D). The rubber dam desiccates the teeth and some of the whiter areas become more vivid, thus evaluation needs to be done when the teeth are wet. It may sometimes be difficult to determine how deep the decalcification is. There is nothing to lose by trying the microabrasion technique first and then continuing on to further treatment such as bleaching or bonding if the former is not successful.
15 Remove the rubber dam.
16 Apply a topical fluoride (neutral sodium fluoride gel) application to the teeth for 4 minutes (e.g. Prevident, Colgate Pharma-

ceuticals; see Figure 10.1C). There are mousse fluoride applications that are used for 1 minute.

17 Re-evaluate the result. More than one visit may be necessary.

18 Review the patient 4–6 weeks later (and take postoperative photographs; see Figure 10.8H).

MICROABRASION AND HOME BLEACHING

Following the microabrasion treatment the teeth can be re-evaluated 6 weeks later, to assess whether any further treatment is required. If home bleaching treatment is to follow, impressions can be taken and bleaching trays made and the patient instructed in how to use the bleach and the trays (see Figure 10.3). The home bleaching treatment would follow the standard protocols as discussed in Chapter 5. Home bleaching following microabrasion can be quite successful (see Figures 10.4–10.6).

MICROABRASION AND ADJUNCTIVE TREATMENT

Deep enamel hypoplastic lesions once removed, leave a tooth form defect which requires a composite restoration. Sometimes the depth of a lesion cannot be ascertained until the tooth is treated (see Figure 10.10). A composite restoration may need to be placed to mask the discoloration. When this is necessary, the enamel surface of the lesion can be roughened with a coarse diamond bur to expose fresh enamel for the phosphoric acid to etch. The enamel surface of the microabraded area should be etched for 60 seconds instead of the usual 15–30 seconds as the mineral pattern and density of the enamel changes.

After the treatment the enamel appears smooth and lustrous (see Figure 10.8F). In many cases the results may be permanent. Remineralization of the enamel surfaces can occur. It appears that the surfaces do not retain plaque and stain as easily. The treated surfaces resist dissolution more easily. They colonize fewer *Streptococcus mutans* bacteria (Segura et al 1997).

BIBLIOGRAPHY

Berg JH, Donly KJ. (1991) The enamel surface and enamel microabrasion. In: Croll TP, editor. *Enamel microabrasion*. Quintessence Publishing: Chicago; 55–60.

Croll TP. (1986) Enamel colour modifications by controlled hydrochloric acid–pumice abrasion. Techniques and examples. *Quintessence Int* **17**:81–7.

Croll TP. (1991a) Enamel microabrasion: the technique. *Quintessence Int* **20**:395–400.

Croll TP. (1991b) *Enamel microabrasion*. Quintessence Publishing: Chicago.

Croll TP. (1997) *J Am Dent Assoc Suppl* **128**(4): 45S–50S.

Croll TP. (1998) Esthetic correction with fluorosis and fluorosis-like enamel dysmineralization. *J Esthet Dent* **10**(1):21–9.

Donly KJ, O'Neill M, Croll TP. (1992) Enamel microabrasion: a microscopic evaluation of the 'abrosion effect' *Quintessence Int* **23**:175–9.

Haywood VB. (1995) Bleaching and microabrasion options. *Esthet Dent Update*. **6**(4):99–100.

McCloskey R. (1984) A technique for removal of fluorosis stains. *J Am Dent Assoc* **109**:63–4.

McEvoy SA. (1998) Combining chemical agents and techniques to remove intrinsic stains from vital teeth. *Gen Dent* March/April:168–73.

Rosenthaler H, Randel H. (1998) Rotary reduction, enamel microabrasion and dental bleaching for tooth colour improvement. *Compend Contin Educ Dent* Jan; **19**(1):62–7.

Segura A, Donly KJ, Wefel JS. (1997) The effects of microabrasion on demineralisation inhibition of enamel surfaces. *Quintessence Int* **28**:463–6.

Touati B, Miara P, Nathanson D. (1999) Treatment of tooth discolouration. In *Esthetic dentistry and ceramic restorations*. Martin Dunitz: London; 83–116.

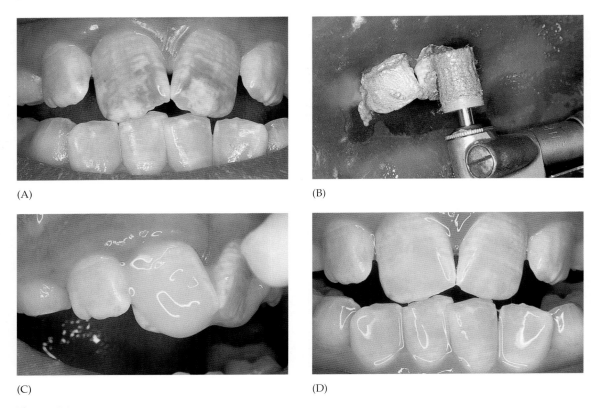

Figure 10.1

(A) Child with white and brown enamel dysmineralization. (B) Prema Compound (Premier Dental Products, King of Prussia, PA USA) is applied with a rubber tip using 10:1 gear reduction angle. (C) After white and brown discoloration has been microabraded, neutral sodium fluoride gel is applied for several minutes. (D) Enamel microabrasion removes superficial brown and white enamel dysmineralization defects. (Courtesy of Dr Ted Croll.)

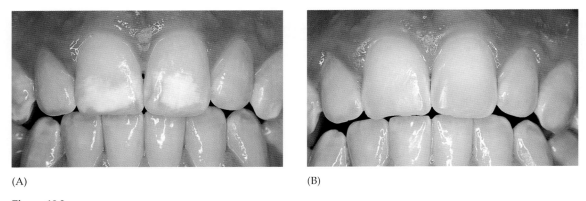

Figure 10.2

(A) Bright white enamel mars appearance of a teenager's central incisors. (B) Several months after enamel microabrasion. (Courtesy of Dr Ted Croll.)

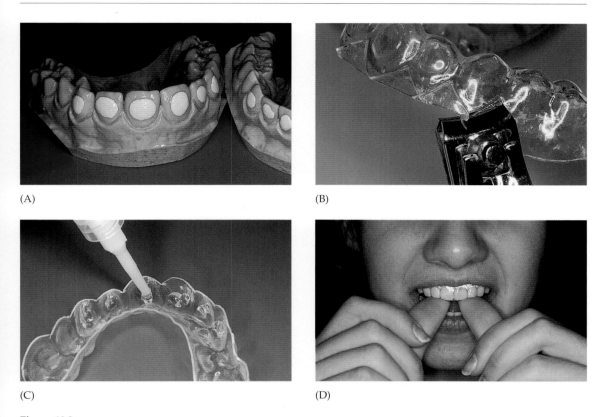

(A)　　　　　　　　　　　　　　　　(B)

(C)　　　　　　　　　　　　　　　　(D)

Figure 10.3

Fabrication of a bleaching tray. (A) Fabrication starts with trimmed dental stone or plaster model. Putty or resin tooth plumpers are placed to create reservoir space for the bleaching gel. (B) Soft vinyl tray material is vacuum formed. Margins of tray are cut with clippers or scissors to coincide with gingival contours. Viscous carbamide peroxide bleaching gel is injected into the tray. (D) Patient seats tray containing bleaching gel. Excess is wiped away. (Courtesy of Dr Ted Croll.)

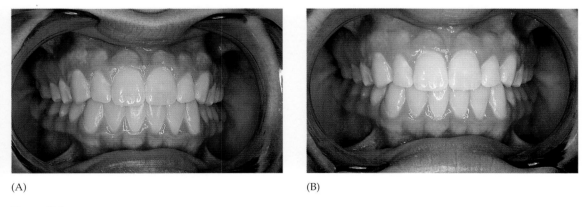

(A)　　　　　　　　　　　　　　　　(B)

Figure 10.4

(A) Teenage patient does not like yellow appearance of the teeth. (B) After 3 weeks of home custom-tray bleaching with 10% carbamide peroxide gel. (Courtesy of Dr Ted Croll.)

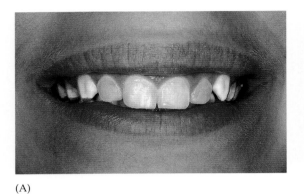

(A)

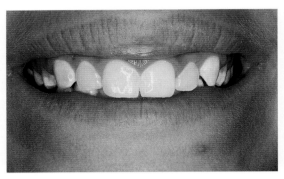

(B)

Figure 10.5

(A) Teenage patient had enamel microabrasion 2 years before. He complained that the maxillary incisors were yellow. (B) After 4 weeks of home custom-tray bleaching, the maxillary teeth appear much whiter. (Courtesy of Dr Ted Croll.)

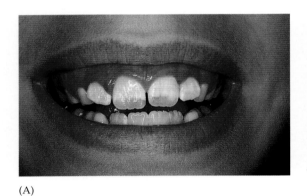

(A)

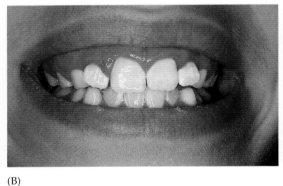

(B)

Figure 10.6

(A) A 12-year-old child had enamel microabrasion immediately followed by a 3-week course of home bleaching. (B) After 6 months home bleaching, tooth colour improvement persists. (Courtesy of Dr Ted Croll.)

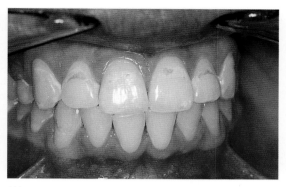

(A)

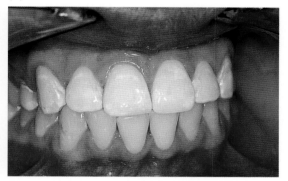

(C)

(B)

Figure 10.7

(A) This patient has small areas of brown and white decalcification following the removal of his fixed braces. (B) The Opalustre microabrasion material is placed on to the areas of the brown discoloration and polished using the special polishing cups supplied with the kit. Rubber 'wedge' strips can be used to hold the rubber dam in place. (C) Microabrasion manages to remove the brown discoloration in one session.

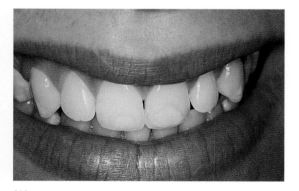

(A)

Figure 10.8

(A) This patient had large areas of white dysmineralization on his two front teeth. Two composite restorations had been placed on his teeth to mask the discoloration, but this was not effective. It was decided to try microabrasion on these front teeth.

continued on the next page

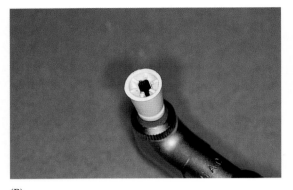

(B)

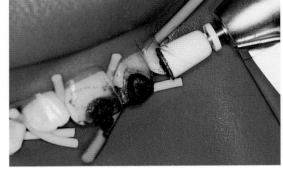

(C)

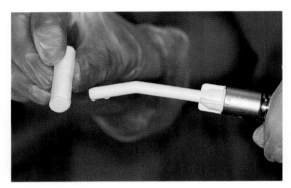

(D)

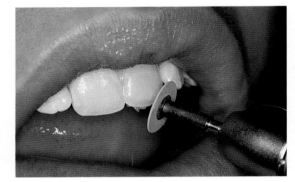

(E)

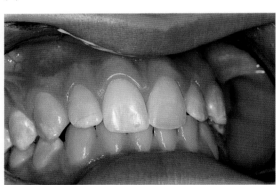

(F)

Figure 10.8 *continued*

(B) A non-latex rubber dam was used for isolation. A stamp on to the rubber dam helped to locate positioning of the teeth under the dam. The specially designed bristle cup for the microabrasion paste (Opalustre, Ultradent). It has internal flutes to retain more material. (C) A gear reduction handpiece was used. The material was applied directly on to the tooth with the syringe. The material was compressed on to the tooth with the use of the bristle cup. (D) As the teeth become dehydrated under the rubber dam, the white dysmineralization areas may become more visible. It may be necessary to use a damp cotton wool roll over the surface of the teeth that have been treated to see if the saliva will mask the dysmineraliza- tion. (E) After the procedure the teeth are polished with a fluoride toothpaste or gel. The areas are smoothed with a polishing disc and polishing paste. (F) The final result showing complete removal of the hypoplastic areas.

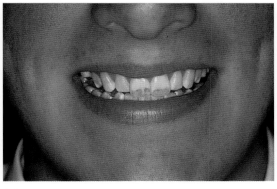

(A)

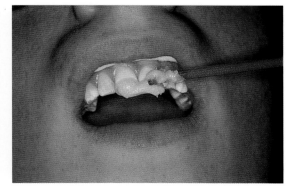

(B)

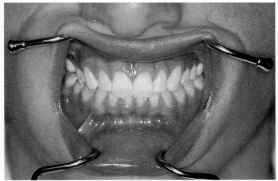

(C)

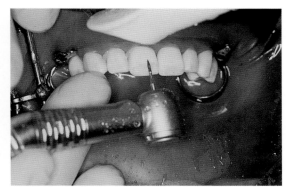

(D)

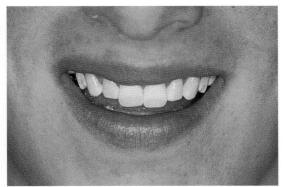

(E)

Figure 10.9

(A) This patient presented with areas of brown discoloration, dysmineralization on the incisal half of his two front teeth. (B) Power bleaching was attempted first. This did not remove the discoloration entirely. (C) This was followed by home bleaching for 1 week, which did lighten the brown discoloration to an extent, but it was not entirely removed. (D) A rubber dam was placed on the teeth and, with a fine tapered bur, microreduction was gently initiated to hasten microabrasion. The reduction was initiated with a fast handpiece under water. A further amount of microreduction was undertaken without water. (E) Polishing with the bristle cups and the microabrasion paste achieved total removal of the brown discoloration. (Courtesy of Dr Martin Kelleher.)

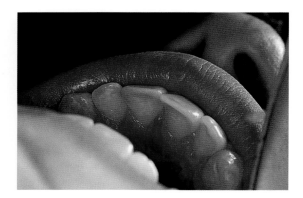

Figure 10.10

It is essential to observe the teeth from the labiolingual direction to ensure that too much enamel is not abraded away. This case shows that too much pressure was used in attempting to remove the discoloration. It is important to only use gentle intermittent pressure when using the bristle cups on the tooth.

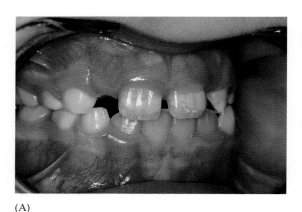

(A)

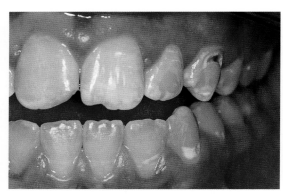

(B)

Figure 10.11

Contraindications to microabrasion. (A) This figure shows areas of deep hypoplastic enamel. This patient is aged 6. She is too young to have microabrasion. As the hypoplastic areas are extensive, it may not be possible to achieve removal of these lesions. As the gingiva still has to mature, it would be prudent to observe and monitor the situation for a few years. (B) This patient has just had his orthodontic brackets removed. There is active caries present which has started cavitating on the upper and lower left canines. Microabrasion is contraindicated for this case.

11

INTEGRATING BLEACHING WITH RESTORATIVE DENTISTRY

INTRODUCTION

The major objective of conservative restorative dentistry is the maximum preservation of sound tooth structure (Magne 1997). Bleaching is quite consistent with this, and in many cases no further restorative dentistry or other invasive techniques are necessary to achieve excellent dental health and aesthetics. However as the uptake of bleaching treatments in practice increases, more patients elect to have further aesthetic dental treatment or continue with simple and complex restorative dentistry. The bleaching treatment motivates patients to seek further aesthetic and restorative dentistry. This chapter will demonstrate numerous ways in which bleaching can be combined with restorative dentistry.

Restorative treatment has to be carefully planned to include further treatments in the correct sequence. Interdisciplinary approaches may be necessary, adding further emphasis to the need for well ordered integration of treatments. Bleaching can easily be incorporated into a restorative treatment plan, regardless of age of the patient. Should bleaching be used before, during or after restorative dentistry? This often depends on the case; the complexity, the time that it will take, and the patient's needs and wishes. Some dentists consider the bleached colour as the baseline from which to start all restorative dentistry. It is normally preferable to first bleach the teeth prior to commencing advanced restorative dentistry

(Williams et al 1992). Bleaching prior to restorative dentistry is undertaken when a change in tooth morphology is required in addition to a shift in shade (Small 1998).

Ask the patient whether he or she is happy with the colour of the teeth at the initial evaluation appointment. Often the patient will express a desire to have lighter teeth. With this information bleaching can be added into the correct sequence of restorative treatment. It is not appropriate to do bleaching treatment during the definitive stage of restorative treatment. It is better to plan for bleaching at the beginning of a treatment plan. Immediately prior to cementing a definitive porcelain crown, the patient may say: 'I really wish I could have all the teeth lighter, but I suppose there is nothing you can do about it'. These days there is something that can be done about it. In this case, it should be explained to the patient that bleaching treatment can be undertaken and a provisional crown can be fitted. The porcelain would have to be stripped from the existing crown and new porcelain placed. If the definitive crown was a strengthened all-porcelain crown such as the Procera or Inceram, it may have to be entirely remade. Another option is for the definitive restoration to be fixed with provisional cement while bleaching treatment is undertaken and the teeth lightened. It is always best to wait a month after bleaching to let the shade 'settle' prior to selecting the new shade of the tooth. Careful pre-planning would prevent a costly crisis from occurring.

SHADE MATCHING THE BLEACHED DENTITION WITH INDIRECT RESTORATIONS

The process of matching fixed restorations to the bleached dentition can be difficult (see Figure 11.7) because sometimes the shade changes so dramatically that it lightens than the lightest shade referenced on the prosthetic shade guide. It is difficult for the dentist to communicate accurately shade selection to the dental technician. The manufacturers have produced bleaching shade guides and bleaching shades of composites in much lighter shades than before to help with the matching of restorations after bleaching. A key to successful aesthetic enhancement requires that dental harmony be maintained when multiple restorative modalities are used (Schwartz 1998).

Building and layering porcelain restorations is more challenging as the optical properties of the adjacent bleached enamel and dentine have to be incorporated into the restoration. External layers of porcelain, which provide light scattering depth potential to the definitive crown restorations need to be built-in correctly. When fabricating porcelain restorations with a bleached enamel appearance, an assortment of external porcelain layers can be utilised to match predictably the shade of the existing enamel (Schwartz 1998). Altering the external surface with the porcelain layers enables the development of transparent zones to give a more natural appearance. While these powders are capable of imparting a bright opalescent colour in porcelain, they do not increase its opacity (see Figure 11.1). By using this porcelain building technique the six upper anterior teeth can be built up in layers to give the appearance of bleached enamel in the laboratory.

SHADE MAINTENANCE OF PORCELAIN RESTORATIONS WITH ADJACENT BLEACHED ENAMEL

To maintain the natural appearance of the bleached dentition with well-matched porcelain restorations, it has been suggested that once per month the teeth should be bleached, to remove the accumulation of stains and maintain the desired tooth colour. A new mouthguard is constructed over the porcelain restorations and the patient is advised to bleach with 16% carbamide peroxide gel for 2 hours once per month. Following the bleaching regime, a 1-minute sodium fluoride rinse is prescribed to remineralize the enamel. However, such maintenance bleaching is not universally recommended.

TEETH REQUIRING SIMPLE RESTORATIVE DENTISTRY

DEFECTIVE RESTORATIONS

Large defective restorations such as open carious cavities should be repaired prior to bleaching treatment to prevent unwanted penetration of the bleaching agent through the open margins, which may exacerbate sensitivity during bleaching treatment. The carbamide peroxide bleaching material does not have any detrimental effect on the existing tooth decay; in fact it may act as a cleansing agent. Small marginal defects can be repaired temporarily, by acid etching the margins and applying a flowable composite into the defective margins. Broken fillings can be repaired.

If the entire restoration needs to be replaced, it is better to wait until after bleaching treatment is completed as a composite shade lighter than the existing dentition can be selected. If the definitive tooth coloured restoration is placed prior to bleaching, the patient should be told that the selected shade is an estimate and that the shade may need to be modified after bleaching. Temporary or provisional fillings can be placed using the standard materials available, such as zinc oxide eugenol dressings or glass ionomer dressings.

PORCELAIN VENEERS

Porcelain veneers are an excellent, clinically proven method for correcting severe colour problems (Calamia 1983, Swift 1997). They are used when the defects on the facial/buccal surfaces are generalized and the majority of the facial surface is defective. Bleaching can be attempted first to assess the potential for whitening of the teeth. If bleaching is successful porcelain veneers may not be necessary. Even if the colour is lightened slightly, it may be sufficient to eliminate the use of opaque porcelains or opaque cements in the final restoration to mask the existing discoloration. This would still give an improved appearance to the veneer (see Figure 11.6). Nevertheless, bleaching is a simple and relatively inexpensive technique to try first. If it is unsuccessful, porcelain veneers are an appropriate next treatment option.

If veneered teeth become darker over time due to colour regression, they can be lightened from the palatal aspect using a bleaching material placed palatally in a nightguard. This procedure is effective because peroxide is able to diffuse freely through the tooth to the unrestored areas. This would be a situation where bleaching was undertaken after restorative dentistry.

Mandibular teeth are more difficult to veneer because of their greater functional demands and it may thus be more appropriate to bleach them. Even if the cervical areas have not bleached as well as the incisal edges, it is satisfactory for many patients. Similarly porcelain veneers may be placed on the maxillary incisors, while the canines are bleached to a lighter shade. In this case it may be advisable to use a bleaching material with a concentration stronger than 10%.

CERAMIC CROWNS

As teeth age, they usually absorb stains and darken. Restorative dentistry that was undertaken 10, 15 or 20 years ago to match the existing adjacent dentition will be noticeably lighter than the age-yellowed teeth (see Figure 11.3). An option for treatment in this situation is to replace the existing crowns and bridges with the new darker shade. This is acceptable if there are problems associated with the existing restorations such as fractured porcelain and secondary caries around the margins (see Figure 11.3). However, if the existing restorative dentistry is acceptable and a lighter shade

is required, it would be more appropriate to undertake bleaching treatment of the adjacent teeth, rather than expensive and extensive restorative dentistry.

Frequently when a single anterior crown is required, the adjacent teeth have a shade that is difficult to match. It may be appropriate to bleach the teeth first, to a shade that can be more easily replicated in porcelain.

COSMETIC RECONTOURING

Many patients choose to have further aesthetic treatment following bleaching. One option is cosmetic contouring which consists of selectively grinding enamel surfaces to produce an improved outline form (Heymann 1997). This can be achieved with fine diamond burs followed by abrasive polishing points and polishing discs. When a patient needs routine anterior restorative dentistry, careful consideration to smile analysis should be undertaken (see Treatment planning sheet). Symmetry and proportionality of the anterior teeth should be evaluated during this time. A diagnostic wax-up can show a patient what can be achieved prior to treatment.

MACROABRASION OR MEGABRASION

Some enamel defects or white spots/opacities on teeth that don't respond to microabrasion and bleaching may respond better to macroabrasion. The discoloured enamel contains an increased amount of organic matrix, which is not an adequate substrate for adhesion of dental materials. The lesion is generally restricted to enamel. Its elimination will not result in exposure of the dentine (Magne 1997). Macroabrasion involves removing the outer layer of the opaque enamel with a fine grit diamond in a fast handpiece with water-air spray. The final finishing and polishing is done with a 30-blade tungsten carbide bur, polishing discs of decreasing coarseness and composite or diamond polishing paste. Although macroabrasion may be faster than microabrasion it should only be used if bleaching and microabrasion have not been effective to remove the enamel defect. There is a greater potential for inadvertent excess removal of tooth structure and the technique should be used with care and caution.

Megabrasion is the more radical removal of enamel to eliminate the defect. As the underlying dentine provides the natural optical effects of the tooth, a neutral translucent composite restoration is placed over the defect to mask the defective enamel (Magne 1997). Coarse diamond instruments used at low speed allow safe and well controlled elimination of enamel. Highspeed handpieces are contraindicated as the vibration may cause enamel microcracks. The prepared surfaces are finished with coarse flexible discs (Sof-Lex, 3M, St Paul, Minnesota). Fine finishing of the surface is not necessary, as the rough enamel represents a good substrate for adhesion. Composite materials can be built-up in different ways according to the adjacent teeth (see Chapter 12). A 'chameleon effect' (Magne 1997) is evident where the composite restoration can blend into the tooth and the adjacent dentition.

TEETH REQUIRING EXTENSIVE RESTORATIVE DENTISTRY

Meticulous treatment planning is essential when undertaking extensive restorative dentistry. If a reorganized approach is chosen where full mouth rehabilitation is the treatment of choice, it may not be necessary to do bleaching treatment first, because all the teeth will be the same colour of porcelain, and the patient and dentist can select a lighter shade of porcelain. However, for those patients who require extensive treatment, but not to all the teeth, it is essential to discuss treatment options, as some prior bleaching treatment may be appropriately undertaken (see for example, Figure 11.2).

Some patients may require provisional restorations or crowns on teeth prior to bleaching to stabilize the occlusion, or may simply prefer to have provisional crowns placed prior to bleaching treatment (see Figure 11.7). Selecting the appropriate shade can be difficult in such a situation. It is best to choose a shade about 1.5–2 shades lighter and explain to the patient that while the teeth are

lightening the colour of the provisional crown may not match the other teeth.

Even if patients are about to embark on a course of extensive restorative dentistry that may take two years to complete, bleaching as an initial therapy may motivate the patient sufficiently to continue and complete the extensive programme of restorative dentistry that lies ahead (see Figure 11.2). The simple shift in shade of the anterior teeth may boost the patient's morale and self-confidence such that they can start to feel better about themselves. This improved morale may help them to improve their oral hygiene techniques and home care, which are essential with advanced restorative dentistry.

BLEACHING IN COMBINATION WITH PERIODONTAL TREATMENT

Bleaching treatment should always follow oral disease control particularly inflammatory periodontal disease. Initial treatment, which may include root planing, curettage and periodontal surgery, should be carried out first (see Chapter 4). It is more appropriate to commence bleaching treatment once periodontal stability has been achieved (see Figure 11.4).

Patients who have extensive gingival recession and gingival clefts, should be assessed by a periodontist first to determine whether the patient would benefit from further procedures such as free gingival grafts and other perioplastic procedures. Bleaching treatment should be delayed until such time as periodontal stability has been achieved which may be 3–6 months and 6–12 weeks after periodontal surgery (see Figure 11.1).

BLEACHING AND ORTHODONTIC TREATMENT

Major orthodontic treatment to improve malocclusion, aesthetics, function and phonetics should be undertaken prior to doing any bleaching treatment. In most cases, orthodontic treatment should be completed prior to commencing bleaching treatment. However, bleaching treatment can motivate a patient to seek further aesthetic dental treatment and thus simple orthodontics may be undertaken after bleaching treatment. For example, after bleaching treatment, patients may suddenly become aware that their lower incisors are overcrowded and ask for treatment options, which may include an orthodontic referral, cosmetic contouring to give the illusion that the teeth are straight, composite bonding, or porcelain laminate veneers. Orthodontic options may include full banding, extraction of one of the crowded incisors, or creating space by disking or stripping a small amount off the width of each lower anterior tooth.

BIBLIOGRAPHY

Calamia JR. (1983) Etched porcelain facial veneers: a new treatment modality based on scientific and clinical evidence. *NY J Dent* **53**:255–9.

Chiche GJ, Pinault A. (1994) *Esthetics of anterior fixed prosthodontics*. Quintessence Publishing: Chicago.

Goldstein RE. (1998) *Esthetics in dentistry*, 2nd edn. Vol 1. BC Decker: Hamilton, Ontario.

Heymann H. (1997) Conservative concepts for achieving anterior aesthetics. *CDA Journal* **25**(6):437–3.

Magne P. (1997) Megabrasion: a conservative strategy for the anterior dentition. *Prac Periodont Aesthet Dent* **9**(4):389–96.

Schwartz JC. (1998) Anterior fixed prosthetic restorations and the bleached dentition: laboratory techniques. *Prac Periodont Aesthet Dent* **10**(8):1049–55.

Small BW. (1998) The application and integration of at-home bleaching into private dental practice. *Compend Contin Educ Dent* **9**(8):799–807.

Smith BGN. (1999) *Planning and making crowns and bridges*, 3rd edn. Martin Dunitz: London.

Swift EJ. (1997) Restorative considerations with vital tooth bleaching. *J Am Dent Assoc Suppl* **128**:60S–4S.

Touati B, Miara P, Nathanson D. (1999) *Esthetic dentistry and ceramic restorations*. Martin Dunitz: London.

Williams HA, Rueggeberg FA, Meister PA. (1992) Bleaching the natural dentition to match the colour of existing restorations: case reports. *Quintessence Int* **23**(10):673–7.

Wise MD. (1995) *Failure in the restored dentition: management and treatment*. Quintessence Publishing: London.

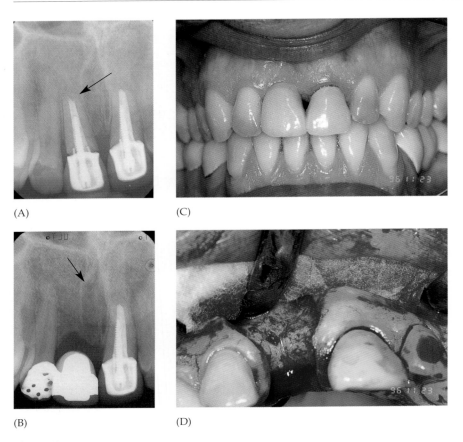

(A)

(C)

(B)

(D)

Figure 11.1

Shows complex restorative dentistry to provide aesthetic treatment for a missing tooth. Treatment involved: extraction of a fractured, endodontically treated tooth; healing; placement of a Gortex membrane to prevent further bone loss of the alveolar ridge, and provisional adhesive bridge placement in the pontic area. Once sufficient healing had taken place and the Gortex membrane had been removed, bleaching treatment was undertaken. This involved assisted bleaching of the upper left lateral incisor which was discoloured, followed by home bleaching of the upper teeth. Cosmetic contouring of the upper canine teeth was undertaken, to make them less pointed and more rounded. The upper teeth were restored with a fixed three-unit bridge of porcelain bonded to metal and a porcelain veneer was placed on the upper left lateral incisor to lengthen the tooth and improve the facial harmony. Treatment for the lower teeth which involved cosmetic contouring and bleaching was undertaken a few months later. (A) The patient had two porcelain fused to metal crowns placed 5 years previously. Both crowns had preformed screws placed into the root canals. These screw-type posts can cause forces to be set up within the root canal which can cause fracture of the root. The existing crown on the right central incisor had become decemented and on further inspection a vertical fracture along the root length was noted (arrow). (B) The tooth was extracted and an immediate adhesive bridge was placed. This was left for 6 months. This radiograph revealed that there had been further vertical loss of bone in the edentulous section. The radiograph also revealed a large nutrient canal (see arrow) which would preclude the placement of an osseointegrated titanium implant in the ideal position. Placement asymmetrically would have a detrimental effect on the lateral tooth. It was thus decided that the best course of action would be to place a three unit bridge in this space after a ridge augmentation. (C) The teeth prior to the augmentation procedure. There was loss of the interdental papilla on the central incisors. The anterior teeth have different colours and shapes. There was shine-through of the right lateral from the adhesive bridge which made the tooth appear grey. The left lateral incisor was discoloured, but still gave a vital response to thermal and electric testing. The lateral incisors have different shapes and the canines are very long. There was recession of the gingiva around the crown margin of the left lateral and central incisor. (D) Reflecting the flap back to commence the ridge augmentation. (Periodontal treatment carried out by periodontists Dr Stephen Smith and Dr Ros O'Leary.)

continued on the next page

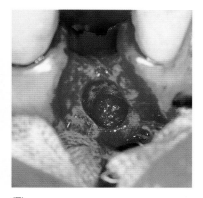

(E)

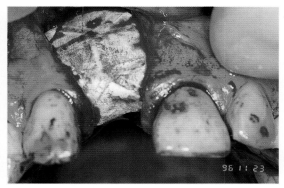

(F)

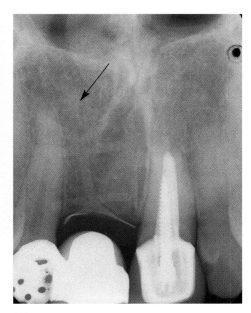

(G)

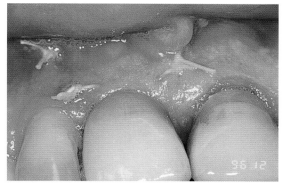

(H)

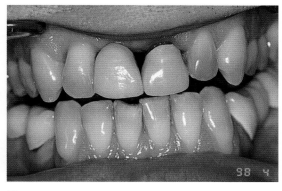

(I)

Figure 11.1 continued

(E) A bone cleft was identified as well as a residual cyst. The cyst was curetted and the site was developed with bone chisels and files laterally and mesially towards the site of the suspected nutrient canals. Bone was harvested from the site. (F) The autogenous bone was placed in the defect and the area was closed with a Gortex membrane. (G) The Gortex membrane was placed and left in situ for a period of 3 months to try to achieve a fill in of new cells and bone: see arrow pointing to its location. Bone loss appears to have reduced and stabilized. (H) The flap was sutured with PTFE sutures. The site after 2 weeks of healing. (I) The appearance of the teeth 18 months after periodontal surgery. Ideally it would have been better to place a connective tissue graft to bulk out the pontic area further, but the patient was happy with the result. There has been further deepening of the black triangle where the incisive papilla has flattened and gingival recession on the left side. The upper canine teeth have been rounded and shortened to improve the proportions of the teeth in the area. A shade is taken and verified for the lateral incisor using the shade guide supplied in the bleaching kit. *continued on the next page*

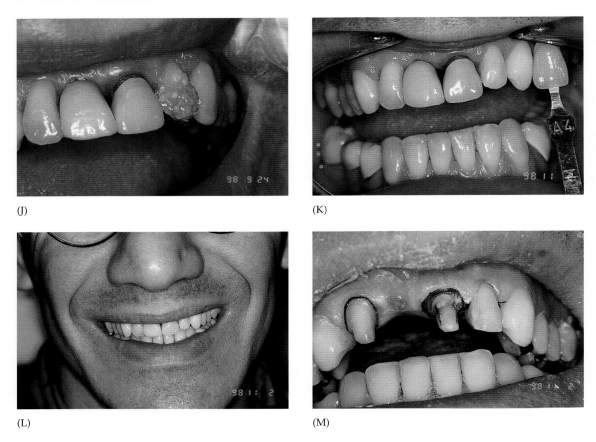

(J)   (K)

(L)   (M)

Figure 11.1 continued

(J) Bleaching treatment was commenced using the assisted-bleaching system whereby a bleaching material is applied on to the teeth at the chairside. This material has a higher concentration of carbamide peroxide (35%) than the home bleach (10%). It was used on a single dark tooth on this occasion as this tooth although it was vital was noticeably darker than the surrounding teeth. The material is designed to be used in-office with the customized tray. However there may be some irritation of the gingivae and it may be better to isolate the teeth using cotton rolls or protective light-cured resins. (K) The appearance of the teeth after 6 weeks of bleaching. The previous shade is shown next to the canine for comparison. The lower teeth have been cosmetically contoured and bonded where necessary to improve the alignment and shape of the lower teeth. (L) The patient's smile demonstrating the new lighter colour of the teeth. As the patient has a lower lipline the defect between the central papilla is not as noticeable. He has a broad smile with a broad buccal corridor. The premolars and molars are visible showing that the teeth are slightly grey from the existing amalgam restoration. These can be replaced at a later stage. (M) The right lateral incisor and the left central incisor were prepared for a three unit fixed bridge of porcelain bonded to metal, while the left lateral incisor was prepared for a porcelain laminate veneer. Retraction cords are in place prior to taking an impression. It can be argued that it was not necessary to veneer the tooth as it was now an excellent colour; however, the issue of the length was not addressed and to create a pleasing harmony it was decided to lengthen this tooth. By bleaching the tooth first, it was easier to achieve a more natural shade of porcelain without having to place opaquers in the porcelain or use an opaque cement to mask the discoloration. The light could reflect through the tooth to create a natural appearance. It can also be argued that the screw post should be removed from the tooth together with the two dentine pins, because the potential for further fracture exists. It would be more ideal to replace the screw post with a cast gold post, however it was decided not to disturb the area as further attempts to remove the screw could cause further damage and fracture of the root and core.

continued on the next page

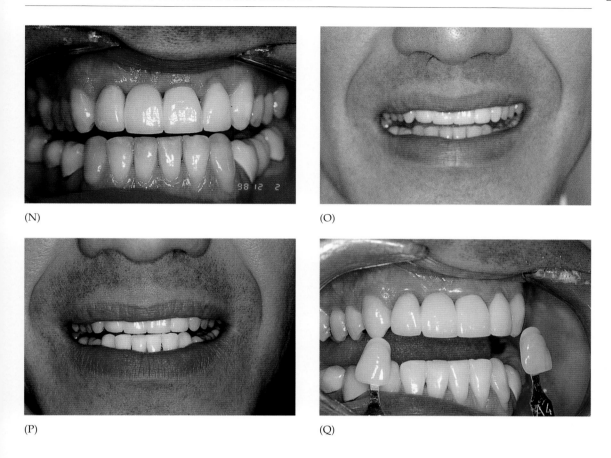

(N)

(O)

(P)

(Q)

Figure 11.1 continued

(N) The appearance of the bridge and porcelain laminate veneer once cemented. Symmetry of length, size and shape of the teeth was created. The canine teeth are now in harmony with the other teeth. The interdental contact points on the two central incisor teeth was taken much higher to reduce the size of the dark triangular space. The margin of the porcelain veneer was left supragingival due to the thin anatomic nature of the gingiva in this area and its tendency to recede. (O) Portrait of the patient after definitive treatment. It is evident that the lower teeth need to be bleached. (P) The patient's smile after bleaching the lower incisor teeth. It may now appear that the lower incisor teeth are lighter than the upper teeth. This photo was taken immediately after completing the bleaching treatment. There is normally a settling down period immediately after the bleaching treatment where there will be a slight shift of one shade so the light colour difference is not a problem. It can be argued that the upper and lower teeth should have been bleached simultaneously, but that does not give a colour control. In this case the patient with his heavy work schedule chose to do further bleaching of the lower teeth in this sequence. (Q) There has been a shade shift from the existing shade of A4 to A1 on the Vita Shade guide. It may be noticeable that the canine teeth are not uniformly white. Due to the large amount of recession on the canine teeth, the patient was advised to only apply the bleaching material on the tips of these teeth. Some patients are concerned that they can see a demarcation line on the lower canine teeth, but they need to be reassured that bleaching will eventually be more even as it penetrates further into the dentine to modify the dentine shades. Bleaching of the lower teeth is normally slower than the upper teeth. However, this is not noticeable when the patient smiles and the patient is delighted with the final result.

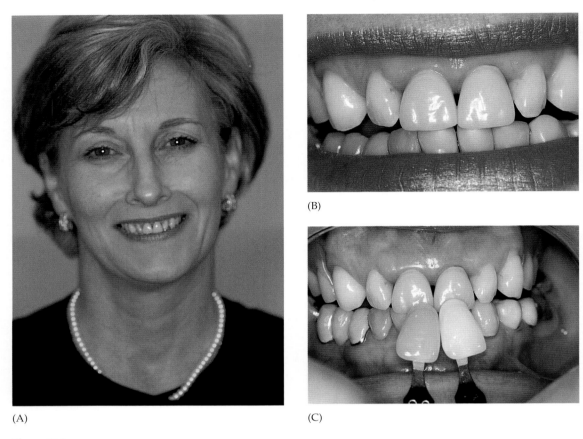

(A)   (C)

(B)

Figure 11.2

A patient who needed extensive restorative dentistry. She has missing upper posterior teeth. Her existing crowns, which are poorly contoured, were made over various occasions and have different colours. The endodontic treatment involves making new cores for all the crowns, re-establishing the occlusal vertical dimension, placing long-term provisional crowns, a bilateral sinus lift procedure and bone grafting to provide adequate bone in the posterior maxilla and placement of titanium fixtures. Following a 6-month healing phase, definitive treatment will be undertaken. It is estimated that treatment will take about two years to complete. In the meantime the upper lateral and canine teeth were bleached using the home bleaching technique. This resulted in a much lighter shade for these teeth. New provisional restorations could be built to the new colour of the natural teeth. The lighter colour of her natural teeth and lighter provisional restorations boosted the patient's self-confidence so that she could be motivated to complete the rest of the extensive treatment. (A) Portrait of patient before treatment. An indication as to whether the patient can have lighter teeth and whether bleaching will be successful is to assess the colour of the patient's white of the eye contrasting with the colour of the teeth. If the natural tooth colour is darker than the white of the eye, bleaching can be successful. (B) The colour of the teeth after bleaching. The existing crowns are poorly fitting and show a dark triangular space between the central incisors. (C) Shows the contrast of the shade before bleaching with the shade after bleaching using the porcelain shade tabs as a guide.

continued on the next page

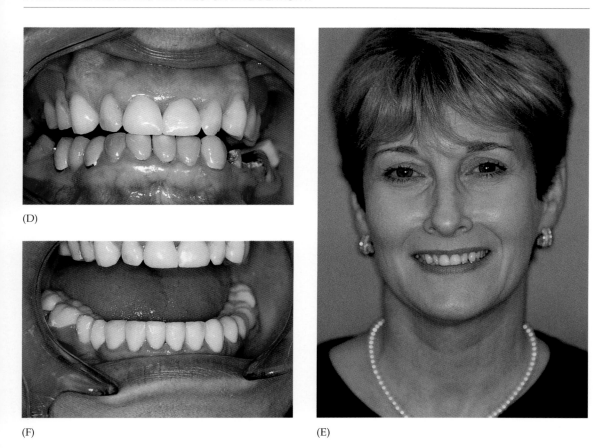

(D)

(F)   (E)

Figure 11.2 continued

(D) The crowns on the central incisors were replaced with provisional ones made from metal and composite resin. These crowns would be durable enough to last until completion of the rest of the treatment. The metal substructure ensured excellent fit and the composite resin gave the teeth a natural appearance. The interdental contacts were moved higher up the tooth to reduce the triangular space. The crowns were shortened and rounded to give a better harmony with the rest of the natural teeth. Further adjustments to the final shape of the definitive crowns will be done to get an even better alignment particularly around the interdental contacts and the line angles related to the lateral incisor teeth. As the patient has a high lip-line it is essential to ensure excellent aesthetics. (E) Portrait of the patient after bleaching treatment. Patient has the long-term provisional restorations in place. The occlusal vertical dimension has been re-established. This was achieved by opening the bite to ensure there is sufficient vertical height posteriorly to provide space to place the implants. The marginal inflammation associated with the previous crowns has resolved and further healing is expected. (F) The lower provisional crowns immediately after cementation in the mouth: the new lower incisor teeth are better aligned than the previous ones as a result of opening the vertical dimension. The teeth on the partial denture were added to on the occlusal surface, to improve the interdigitation with the lower provisional restorations.

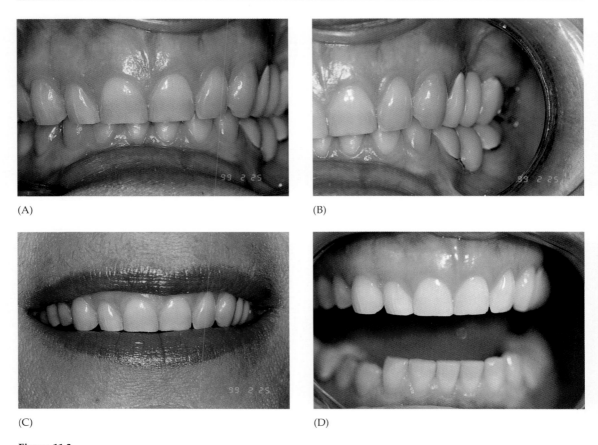

(A)

(B)

(C)

(D)

Figure 11.3

This patient had age-yellowed teeth. She went on to have an oseointegrated implant placed, bone augmentation and two crowns of porcelain bonded to metal. She had healthy anterior teeth which had discoloured from drinking coffee and tea. The teeth were bleached using the power bleach system on the maxillary and mandibular teeth over two sessions. The patient continued with home bleaching trays for 2 weeks on the upper teeth and 3 weeks on the lower teeth. The upper teeth were bleached first to have a colour control. At the end of treatment the upper teeth matched the shade of the old bridge which had been in place for 20 years. However the old bridge had deteriorated and decay was present distally. Porcelain had chipped off the occlusal surface over the years. The patient was concerned with the bony concavity that had developed in the edentulous space where a tooth had been extracted. It was decided to remove the existing bridge, place a provisional bridge while the patient had a bone augmentation procedure followed by an implant to maintain the bone in this area. (A) Appearance of the teeth prior to bleaching treatment. (B) Shows the discrepancy in colour between the canine tooth and the existing bridge. The bony concavity in the pontic area is of concern to the patient. (C) The patient has developed a smile to avoid the bony concavity where the second premolar should be. (D) After bleaching of the upper teeth: note the difference in the shade between the upper and lower teeth.

continued on the next page

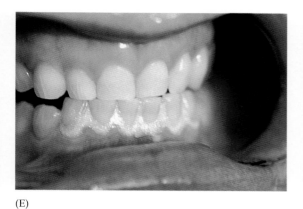

(E)

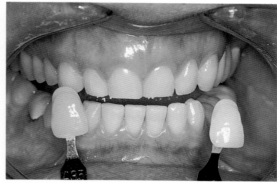

(F)

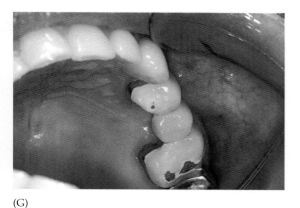

(G)

Figure 11.3 continued

(E) The lower teeth were bleached using the in-office technique. The teeth were isolated using the light-cured gingival protectant. The power gel consisting of 35% hydrogen peroxide was placed on to the teeth for three 10-minute sessions to lighten the teeth. (F) Successful lightening has been achieved of both the upper and lower teeth. The lighter shade matches the upper bridge which is twenty years old. (G) The occlusal surface of the upper bridge. The porcelain has worn through and the underlying metal is exposed. (H) The bony concavity when the flap is raised. (I) The flap is repositioned after the implant fixture is placed and bone is augmented around the defect. (Surgeon, Dr Oded Bahat.)

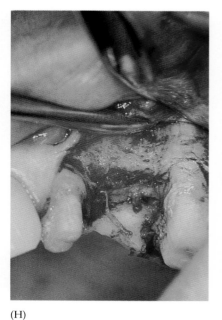

(H)

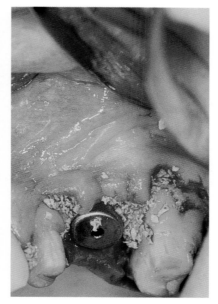

(I)

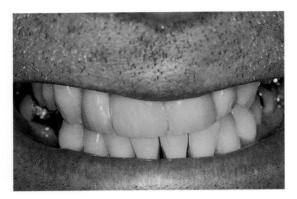

(A)

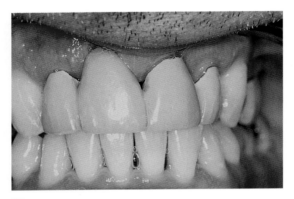

(B)

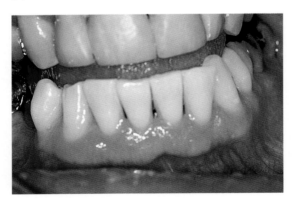

(C)

Figure 11.4

This patient had periodontal problems and was undergoing a course of periodontal treatment. There was severe bone loss around the two central incisors such that the upper right central incisor became so loose that it had to be extracted. An immediate fixed temporary bridge was placed while a metal composite provisional bridge was made in the laboratory. After periodontal healing and during the maintenance phase of his treatment the patient expressed a desire to have the lower incisor teeth lightened. An impression was taken to make a home bleaching tray for the lower teeth. The tray was fitted and checked and the patient given the bleaching material to take home. Successful bleaching treatment was achieved using the home bleach technique. The patient had previously been a smoker but had given up smoking 1 month before the tooth was extracted. The provisional bridge was an adequate match before bleaching treatment. After bleaching treatment it became evident that there had been lightening of the lower teeth and the colour of the provisional bridge did not match. The provisional bridge was to be used for a further period of stability while the pontic area healed and the bridge was extensively reshaped in this area. Definitive treatment will only commence once excellent healing of the periodontium has been achieved and the periodontal disease stabilized. (A) The patient has a low lip-line. (B) The provisional bridge before bleaching treatment was undertaken for the lower teeth. Extensive bone loss in the area shows that the pontic had to be shaped much longer in the vertical bone defect. (C) The appearance of the teeth after home bleaching treatment on the lower teeth: note the contrast in colours of the upper bridge to the new lower incisors.

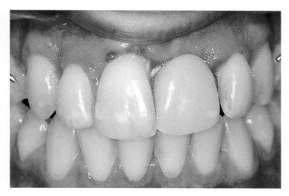

(A)

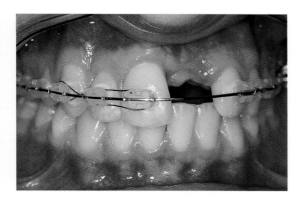

(B)

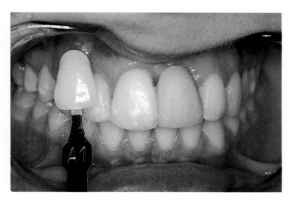

(C)

Figure 11.5

This young girl, who had recently completed a course of orthodontic treatment, was involved in a motor vehicle accident and lost her upper left central incisor. She had sustained head and facial injuries and fractures of her maxilla and nose. (A) A provisional partial denture was fitted. It became obvious that the fracture of the maxilla had altered the alignment of the anterior teeth and the edentulous space. The patient had to undergo further orthodontic treatment to realign the anterior teeth and reduce the width of the edentulous space and so to improve the symmetry of the central incisors. The partial denture was used during the orthodontic treatment so that the acrylic tooth could be adjusted to correct the midline. (Orthodontist, Dr Brian Miller.) (B) During orthodontic alignment the edentulous space was measured to assess whether sufficient space had been reduced and whether the anterior posterior alignment had corrected. The Golden Proportion gauge was used to assess the teeth were achieving the correct proportions (see Figure 4.10). (C) After orthodontic treatment an adhesive bridge was fitted in this area. During this maintenance phase where the bridge acted as a retainer, the patient expressed a concern that the teeth appeared yellow and requested that the teeth be bleached. An impression was taken and a home bleach tray was made. The patient bleached every night for 2 weeks and achieved a colour change from shade A3.5 to A1. The adhesive bridge which originally matched the other teeth now appeared yellow.

continued on the next page

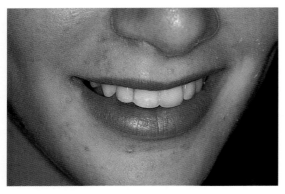

(D)

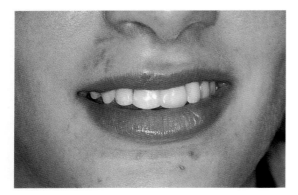

(E)

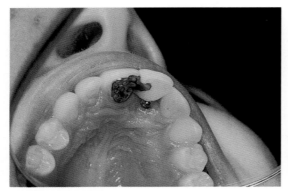

(F)

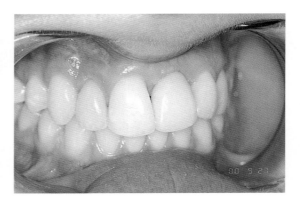

(G)

Figure 11.5 continued

(D) The adhesive bridge was removed and sent to the laboratory to have the porcelain stripped and replaced with a new lighter shade. The patient's smile after the bridge was refitted shows the new lighter shade of porcelain. (E) The patient has also had microabrasion to remove some of the white spots on the central and lateral incisor teeth. (F) Mirror view. Titanium implant has now been placed into the edentulous space to reduce further bone loss while the adhesive bridge had been adjusted palatally to accommodate the fixture. She is now in the healing phase while the implant integrates. (G) Provisional composite metal crown, which will remain in place for 3 years, prior to placing definitive (porcelain bonded to metal) crown: since the patient is in her late teens, one must allow time for further maturation of the gingiva.

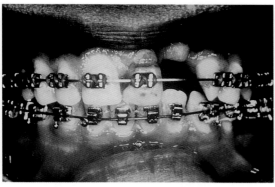

(A)

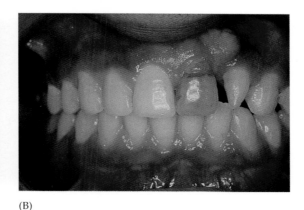

(B)

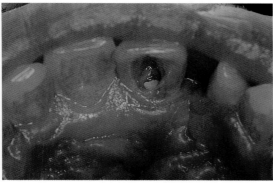

(C)

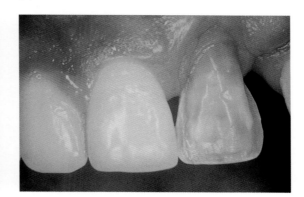

(D)

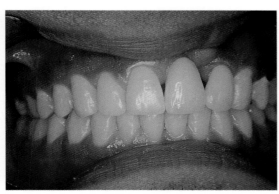

(E)

Figure 11.6

This patient presents with a cleft palate and lip which had been repaired. A non-vital discoloured central incisor was adjacent to a peg-shaped lateral incisor. Treatment included orthodontic treatment to align the teeth and midline, endodontic treatment, bleaching treatment using the inside/outside technique. (Courtesy of Dr Martin Kelleher.) (A) shows the patient with fixed banding during orthodontic treatment. The teeth were realigned to correct the midline discrepancies. (B) The appearance of the teeth following completion of the orthodontic treatment prior to commencing bleaching treatment. (C) Following successful endodontic treatment, the access cavity was cleaned. The gutta-percha was removed to below the cemento-enamel junction. A glass ionomer barrier was placed to seal the gutta-percha from the bleaching material. (D) Two months following successful bleaching treatment, where the tooth had lightened considerably, porcelain veneers were prepared for the central and lateral incisors to close the diastema between these teeth and to improve the proportions of these two teeth. (E) The veneer on the central incisor was prepared supragingivally as the patient had a low lipline.

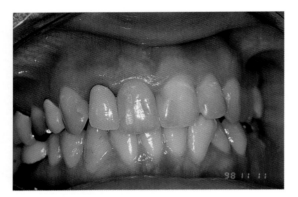

(A)

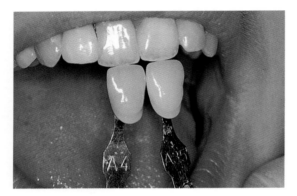

(B)

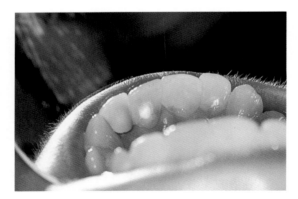

(C)

Figure 11.7

Shows the difficulty which can arise in shade selection for porcelain crowns following bleaching treatment. (A) This patient had discoloration of her upper anterior teeth. There were multiple colours of the teeth which gave an unaesthetic appearance. The upper central incisor was non-vital and needed to have endodontic treatment. The crown on the upper right premolar was ill-fitting. The crown on the upper first molar was ill-fitting. There were multiple areas around the previous root treatment. The gold onlay was leaking around the margins and the amalgam core had stained the enamel. (B) A provisional crown was made for the upper right lateral incisor as the patient did not wish to continue with the existing crown. This provisional restoration was used during the bleaching treatment and for 1 month afterwards once the shade had settled. Selecting the shade of the existing teeth was difficult as the teeth had different colours. The different colours are recorded on the bleaching record sheet. (C) The access cavity was left with a temporary filling for a period of four weeks while endodontic healing took place. After this time a barrier was placed and bleaching treatment was undertaken using the inside/outside technique for this tooth.

continued on the next page

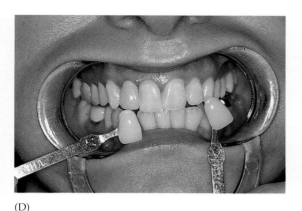

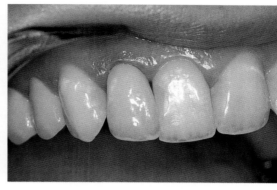

(D)   (E)

Figure 11.7 continued

(D) The appearance of the teeth after 2 weeks of bleaching. The access cavity was closed after 2 days of the inside/outside bleaching. There is now a discrepancy in the shade of the provisional restoration. It now appears too yellow. The patient has a high lip line which is a difficulty for margin placement. Her gingivae are thin which can lead to further recession. (E) The Procera crown tried on to the lateral tooth. This crown appeared a little grey in comparison to the lateral and central incisor which both have different colours. The composite on the central incisor should be replaced as it is much darker than the new bleached shade. The posterior teeth were restored with new porcelain bonded to metal crowns. Shade management of these crowns was also difficult, but it was not as crucial because of the posterior location. These restorations were fixed with temporary cement during 6 months to let the shade of the bleached teeth settle before eventual modification of the final shade. The anterior restoration was cemented on to the tooth with trial cement for 6 months to assess whether there would be a further shade shift following bleaching treatment.

12

COMBINING BLEACHING WITH DIRECT COMPOSITE RESIN RESTORATIONS

Valeria V Gordan

INTRODUCTION

Discoloured anterior teeth may be treated with porcelain veneers, all-ceramic crowns or PFM (porcelain-fused-to-metal) restorations to restore aesthetics. These treatment alternatives may be indicated when patients require and desire realignment or reshaping of the teeth. However, it is a legitimate concern that some patients may receive extensive, irreversible treatment when correcting minor discrepancies. Non-invasive bleaching or tooth whitening may be a more attractive alternative to treat discoloured teeth.

The conservation of tooth structure allied with quality and life-long management of the teeth should be the main goal when correcting tooth colour. Today, with adhesive technology and bleaching regimens it is possible to provide conservative approaches for treatment of stained, mis-shaped and mal-positioned teeth.

Enamel and dentine bonding systems have gradually been improved and have a higher level of consistency than previously. In addition, more reliable results have been obtained when bonding different substrates to tooth structure. The techniques are also becoming simpler and more user-friendly.

An approach involving a combination of bleaching and composite resin restoration is more conservative and less expensive than treatment with porcelain laminates or crowns. Composite restorations may also be repaired or replaced with minimal difficulty and little loss of tooth structure.

This chapter will describe the importance of understanding patients' expectations, shade selection, techniques to bond to bleached teeth, the achievement of optimal aesthetics by combining bleaching with composite resin restorations, and maintenance of the combined treatment.

ESTABLISHING A GOOD START

After a treatment plan (see Chapter 4) has been established, including full mouth radiographs, scaling and polishing, periodontal screening, oral hygiene instructions, oral and medical history review, temporo-mandibular joint and occlusal examination, study models should then be prepared and a tooth shade examination should be performed. It is important to decide if any change in shade of teeth is to be performed before any final treatment plan is given to the patient. This will avoid future replacement of restorations saving both clinician's and patient's time and also prevent wrong assessment and false expectations about the completion of the treatment.

Patients should be informed that the bleaching will change the colour of the tooth structure only. This may pose a problem if the patient has several composite or porcelain restorations. Furthermore, the replacement of such restorations should be a consideration prior to bleaching treatment.

The shade examination should be done with the patient sitting in an upright position, with the light of the dental unit turned off. If colour corrected fluorescent light is not available in the office, the patient should be brought close to a natural light source, e.g. a window. However, with today's lifestyle it is common for many people to stay inside with artificial light source most of the time.

Surrounding colours cause distractions, therefore remove any lipstick or other external factors. One alternative is to have a small piece of neutral grey cardboard with a cut-out window in the centre of approximately the size of a maxillary central incisor. This device helps to eliminate any colour interference when the shade is being taken.

After the tooth shade has been established, a decision must be made as to whether the discoloration or change in colour can be corrected with vital or non-vital bleaching. The advantage of home bleaching before the placement of composite resin restorations is that it enables the practitioner to have a relative control over the colour of the teeth. If tooth reduction is necessary for restoration adjustment, the underlying dentine shade may be less noticeable and more easily covered after bleaching.

BONDING TO BLEACHED TEETH

After the bleaching is done, shade matching may be a challenge because both vital and non-vital bleaching may leave a somewhat opaque shade. Even though an increase in shade value may occur, it will not be enough to cover white spots caused by demineralization or fluorosis. Enamelplasty or microabrasion (see Chapter 10) may sometimes be the best treatment option for improved results with white spots or bands caused by demineralization (Figure 12.1).

It is important to bear in mind that the bleaching can produce a lighter shade than that of the colour guide provided by most manufacturers, and thus create a problem if composite or porcelain restorations are to be placed. The recommendation is to monitor patients on a weekly basis to prevent teeth becoming bleached to an extent that makes their colour difficult to match for restorative therapy.

Placement of restorations should be delayed for at least 24 hours after completion of the bleaching (Titley et al 1992, Dishman et al 1994). Ideally, it should be postponed for 1 week after the bleaching treatment (Torneck et al 1991, McGuckin et al 1992, Miles et al 1994). Several studies have shown a decrease in bond strength for teeth bonded immediately after bleaching (Titley et al 1988, Titley et al 1992, Stokes et al 1992, Garcia-Godoy et al 1993, Dishman et al 1994, Ben-Amar et al 1995). Bond strength results are not related to morphological or chemical changes in the enamel (Ruse et al 1990), although studies have shown shorter and less defined resin tags in bleached enamel when compared to unbleached enamel (Titley et al 1991). This may be related to the fact that hydrogen peroxide, a by-product of the carbamide peroxide bleaching reaction, releases oxygen which will not be completely removed from the enamel immediately after the bleaching treatment is finished. Hydrogen peroxide and oxygen are soluble in water and can readily reach the dentinal fluid through enamel and be released later through surface diffusion (Torneck et al 1990). The remaining oxygen can be a barrier for the bonding process, by forming an oxygen inhibition layer. Such interference with the polymerization of resin bonding systems is crucial. Optimal results cannot be achieved in the presence of oxygen during curing (Kalili et al 1991, McGuckin et al 1992, Titley et al 1992). Some studies have shown that the use of acetone or ethanol solution or acetone-based adhesive system can prevent the adverse effects of bleaching on enamel bond strengths (Kalili et al 1993, Barghi and Godwin 1994). These volatile chemicals will prevent the presence of oxygen in the immediate vicinity of polymerization. Delaying bonding procedures is also important to compensate for the possible shade relapse after the bleaching treatment is completed. Bleached teeth may become slightly darker after the first week following the treatment (Haywood 1996).

DIRECT RESIN VENEER AND RESHAPING

Many patients expect superior aesthetics from restorations placed in anterior teeth. An aesthetic restorative material must simulate the appearance of the tooth in colour, translucency, texture, shape and still present adequate strength and wear characteristics, good marginal adaptation, sealing, insolubility, and biocompatibility (Lambrechts et al 1990).

Direct composite resin veneers offer several advantages over ceramic veneers. They can be placed in only one session without laboratory involvement consequently featuring reduced cost. The elimination of laboratory involvement also favours an easier colour matching with the adjacent teeth, especially as compared to single ceramic restorations. It is possible to achieve an overall evaluation of the results if a mock-up of the composite resin shape and colour is done prior to the placement of the restoration. However, the conservation of tooth structure is the major advantage of direct composite resin restorations, in some cases little or no enamel removal is required.

In order to match the colour of adjacent teeth properly, tints and opaquers may be applied to simulate natural colour and stain. A colour map should be established before the restoration placement including the mapping of all the different stains, shade variations, craze lines, and other details (Figure 12.2). The colour mapping should follow the same guidelines as for shade selection before the teeth are dehydrated. It should be kept in mind that not only colour, but also texture, shape and contour are necessary for a successful reproduction and characterization of teeth.

The degree of tooth roughness can be appreciated when the light is reflected and deflected from its surfaces. Anatomic grooves, facets and prominences play an important role in this context (Figure 12.3). Smooth glossy surfaces enhance the appearance of restorations and may also mimic that of enamel.

DIASTEMA CLOSURE

Multiple maxillary diastemas can pose a difficult aesthetic management problem, especially in adult patients (Figure 12.4). In patients with irregular spaces between maxillary anterior teeth owing to tooth-size/alveolar bone discrepancies, composite resin restorations may be used as a conservative technique for the correction of minor alignment of teeth with improvement in tooth size and shape. If a change in shade is desired, bleaching should be completed prior to restoration.

Composite resin restorations are classified according to the filler particle in hybrid and microfill. Hybrid composites contain more than one type of filler particle. These particles typically consist of a glass in the 0.6–3 μm range and 0.04 μm particles of silica. Hybrids are stronger than microfill composites and they are less likely to fracture in high stress areas. They are the prime choice for core dentine build-up. Microfill composites, however, have a small particle size, in the range of 0.01 μm. This particular characteristic allows the materials to be polished easily to a high gloss. They are the most aesthetic direct enamel replacement material. In addition, they have a higher percentage of unfilled resin, and lower volume percentage of filler. These features make the microfill composites more elastic (low Young's modulus) than hybrids. Microfill composites are particularly recommended for Class V abfraction type of restorations because they are less likely to be dislodged from the cavity preparation if the tooth is under occlusal stress. They are also the best option for veneering of restorations.

For small diastemas, microfill composite resin alone can be used (Figure 12.5). If the diastema exceeds 2 mm, a combination of hybrid and microfills must be used for proper strength and aesthetics of the restoration.

When diastema closure is performed, occlusal relationships, as well as overall facial aesthetics, must be considered. The 'golden rule proportion' (Levin 1978) or the 'harmony law of proportion' (Williams 1914) must be applied for optimal aesthetics results to be achieved. Golden Proportion is an old rule that was formulated by early Greek philosophers as a numerical value (1.618 : 1) used in aesthetic appraisal and is explained in Chapter 4. As developed by Levin, aesthetically pleasing dentitions viewed from the front show the width of the incisors and anterior canine to be in golden proportion. Also dental, dento-facial and facial compositions have a variety of relationships that can be evaluated by this proportion. It is the proportion or ratio of these dimensions that produce harmony rather than the absolute size of any particular feature.

When anterior teeth are widened, it may also be necessary to lengthen them to preserve natural anatomic proportions. If the occlusal relationship allows tooth lengthening, this can be established by adding composite to the incisal edge.

Pleasing proportions of the central incisors are expressed in a width-to-length ratio of approximately 75 to 80 (Figure 12.6). Short square incisors are inappropriate because their width-to-length ratio exceeds 85 (Figures 12.7 and 12.8). They can be corrected by elongation through surgical procedure or by increasing the incisal crown length as long as it does not interfere with the occlusion. Conversely, a width-to-length ratio lower than 70 could lead to incisors that are unpleasantly long (Figure 12.9).

A diastema between the maxillary central incisors is the most frequently encountered space to which patients object. A gap of 2 mm or more is difficult to close without making the teeth look abnormally large, and there is also grave danger of compressing the interdental papilla. It is advisable to construct a mock-up in the mouth of the patient for a good prognosis.

The composite should be built to slightly oversized proportions and then finished to the proper contour. An overlap is not so critical in this situation, as long as it has been properly shaped. If the area has been properly etched and bonded, the overlap can actually be an advantage because it can increase the area of bonding to enamel, thereby increasing the composite resin bond strength and decreasing the possibility of leakage. The overlap can also disguise the line of bonding, producing a better transition from the tooth structure to the restorative material.

The restoration should follow the average dimensional values for mesio-distal width. For example, a reduction of the mesio-distal width is a sign of ageing (Lammie and Posselt 1965). It is also race and sex dependent. The inciso-gingival height is less critical than mesio-distal width, and it is dependent on the vertical dimension and free space for phonetics and function.

Contact points are important for the re-establishment of a natural smile. In the anterior segment the contacts are situated from the incisal towards the cervical and from the central incisors toward the canines. The contact between the central incisors is at the incisal angle. The lip, incisal and contact lines are related and should be maintained in harmony. The anatomy of the contact point is influenced by the morphology, width and arrangement of the teeth. The absence of a contact point produces an absence of a col. The gingival embrasures help to shape the col. The interdental gingiva largely follows the shape of the bone. This shape varies dependent on location: in the anterior area it is convex, producing a pyramidal shape, and it becomes more flat in the posterior area.

ART OF ILLUSION

When there is insufficient space for correction of shape, contour and position of teeth, optical illusions of size and shape can be created to solve or hide an aesthetic problem. Visual perception is possible only if objects contrast in colour and shape. The perception of the contour of objects depends on the deflection or reflection of the light that reaches them because the surface form of these objects is responsible for light reflection. The control of light reflections and colour contrast will create an illusion and re-establish proportions (Rufenacht 1990).

Illusion works on the following principles: increased contrast and light reflection increases visibility, whereas increased light deflection diminishes visibility. These principles are better explained by observing the following points: shadows create depth, light creates prominences, vertical lines accent length, and horizontal lines accentuate width (Chiche and Pinault 1994). Another technique can be used when trying to match a recontoured tooth to its adjacent natural tooth: the visible contours are divided into sections that include the facial surfaces and the labial aspects of the mesial and distal surfaces (Chiche and Pinault 1994). These sections are separated by the mesial and distal line angles, which should be outlined in pencil.

Improvement in tooth contour should not be made at the expense of periodontal health. For example, vertical correction should be undertaken with great care since encroachment upon the interocclusal space may cause damage to the dentition. Orthodontic consultation should always be sought before attempting to correct gross changes in shape and position.

MAINTENANCE OF THE COMBINED TREATMENT

Using the existing composite technology, with excellent materials strength and shade selection, it is possible to create enamel-like and life-like restorations. Paying attention to essential elements such as cavity preparation, rubber dam isolation, correct understanding of the tooth substrate, bonding agents and composite resin material, proper case selection, and maximal finishing and polishing will lead to good, long-term clinical results. Both patients and dentists must participate in this process.

The success of any restoration depends on patient compliance. It is important that the patient be educated after a restoration has been placed. Maintenance is a part of this education process followed by explanations of the aetiology of caries and preventive measures.

Manufacturers' instructions should be followed in every case. Even though they are similar for most materials, some companies have different technology, which could affect the final results if some details are not followed.

Adequate case selection is important for maximal results and preservation of the restorations which should be matched according to the different properties of the composite resins. The use of a hybrid composite resin for stress bearing areas is required for optimal strength. Veneering with a microfill material will provide smooth, glossy restorations.

Composite resin adaptation is also important. Attaching the composite properly to the tooth surface will avoid air bubbles incorporation and prevent future staining (Figure 12.10). The handling of the composite resin should be done in as few steps as possible. Two points should be observed to avoid air bubbles being incorporated into the restoration. When removing the composite from the syringe it is preferable to slice it instead of smearing it (Figure 12.11). For direct veneers that do not require more than 1.5 mm in thickness, ideally the material should be placed in only one piece on to the tooth surface. Incremental placement of the composite is prone to provide air bubbles.

The use of spatulas and soft bristle brushes is indicated for proper attachment, smooth transition, anatomical shaping, and good texture of the restoration (Figure 12.12).

Light curing the composite is probably one of the most critical steps. The output of the curing lights should be checked regularly with a radiometer. The light tip and filters should be systematically cleaned.

Finishing is the second most critical step. A smooth finishing is expected to improve the life-time of the restoration. The use of aluminium oxide finishing disks of 3–60 μm particle size (Figure 12.13) and the use of silicon dioxide and diamond acrylic rubber polishing points and cups of 4–30 μm particle size with felt disks (Figure 12.14) are recommended. Aluminium oxide polishing paste of 1 μm particle size with felt disks (Figure 12.15) provide a highly polished, glossy surface.

The application of surface penetrating sealant or adhesive after the restoration is completed can promote a better seal of the restoration, decreasing the risk for marginal staining and leakage. Both restoration and tooth surface should be acid-etched before the sealing procedure.

For professional oral hygiene of Class V type of restorations, or restorations that are close to the cemento-enamel junction, curettes are preferred over ultrasonic scalers which have a great potential to damage composite materials. Air-abrasive units and regular prophylaxis pastes can scratch the composite surface and make them prone to further stain accumulation. Following professional cleaning, polishing pastes of aluminium oxide base and small particle size should be used in areas of composite resin restorations.

One of the goals of maintenance treatment is to make sure that the patient understands the limitations of the restorative material and what he or she can do to increase the life-time of the restoration. Oral and written instructions are recommended for this phase of the treatment.

The use of mouth-rinses that contain alcohol (ethanol) in their composition should be avoided. Ethanol plasticizes the matrix of the composite resin accelerating its wear rate. Some commercial chlorhexidine solutions, besides containing alcohol in their composition, also have a great potential to stain teeth and composite resin restorations (Nathoo and Gaffar 1994). If it is established that the use of chlorhexidine is necessary, it should be a part of the treatment plan and it must be used before any bleaching or tooth coloured restorations are placed.

It is recommended to refrain from using fluoride containing rinse or gel with a 3–5 pH value. If topical fluoride treatment is indicated, neutral sodium fluoride is the choice for patients with aesthetic restorations. The low pH of acidulated or stannous types of fluoride can etch, erode or stain composite resin materials.

Patients should be recommended to use a soft toothbrush and non-abrasive toothpastes. Some types of whitening toothpaste can have large particle size and roughen the restoration surface (see also Chapter 3).

Non-coloured toothpaste and mouth-rinse should be used whenever possible to avoid long-term staining. Tobacco, coffee, tea, soft drinks, wine, berries can stain the tooth surface (Vogel 1975) and particularly the restoration. Patients should be advised about staining from these agents and they should be urged to decrease the frequency of intake if possible. The oral education allied with improved aesthetic result work as high motivation factors for a change in attitude of tobacco users and other damaging oral habits.

For minor relapse in the colour of the teeth after the treatment is completed, new impressions and bleaching trays can be manufactured and a 'touch-up' of the shade may be done with home-bleaching technique. This 'touch-up' treatment only takes 3–4 days to achieve the desired result. Maximum treatment should be 7–10 days.

CASE REPORT 1

A 19-year-old woman was referred for PFM restorations for correction of discoloration and slight rotation of maxillary central incisors. The patient had significant loss of tooth structure because of a physical trauma. The teeth had also received root canal treatment (Figure 12.16A). Both teeth presented slight discoloration of the composite restorations and some intrinsic staining. Adjacent teeth also had moderate extrinsic staining (Figure 12.16B). Maxillary lateral incisors presented with mesio-labial version.

CLINICAL PROCEDURE

A conservative approach involving a combination of bleaching and direct composite resin restorations was explained to the patient. The conservation of tooth structure was appealing to the patient who immediately agreed to the new treatment plan. The initial treatment involved a home bleaching technique with carbamide peroxide.

After cleaning the teeth with fine pumice and rubber cup, an alginate impression was made of the maxillary and mandibular arches and poured-in dental stone. A light-cured spacer (LC Block-out resin, Ultradent Products, Inc, South Jordan, UT) was painted on the facial surfaces of the casts of all anterior teeth to provide space for the bleaching agent. Custom bleaching trays were vacuum-formed with 2-mm soft vinyl mouthguard material. The trays were trimmed to the gingival margin to minimize soft tissue contact with the bleaching gel. A high viscosity, 10% carbamide peroxide bleaching gel (Opalescence, Ultradent Products, Inc, South Jordan, UT) was selected for this case to ensure retention of the gel inside the tray. The patient was instructed to apply the bleaching gel using the soft vinyl trays for 8 hours daily. The home bleaching regimen was followed for 3 weeks. The patient came for a control examination every week.

The vital bleaching technique eliminated the external discoloration from the teeth. The colour of the teeth changed from shade D-3 (Vita Shade Guide, Lumin® Vacuum-Farbskala, Vita Zahnfabrik, Bad Säckingen, Germany) to a final shade of B-1. Maxillary central incisors remained as C-3 shade (Figure 12.16C).

A non-vital intrinsic bleaching technique with 35% hydrogen peroxide was used on both maxillary central incisors. The teeth were isolated with rubber dam. Vaseline and dental floss were tied around the teeth to ensure proper isolation. The access to the root canal was obtained (Figure 12.16D). A glass ionomer base (Vitrabond, 3M Dental Products Division, St Paul, MN) approximately 2-mm thick was used to cover the gutta-percha (Heymann et al 1994). A paste of 35% hydrogen peroxide and sodium perborate (Superoxol, Sultan Chemist, Englewood, NJ) was mixed and applied inside the pulp chamber (Figure 12.16E). A glass syringe with hydrogen peroxide was used to rinse the paste which was reapplied four times. At the last application, the paste was left inside the coronal part of the teeth and temporary restorations were placed. The patient returned after 5 days and the procedure was repeated. Following the second 5-day treatment an improvement could be observed. The two maxillary central incisors were shade B-1 (Figure 12.16F).

SHADE SELECTION OF TEETH AND RESTORATION

The shade of patient's teeth was established and ready to receive the final restorations. A shade map was drawn before the teeth were isolated, for proper shade characterization. The detailed colour map included mainly the location of minor white spots, extent of the enamel translucency, and cervical opacity (Figure 12.2). Lateral incisors were used as a reference guide for the colour mapping. Morphological and optical characteristics were collected and recorded. Primary and secondary anatomy were projected, and the form of the lobes, depth and length of the developmental grooves, and surface texture were planned. Even though the shape and positioning of maxillary lateral incisors could be improved, the patient did not wish to change the shape and contour of these teeth.

Tooth contour was determined according to the appropriate proximal and occlusal space

and a width-to-length ratio of 80 was chosen. Colour shade selection was done. It is mandatory that the colour shade selection be performed before isolation as tooth dehydration may result in an elevated value and lead to an incorrect shade selection.

The colour was selected according to the three dimensions of colour. The selection of the enamel substitute, a microfilled composite resin (Durafill, shade B-1, Heraeus-Kulzer, Wehrheim, Germany), was made by applying a small increment of the selected shade into the facial surface of the teeth and close to the adjacent teeth surfaces. After polymerization, the resin was moistened with the patient's own saliva to simulate the final result. It is important to polymerize the resin at this stage because microfilled composites are usually of lower value and higher chroma prior to polymerization.

The dentine core shade was chosen by using one chroma shade higher than the enamel shade. Because the dentine substitute material was the core of the restoration, a hybrid composite resin (Herculite, B-2 shade, Kerr Corporation, West Collins Orange, CA) was chosen for appropriate strength of the restoration. The incisal shade was also chosen (Herculite, Light Incisal shade, Kerr Corporation, West Collins Orange, CA).

The old composite resin restoration was removed with a high speed drill under an abundant water spray. Facial and lingual bevels were placed with a medium grit diamond stone at slow speed (Figure 12.16G). Isolation was accomplished with cheek and lip retractors (Expandex, Henry Schein Inc, Port Washington, NY) in conjunction with cotton rolls and gauze.

After etching with 35% phosphoric acid, a bonding agent was applied following the manufacturer's instructions (Scotchbond Multi-Purpose, 3M Dental Products Division, St. Paul, MN). The hybrid composite was applied in increments no thicker than 2.0 mm. Each increment was polymerised for 20 seconds with a visible light-curing unit (Optilux 401, Demetron a Division of Kerr Corporation, Danbury, CT). Mamelons were created and shaped with spatulas (Figure 12.16H). (An alternative to the use of spatulas is to build-up a large incisal edge and cut it back to simulate the shape of mamelons. However, after the reduction of the composite, the bonding agent must be re-applied.) The artificial dentine and mamelons must be slightly feathered at the facial and lingual surfaces to allow a transitional blending of the artificial enamel.

It is important to leave appropriate space for the enamel part. Ideally, no reduction of the dentine core should be done after light polymerization. The oxygen-inhibited layer that is left after resin polymerization can be used for application of the artificial enamel. If a reduction of the dentine core is required, the bonding agent should be reapplied, including the etchant and adhesive application.

A translucent hybrid composite incisal shade (Herculite XRV light incisal shade, Kerr Corporation, West Collins Orange, CA) was applied, covering the space between the mamelons and overlapping the artificial dentine for a good colour transition (Figure 12.16I).

After the polymerization of the incisal hybrid resin, a microfill composite resin (Durafill B-1 shade, Heraeus-Kulzer, Inc., Wehrheim, Germany) was used to veneer the underlying dentine frame of the restoration. Spatulas were used (Gold-microfill instrument, Almore International Inc, Portland, OR) to create proper contour, and soft sable brushes were used for blending of the microfill into the hybrid and the tooth surfaces. Before the finishing of the restoration, proper polymerization was accomplished, followed by examination of the surfaces. Detailed examination is recommended to determine if sufficient material is present on the facial and lingual surfaces and at the line angles of the restoration.

It is important to finish one of the restorations completely before starting the other. This will avoid bonding the restorations together. Initial finishing was accomplished with aluminium oxide disks (Sof-Lex XT, 3M Dental Products Division, St Paul, MN) observing morphology, width-to-length ratio and embrasure forms. After the primary anatomy was created, the excess of the material was removed from the cervical margins and line angles with a scalpel blade (No. 12 or 12b, Becton Dickinson, Franklin

Lakes, NJ). The interproximal areas were finished and polished with different grades of aluminium oxide strips (Epitex strip, G.C. America, Inc, Chicago, IL).

Secondary anatomy and surface texture were created with a 12-fluted carbide finishing bur (Midwest Dental Products Corporation, Des Plaines, IL). At this stage it is recommended to observe the light reflection from the tooth surface. The drawing of guide lines on the restoration can aid to detect incorrect positioning of the line angles which will reflect the light asymmetrically.

Finally, the restoration was polished with different grades of silicon dioxide rubber cups and points (Vivadent Politip F-P, Ivoclaire Vivadent, Ivoclar North America, Inc, Amherst, NY) (Figure 12.16J). For a shiny and enamel-like surface a felt buffing disk (Flexibuff, Cosmedent Inc, Chicago, IL) was used in conjunction with a fine polishing paste (Proxyt, Ivoclaire Vivadent, Ivoclar North America, Inc, Amherst, NY). Both restorations were checked for occlusal contacts in functional and para-functional movements.

CONCLUSION

A distinct change occurred in the anterior aesthetic design of this case. The combination of bleaching and composite resin restoration offered the clinician an opportunity to provide the patient with an aesthetic conservative restoration with minimal tooth reduction. This combination is especially appropriate for restorations where the colour and shape of the teeth are critical and to patients for whom cost is a significant factor.

CASE REPORT 2

A 20-year-old woman presented with the maxillary right central incisor severely discoloured. The patient reported that a tooth coloured restoration had been placed following physical trauma, which had occurred a few years previously (Figure 12.17A).

CLINICAL PROCEDURE

After radiographs, a tooth vitality examination indicated that a vital pulp was present. A conservative approach with vital bleaching was proposed to the patient. Further treatment might be necessary if home bleaching results were not satisfactory.

A regimen of 2 weeks of single tooth home bleaching with carbamide peroxide (Opalescence, Ultradent Products, Inc, South Jordan, UT) was indicated. Impressions were taken and plastic trays were made and a window was cut to avoid contact of bleaching gel with the adjacent teeth. The patient was instructed to apply the bleaching gel in the region of the discoloured tooth only.

A dramatic change was observed after the 2-week regimen. The tooth colour changed from a low value and high chroma to a high value and low chroma (Figure 12.17B). Even though an improvement was accomplished in the composite colour, the contour and surface roughness still required further treatment.

The restoration was replaced with a combination of hybrid and microfill composites using a similar technique to that described in case report 1 (p. 229).

The new restoration with proper contour and surface texture gave the maxillary right central incisor more natural appearance and excellent blending with the adjacent teeth (Figure 12.17C).

CASE REPORT 3

An 18-year-old female patient presented with small diastemas between the maxillary anterior teeth.

Upon shade evaluation it was observed that the teeth had extrinsic stains of low value as well as localized stains of high value mainly at the incisal region of the maxillary canines, lateral and central incisors (Figure 12.18A).

CLINICAL PROCEDURE

A home bleaching regimen of 2 weeks with 10% carbamide peroxide was recommended for the patient prior to diastema closure. The patient was advised that the vital bleaching technique could improve the low value discoloration; however, microabrasion or localized enamel removal treatment may be necessary for proper removal of the high value stains. The home bleaching treatment of the maxillary arch was extended for an additional week. After 3 weeks, a distinct improvement in the colour of the maxillary teeth could be observed. The overall shade of the maxillary teeth had achieved a pleasant colour blending (Figure 12.18B).

It is important to bleach one arch at the time. This will allow both the clinician and the patient a better shade control. It is especially relevant for patients to observe the improvements of the bleaching treatment. It is also important for patients that have temporomandibular joint problems. The thickness of each bleaching tray is about 2 mm and it may create a discomfort if both trays are used at the same time.

A 2-week home bleaching regimen was followed for the mandibular arch with positive results and shade colour matching with the maxillary arch. Diastema closure was performed at the mesial surface of the maxillary right canine, mesial and distal surfaces to the right lateral, and mesial surfaces of both right and left central incisors with a microfilled composite resin. The lingual surface of the maxillary left canine was restored with a hybrid composite for proper contour (Figure 12.18C).

Further treatment was suggested to the patient for elimination of the white discoloration, but she was pleased with the results and did not want to correct the white stain at the facial surface of the mandibular right central incisor.

CASE REPORT 4

A 21-year-old woman presented with discoloration of the maxillary and mandibular teeth (Shade A-3, Vita Shade Guide, Lumin®

Vacuum – Farbskala, Vita Zahnfabrik, Bad Säckingen, Germany).

The patient was missing the maxillary right lateral incisor. The adjacent canine had been reshaped with a direct composite resin veneer to mimic the shape of a lateral incisal. The patient also had diastema closure of the maxillary left lateral incisor (Figure 12.19A). In addition a small diastema and minor defects at the incisal edge of both maxillary central incisors were noted.

CLINICAL PROCEDURE

After complete examination of the patient, a 1-week regimen of home bleaching with 10% carbamide peroxide on the maxillary arch followed by 1 week bleaching regimen on the mandibular arch was recommended.

The patient was pleased with the colour of the teeth (Shade B-1, Vita Shade Guide, Lumin® Vacuum – Farbskala, Vita Zahnfabrik, Bad Säckingen, Germany) but the replacement of the old direct resin veneers as well as the minor reshaping was still required.

Each maxillary anterior tooth was examined for width-to-length ratio and proportion to the adjacent teeth. It was observed that the maxillary left lateral incisor was not in proportion to the adjacent teeth: the width to length ratio was below 70. This gave the tooth a narrow appearance. The patient was referred to a periodontist for recontouring of the maxillary lateral incisor.

After healing, the old restorations were replaced with direct composite resin veneers on the maxillary left lateral incisor and the maxillary right canine. A hybrid composite resin was used to restore the incisal areas and a microfill was used to directly veneer the facial surfaces of both teeth. The maxillary right canine was contoured to simulate the appearance of a maxillary right lateral incisor.

A hybrid composite was placed at the incisal edge of the maxillary central incisor to reshape the length of the tooth. Closure of the small diastema was achieved using a microfill composite (Figure 12.19B).

CASE REPORT 5

A 55-year-old woman presented with overall discoloration of both maxillary and mandibular teeth. The maxillary left central incisor had a superficial crack which was severely stained (Figure 12.20A). The patient reported that her teeth always had a dark shade. However, the discoloration had become worse in the last few years. The patient was a cigarette smoker and was accustomed to drink 4 cups of coffee per day.

During clinical examination the patient was diagnosed with cervical caries lesions on both maxillary canines and the mandibular right first premolar. The patient also had multiple small diastemas on both maxillary and mandibular front teeth. Assessment of tooth contour, width-to-length ratio and proportion among the different teeth revealed asymmetry in both tooth shape and proportion. The patient was shade C-4 on Vita Shade Guide (Vita Shade Guide, Lumin® Vacuum-Farbskala, Vita Zahnfabrik, Bad Säckingen, Germany).

CLINICAL PROCEDURE

An initial 4-week regimen of home bleaching with 10% carbamide peroxide was recommended. After the 4-week period, discoloration of the crack in the maxillary left central incisor had disappeared. However the bleaching regimen was extended for another 2 weeks until the patient had reached a higher shade value and lower shade chroma than the one that was originally observed for all teeth.

One week after the bleaching was completed, the diastemas in the maxillary and mandibular front teeth were restored with a combination of hybrid and microfill composite as described previously. The A-1 shade of the Vita Shade Guide was selected to match the tooth structure after bleaching.

After width-to-length ratio examination, it was decided that direct composite veneers were appropriate to increase the length of both maxillary lateral incisors. The cervical lesions were restored with a microfill composite resin in one chroma shade higher than the remaining restoration.

After occlusal examination, a space was observed at the lingual surface of the maxillary left canine. A hybrid composite resin was added to close the black hole effect created by the presence of the space.

CONCLUSION

An excellent improvement was accomplished with the combination of the home-bleaching and composite resin restoration (Figure 12.20B). The underlying tooth structure was maintained intact with no tooth reduction necessary.

The patient was highly motivated after treatment and discontinued the tobacco habit. On a recall examination patient also reported to have reduced the coffee intake to 1 cup per day.

CASE REPORT 6

A 17-year-old woman presented with maxillary diastemas on both lateral incisors. The patient also had a mixture of orange and white stains at the facial surfaces of the maxillary front teeth (Figure 12.21A).

CLINICAL PROCEDURE

A home bleaching technique was proposed to the patient as the most conservative treatment for correction of the white stains. Although white stains often do not respond well to this type of treatment, a regimen of 2 weeks with 10% carbamide peroxide was recommended. After 2 weeks a remarkable colour change could be observed in the colour of the maxillary front teeth. However, there was no improvement of the white stains (Figure 12.21B). Micro-abrasion was proposed as a tentative treatment for the correction of the white stains but this was not appealing to the patient.

A combination of hybrid and microfill composite resin restorations was used to place direct veneers on both maxillary lateral incisors. The contour, shape, colour, and proportion of both teeth were improved by the treatment. Additionally, no tooth reduction was necessary.

CONCLUSION

The final result achieved a better colour blending and smooth transition of the maxillary front teeth (Figure 12.21C), but the white spots remained.

CASE REPORT 7

A 52-year-old woman presented with generalized discrepancies in tooth position and shape. The patient was not pleased with the colour of her teeth (Figure 12.22A).

CLINICAL PROCEDURE

After 3 weeks of home bleaching with 10% carbamide peroxide, direct composite resin veneers were used to restore the maxillary incisors.

A mock-up with composite resin was used to evaluate how much reduction of tooth structure would be necessary for proper correction of the labio-version of both lateral incisors. Only the mesial–buccal line angles were slightly reduced. It is important to leave the mock-up in place during the tooth reduction. The mock-up functions as a guide for proper tooth reduction.

After the mock-up was removed, direct composite resin veneers were used to correct the width-to-length ratio of the maxillary incisors (Figure 12.22B).

REFERENCES

Barghi N, Godwin JM. (1994) Reducing the adverse effect of bleaching on composite enamel bond strength. *J Esthet Dent* **6**:157–61.

Ben-Amar A, Liberman R, Gorfil C, Bernstein Y. (1995) Effect of mouthguard bleaching on enamel surface. *Am J Dent* **8**:29–32.

Chiche GJ, Pinault A. (1994) Artistic and scientific principles applied to esthetic dentistry. In *Esthetics of anterior fixed prosthodontics.* Quintessence Publishing: Chicago. 13–32.

Dishman MV, Covey DA, Baughan LW. (1994) The effects of peroxide bleaching on composite to enamel bond strength. *Dental Materials* **10**:33–6.

Garcia-Godoy F, Dodge WW, Donohue M, O'Quinn JA. (1993) Composite resin bond strength after enamel bleaching. *Operative Dentistry* **18**:144–7.

Haywood VB. (1996) Achieving, maintaining, and recovering successful tooth bleaching. *J Esthet Dent* **8**:31–8.

Heymann HO, Sockwell CL, Haywood VB. (1994) Additional conservative esthetics procedures. In Sturdevant C, Robertson T, Heymann H, editors. *The art and science of operative dentistry.* Mosby: St Louis; 643–4.

Kalili KT, Caputo AA, Mito R, Sperbeck G, Matyas J. (1991) In vitro toothbrush abrasion and bond strength of bleached enamel. *Prac Periodont Aesthet Dent* **3**:22–4.

Kalili KT, Caputo AA, Yoshida K. (1993) Effect of alcohol on composite bond strength to bleached enamel. *J Dent Res* **72** (Special Issue):285 [abstract 1140].

Lambrechts PP, Willems G, Vanherle G, Braem M. (1990) Aesthetic limits of light-cured composites in anterior teeth. *Int Dent J* **40**:140–58.

Lammie GA, Posselt U. (1965) Progression changes in the dentition adults. *J Periodontol* **36**:443–54.

Levin EI. (1978) Dental esthetics and the golden proportion. *J Prosthet Dent* **40**:244–52.

McGuckin RS, Thurmond BA, Osovitz S. (1992) Enamel shear bond strength after vital bleaching. *Am J Dent* **5**:216–22.

Miles PG, Pontier JP, Bahiraei D, Close J. (1994) The effect of carbamide peroxide bleach on the tensile bond strength of ceramic brackets: an in-vitro study. *Am J Orthodont Dentofacial Orthoped* **106**:371–5.

Nathoo SA, Gaffar A. (1994) Studies on dental stains induced by antibacterial agents and rational approaches for bleaching dental stains. *Adv Dent Res* **9**:462–70.

Rufenacht CR. (1990) Physical components. In *Fundamentals of esthetics.* Quintessence Publishing: Chicago; 127–34.

Ruse ND, Smith DC, Torneck CD, Titley KC. (1990) Preliminary surface analysis of etched, bleached, and normal bovine enamel. *J Dent Res* 1610–13.

Stokes AN, Hood JAA, Dhariwal D, Patel K. (1992) Effect of peroxide bleaches on resin-enamel bonds. *Quintessence Int* **23**:769–71.

Titley KC, Torneck CD, Smith DC, Adibfar A. (1988) Adhesion of composite resin to bleached and unbleached bovine enamel. *J Dent Res* **67**:1523–8.

Titley KC, Torneck CD, Smith DC, Chernecky R, Adibfar A. (1991) Scanning electron microscopy observation on the penetration and structure of resin tags in bleached and unbleached bovine enamel. *J Endodont* **17**:72–5.

Titley KC, Torneck CD, Ruse ND. (1992) The effect of carbamide peroxide gel on the shear bond strength of a microfil resin to bovine enamel. *J Dent Res* **71**:20–4.

Torneck CD, Titley KC, Smith DC, Adibfar A. (1990) The influence of time of hydrogen peroxide exposure on the adhesion of composite resin to bleached bovine enamel. *J Endodont* **16**:123–8.

Torneck CD, Titley KC, Smith DC, Adibfar A. (1991) Effect of water leaching on the adhesion of composite resin to bleached and unbleached bovine enamel. *J Endodont* **17**:156–60.

Vogel RI. (1975) Intrinsic and extrinsic discoloration of the dentition (a literature review). *J Oral Med* **30**:99–104.

Williams JL. (1914) A new classification of human tooth forms with special reference to a new system of artificial teeth. *Dent Cosmos* **56**:627.

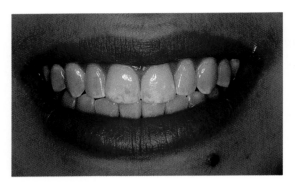

Figure 12.1

Female patient with white hypocalcified areas at the incisal of maxillary teeth.

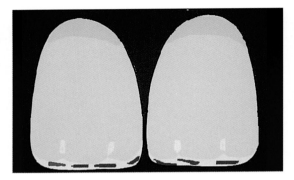

Figure 12.2

Colour mapping containing detailed information that will help on guiding the teeth reconstruction with composite resin.

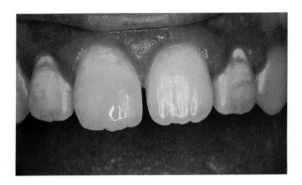

Figure 12.3

Young patient with composite resin restorations. Note that with the light reflection it is possible to observe the natural texture and characterisation of both maxillary central incisors.

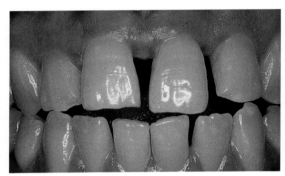

Figure 12.4

Adult female patient with general diastemas on both maxillary and mandibular incisors.

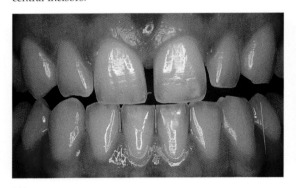

(A)

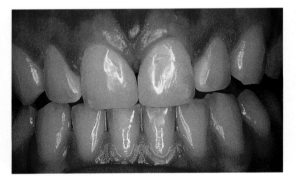

(B)

Figure 12.5

(A) Pre-operative photograph of small general diastemas on maxillary incisors. (B) Post-operative photograph of general diastemas restored with a microfill composite resin (Durafill A-1 shade, Heraeus-Kulzer, Inc, Wehrheim, Germany).

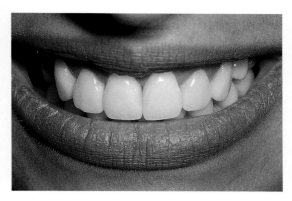

Figure 12.6

Maxillary incisors in width-to-length ratio of 75 and in constant proportion with the adjacent teeth.

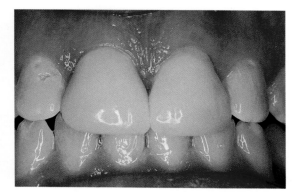

Figure 12.7

Photograph of maxillary central incisors which had received direct veneer for diastema closure. The result was a width-to-length ratio exceeding 90, which gave a fat unpleasant appearance to both incisors.

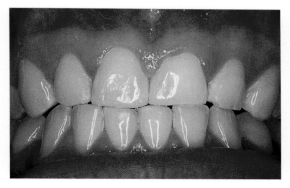

Figure 12.8

Maxillary central incisor with wear at the incisal. The occlusal wear resulted in width-to-length ratio exceeding 100.

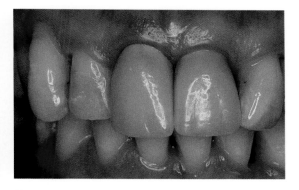

Figure 12.9

Long maxillary central incisors in width-to-length ratio of 65.

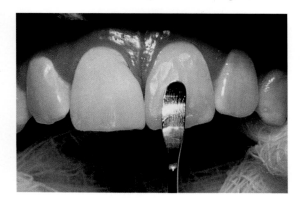

Figure 12.10

Composite resin adaptation with spatula (Almore International Inc, Portland, OR).

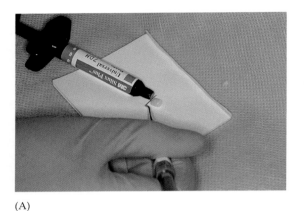

(A)

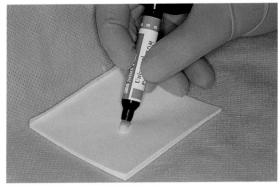

(B)

Figure 12.11

(A) Composite resin removed from the syringe with a flat instrument (Interproximal Carver, American Eagle Instruments Inc, Missoula, MT). (B) Composite resin inappropriately removed from the syringe.

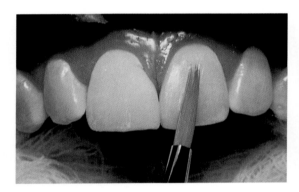

Figure 12.12

Soft bristle brush used to blend the composite resin to the tooth surface.

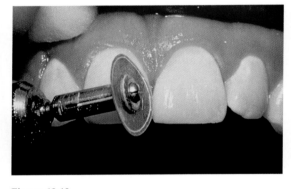

Figure 12.13

Aluminium oxide finishing disk used to open embrasures.

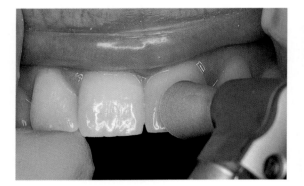

Figure 12.14

Silicon dioxide polishing cup used to achieve a glossy surface.

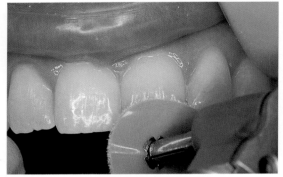

Figure 12.15

Felt disk to be used for enhancement of the polishing procedure and the achievement of a highly polished surface.

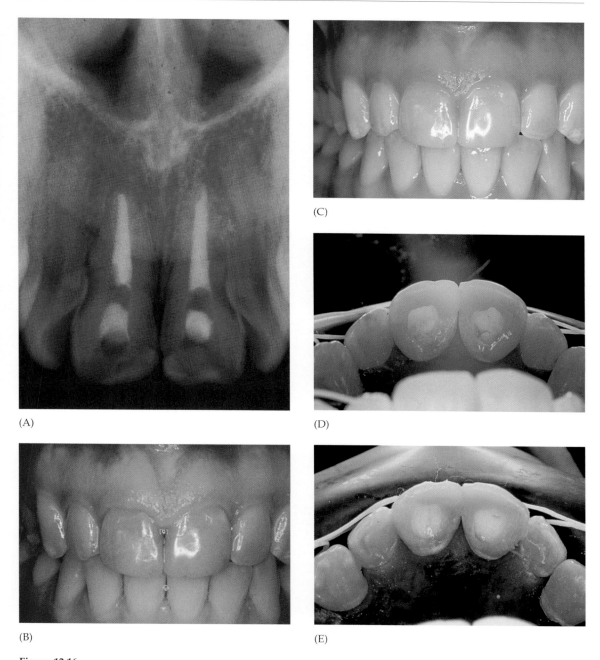

Figure 12.16

(A) Periapical radiograph showing the extent of old composite resin restoration and the apical condition of the teeth. (B) Pre-operative photograph of maxillary central incisors. (C) Post-operative photograph of maxillary central incisors and adjacent teeth after home bleaching with 10% carbamide peroxide. Significant improvement can be seen in the colour of the teeth adjacent to the maxillary central incisors; however, no difference could be observed in these incisors. (D) Coronal access of maxillary central incisors for non-vital bleaching treatment. (E) A paste of 35% hydrogen peroxide and sodium perborate being applied inside the pulp chamber. *continued on the next page*

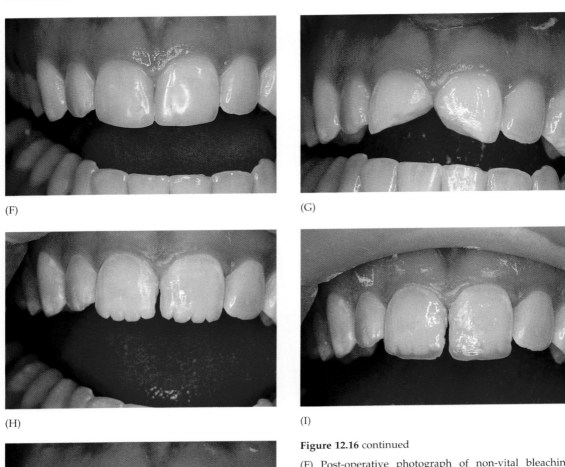

(F)

(G)

(H)

(I)

Figure 12.16 continued

(F) Post-operative photograph of non-vital bleaching results. A shade improvement can be observed on both maxillary central incisors. (G) Long facial and lingual bevels were placed on tooth surface after the removal of the old composite resin. (H) Composite resin dentine core illustrating mamelons and adequate space left for the enamel reconstruction part. (I) Light incisal shade hybrid composite resin applied at the incisal surfaces of both maxillary incisors. (J) Final result after microfill composite was finished and polished. Note the highly glossed surface.

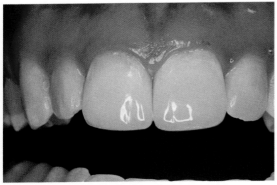

(J)

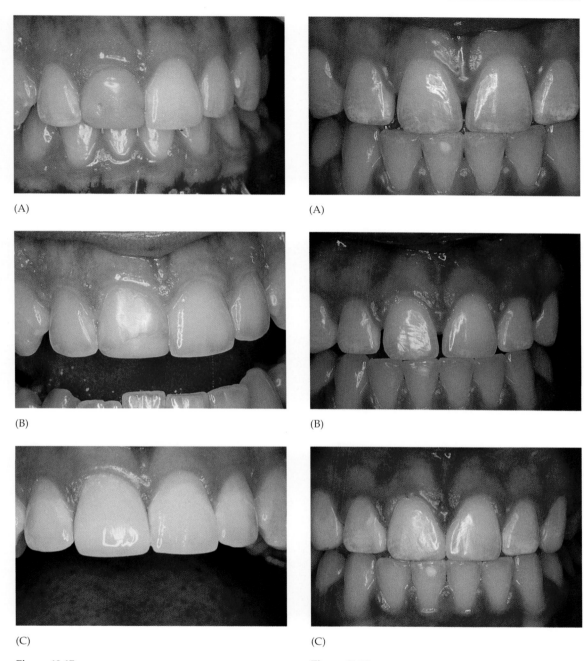

(A)

(A)

(B)

(B)

(C)

(C)

Figure 12.17

(A) Pre-operative front photograph of discoloured right maxillary central incisor. (B) Post-operative photograph of the right maxillary central incisor after home bleaching with 10% carbamide peroxide. (C) Final result after composite resin replacement of a Class IV restoration on the right maxillary central incisor.

Figure 12.18

(A) Pre-operative photograph of general diastemas on maxillary teeth and discoloration of both maxillary and mandibular teeth. (B) Post-operative photograph of maxillary and mandibular teeth after 2 weeks of home bleaching with 10% carbamide peroxide. (C) Final results after diastema closure of maxillary incisor teeth.

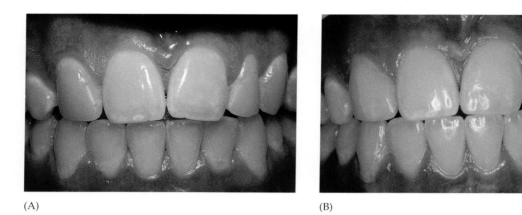

(A)   (B)

Figure 12.19

(A) Pre-operative photograph of discoloured maxillary and mandibular teeth. Note the discoloration of the composite resin veneers on both lateral incisors. (B) Post-operative photograph after home bleaching and direct composite resin restorations.

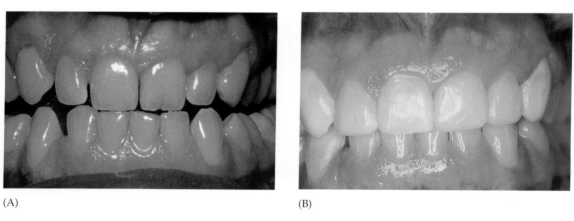

(A)   (B)

Figure 12.20

(A) Pre-operative photograph of discoloured maxillary and mandibular teeth. Note the general diastemas and the lack of proportion (barrel shape) of the maxillary incisors. (B) Final results after home bleaching and direct composite resin restorations.

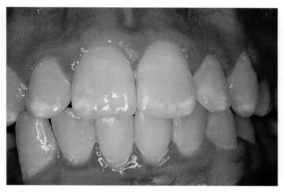
(A)

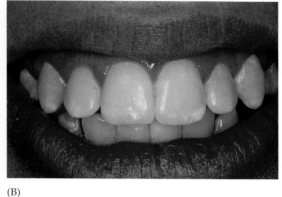
(B)

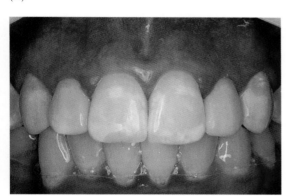
(C)

Figure 12.21

(A) Pre-operative photograph of discoloured maxillary and mandibular teeth. Note the high value stains on the maxillary teeth. (B) Post-operative photograph of maxillary teeth after home bleaching. (C) Final result after direct composite resin veneers were used to restore the maxillary lateral incisors.

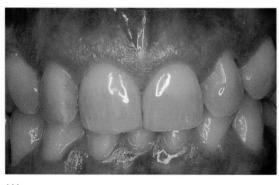
(A)

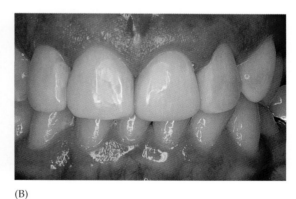
(B)

Figure 12.22

(A) Pre-operative photograph of discoloured and mis-shaped maxillary teeth. (B) Post-operative photograph of maxillary teeth after home bleaching and direct composite resin veneers.

13   SAFETY ISSUES*

Martin Kelleher

INTRODUCTION

Fears that the dentist-supervised use of a product that contains carbamide peroxide and emits hydrogen peroxide might not be safe from the viewpoints of toxicity and cancer risk were engendered by unrealistic animal tests.

In general the small amounts of hydrogen peroxide used in Nightguard Vital Bleaching pose no concern on the grounds of potential general toxicity or carcinogenicity. When used appropriately dental bleaching is free from adverse effects on teeth and the soft tissues of the mouth.

QUESTIONS CONCERNING GENERAL TOXICITY, POSSIBLE MUTAGENICITY AND CANCER RISK

IS THERE ANY RISK OF LOCAL OR SYSTEMIC TOXICITY FROM THE USE OF CARBAMIDE PEROXIDE?

Unless the dose is taken into account, nothing to which humans are exposed can be said to be entirely free of the risk of toxicity. Thus, there is an expression which is well known to toxicologists: 'The dose makes the poison' (Ottoboni 1989).

Carbamide peroxide is formed from urea and hydrogen peroxide. Urea is a normal body constituent and in the doses of carbamide peroxide administered by dentists in the course of Nightguard Vital Bleaching the urea moiety of the molecule is of no toxicological consequence (Haywood and Heymann 1989).

Following the application of carbamide peroxide to teeth, hydrogen peroxide is slowly emitted and absorbed into teeth, resulting in their being bleached. The question arises therefore: Is there any risk of local or general toxicity from the hydrogen peroxide that is emitted from the carbamide peroxide?

The toxicology of hydrogen peroxide (H_2O_2) was thoroughly reviewed by the European Centre for Ecotoxicology and Toxicology of Chemicals (ECETOC 1993) and later by Li (1996, 1998). The main points made in the ECETOC review are as follows. (a) Humans are exposed to H_2O_2 in food. Up to $8000\,g/L$ have been found in some vegetables. (b) H_2O_2 is produced during normal aerobic cell metabolism. It involves a number of enzymatic reactions, especially superoxide dimutase. (c) H_2O_2 is decomposed to oxygen and water by enzymes such as catalase, peroxidases and selenium-dependent glutathione peroxidases. (d) Human deaths have resulted from accidental ingestion of unknown quantities of 30–40% solutions. Toxic effects were generally related to the corrosive action on the gastrointestinal tract. (e) Dermal toxicity is low: H_2O_2 solutions of less than 35% are not classified as irritant to the rabbit skin; solutions of 50% and higher are corrosive. (f) Mouth washes with up to 3% neutralized H_2O_2 did not cause mucosal irritation in humans. (g) Systemic toxicity following exposure to exogenous H_2O_2 is difficult to detect and measure because H_2O_2 is so quickly and efficiently decomposed to oxygen and water at the exposure site.

*This chapter was originally published as Kelleher and Roe 1999 and is reproduced by kind permission of the British Dental Journal.

As pointed out above, the process of the conversion of normal foodstuffs to the energy required for the growth, movement and survival of animals, including humans, involves the production of oxygen free-radicals, including H_2O_2. Consequently, H_2O_2 can be found in all body cells as an endogenous metabolite. Boveris (1972) calculated that the human liver – the principal site of metabolism – produces 270 mg H_2O_2 per hour. An important reason why there are no bad consequences of this generation of H_2O_2 is the effective way in which H_2O_2 is decomposed by enzymes, particularly catalase and various peroxidases. All body cells contain these enzymes, but the highest levels are found in the duodenum, liver, spleen, kidney, blood and mucous membranes. In the blood, most of the catalase is found in red blood cells and within just a few minutes the erythrocytes can degrade gram quantities of H_2O_2 (IARC 1985).

IS THERE A RISK OF MUTAGENESIS FROM EXPOSURE TO HYDROGEN PEROXIDE?

No such risk is supported by the best available scientific evidence. A balanced and thorough review of the scientific evidence indicates that clinically useful concentrations and applications of hydrogen peroxide do not entail a risk of mutagenesis in humans (see further Kelleher and Roe 1999). Original questions about the role of hydrogen peroxide in mutagenesis were raised on the basis of certain in-vitro testing results, which have not been reproduced under in-vivo testing conditions (Kawachi et al 1980, Ito 1981, 1984).

IS THERE ANY RISK OF CARCINOGENESIS AS A CONSEQUENCE OF THE EXPOSURE TO CARBAMIDE PEROXIDE?

Major advances in knowledge concerning mechanisms involved in carcinogenesis have occurred during the last 10–15 years (see Roe 1998). Ames (1985) pointed out that the human diet contains a wide variety of natural mutagens and carcinogens, and also many ingredients which, when metabolized, generate potentially mutagenic oxygen radicals. Endogenous mutagens so formed cause massive DNA damage (i.e. by the formation of oxidative and other adducts) that can be converted to stable mutations during cell division (Ames and Gold 1990). These investigators estimated that, on average, the DNA of each cell in the human body suffers 10 000 hits per day from endogenous oxidants. Almost all of this damage is quickly and effectively repaired. However, there is a brief stage in the process of cell division when the normally double-stranded DNA is only single stranded. During this stage DNA repair is impeded. It follows that agents (e.g. irritants, hormones) which stimulate cell division (i.e. mitosis) increase the risk that DNA damage will be transferred to daughter cells. Ames and Gold (1990) coined the expression 'mitosis increases mutagenesis' to describe this phenomenon. In the light of this it becomes easy to see how non-mutagenic agents, which stimulate cell division, might increase the risk of cancer development.

QUESTIONS OF SAFETY OF PARTICULAR RELEVANCE TO DENTISTS

DOES EXPOSURE TO CARBAMIDE PEROXIDE INCREASE RESORPTION?

Resorption frequently occurs as a result of trauma to teeth. The severity of resorption is related inter alia to the type of injury the tooth has sustained, the force involved and whether the tooth is dislodged from its socket. Thus, resorption can and does occur without any exposure to internal bleaching involving H_2O_2.

Invasive cervical resorption is seen very occasionally in bleached root-filled teeth (Fasararo 1992), and has been attributed to a combination of trauma to the tooth followed by the use of heat and very high concentrations of hydrogen peroxide, e.g. 30% (Friedman 1997). Heithersay et al (1994) studied the radiographs and records of 204 teeth in 158 patients, whose bleaching treatment had been carried out in a specialist endodontic practice over periods of 1 to 19 years. In 78% of patients there was a history of traumatic injury. All teeth had been treated with a combination of thermocatalytic (heat-activated) 30% H_2O_2 and 'walking bleach' procedures. It was found that a total of four teeth from the sample group (2%) had developed invasive cervical resorption during the review period. All of these teeth had a history of traumatic injury and the level of root filling was at the cemento-enamel junction.

Resorption appears to be more a function of the application of heat and of high concentrations of H_2O_2. There appears to be no evidence in the scientific literature implicating the use of H_2O_2 in resorption when heat is not used or when only low concentrations of H_2O_2 (i.e. 3%) are used. In other words, it is only when a combination of high concentrations of H_2O_2 and heat are used on teeth with a history of trauma that resorption very occasionally results. Incidentally, there are no reported cases of resorption with carbamide peroxide used for either internal or external bleaching.

DOES INCREASED TOOTH SENSITIVITY ASSOCIATED WITH THE USE OF CARBAMIDE PEROXIDE CONSTITUTE A SERIOUS PROBLEM?

Schulte and Morrisette (1994) reported a clinical study of 28 patients, who had used home bleaching with 10% carbamide peroxide. Four of these discontinued the procedure because of thermal sensitivity. Of the remaining patients there was no difference between the pulpal readings recorded before the use of the gel and those at any point during the study. During a 3-week trial by Sterrett et al (1995) it was reported that mild transient sensitivity was common in all participants. The consensus view from these and other trials was that this mild sensitivity ceased on stopping treatment.

From these studies and from other reports of bleaching by traditional methods using hydrogen peroxide it is clear that increased sensitivity is mainly associated with the use of heat and high concentrations of H_2O_2 (Cohen and Parkins 1970, Cohen and Chase 1979, Nathanson and Parra 1987). Neither heat nor high concentrations of H_2O_2 are involved in the use of carbamide peroxide gels for Nightguard Vital Bleaching.

DOES BLEACHING ADVERSELY AFFECT THE HARDNESS OF TEETH?

Lewinstein and Hirschfeld (1994) claimed that hydrogen peroxide might reduce the hardness of enamel. However, their study was flawed because they used H_2O_2 with a pH of 3. This would, in effect, acid-etch the enamel surface of teeth. In this context most carbamide peroxide gels have a pH near neutral and would not give rise to acid etching. In any case, the apparent small decreases in micro-hardness were only on the borderline of statistical significance. If, indeed, there are any changes in tooth hardness following bleaching they are certainly likely to be far less than those resulting from the removal of the enamel prior to the application of veneers or those associated with microabrasion (Haywood 1992, 1997, Shannon et al 1993).

CAN CARBAMIDE PEROXIDE BE SAFELY USED FOR THE INTERNAL BLEACHING OF TEETH?

The yellow or brown/grey staining attributable to tetracycline is located deep in the dentine, that is to say at some distance from the enamel surface of the tooth. Hydrogen peroxide emitted from carbamide peroxide applied to the surface of teeth has to penetrate the enamel and dentine for the bleaching of tetracycline-stained teeth to be effective (Haywood 1997).

When carbamide peroxide is simply applied to the exterior of a discoloured tooth, the benefit it achieves may be wholly or partly brought about by bleaching stains or other compounds within the substance of the tooth as distinct from removal of mere surface discoloration (Haywood and Heymann 1989).

In any event, it is clear that carbamide peroxide can be safely used for the internal bleaching of teeth provided that care is taken to avoid the introduction of bacteria into the root canal.

DOES DAMAGE TO THE SOFT TISSUES OF THE MOUTH OCCUR DURING OVERNIGHT BLEACHING WITH CARBAMIDE PEROXIDE GELS?

The American Dental Association (ADA) guidelines for the acceptance of peroxide products (JADA 1994) require inter alia an evaluation of the effects of treatment with carbamide peroxide gels on the soft tissues of the mouth, including the gingivae, tongue, lips and palate. The results of double blind controlled clinical trials have been reported (Sterrett et al 1995, Curtis et al 1996, Russell et al 1996). In none of these studies has soft tissue damage of concern been observed. Furthermore, where transient damage to gingivae was seen, it appeared to be related to poorly fitting trays rather than to the carbamide peroxide gel which they contained.

IS TOOTH BLEACHING WITH CARBAMIDE PEROXIDE GELS EFFECTIVE AND LONG-LASTING?

The ADA guidelines (JADA 1994), which are very strict, require companies seeking approval for their products to demonstrate both the safety-in-use of products and their efficacy.

In relation to efficacy, the data required included: (i) two double blind trials, involving the comparison of the test material with a non-active control material; (ii) the assessment of the effects of treatment over periods of from 2 to 6 weeks; (iii) the measurement of tooth colour at the start and at the end of treatment using two different systems of colour measurement, and (iv) colour duration measurements

of 3 to 6 months to assess whether colour improvement was maintained.

Following extensive evaluation, six products have been given the ADA Seal of Approval (JADA 1997). This demonstrates that the ADA was satisfied that efficacy had been convincingly demonstrated.

Other reviews of the safety and efficacy of tooth-bleaching by carbamide peroxide have been provided by Haywood et al (1994) and by Goldstein (1997).

CONCLUSIONS

1 Noticeable discoloration of teeth can amount to a physical handicap which impacts on a person's self-image, self-confidence, attractiveness and employability. It should not therefore be dismissed as a matter of no more than cosmetic importance.
2 Hydrogen peroxide liberated from carbamide peroxide is effective in bleaching teeth because it penetrates through the enamel and into the dentine. Bleaching is not achieved solely or mainly by a surface effect.
3 Low concentration carbamide peroxide gels, when used under the supervision of dentists within customized trays, are completely safe from the viewpoint of general toxicity, risk of mutation and risk of carcinogenesis.
4 When properly used, there are no more than minimal adverse effects on dental pulps or the soft tissues of the mouth, and these are very transitory.

BIBLIOGRAPHY

Ames BN. (1985) Dietary carcinogens and anticarcinogens: oxygen radicals and degenerative diseases. *Science* **211**:1256–64.

Ames BN, Gold LS. (1990) Too many rodent carcinogens: mitogenesis increases mutagenesis. *Science* **249**:970–1.

Boveris A, Oshino N, Chance B. (1972) The cellular production of hydrogen peroxide. *Biochem J* **128**:617–30.

Cohen SC, Parkins FM. (1970) Bleaching tetracycline-stained vital teeth. *Oral Surg* **29**:465–71.

Cohen SC, Chase C. (1979) Human pulpal response to bleaching procedures on vital teeth. *J Endodont* **5**:134–8.

Curtis JW, Dickinson GL, Doney MC, et al. (1996) Assessing the effects of 10% carbamide peroxide on oral soft tissues. *J Am Dent Assoc* **127**:1218–23.

ECETOC. (1993) Joint Assessment of Commodity Chemicals No. 22: Hydrogen peroxide [CAS No. 7722-84-1]. European Centre for Ecotoxicology and Toxicology of Chemicals: Chipping Sodbury.

Fasanaro TS. (1992) Bleaching teeth: history, chemicals and methods used for common tooth discoloration. *J Esthet Dent* **4**:71–8.

Friedman S. (1997) Internal bleaching: long-term outcomes and complications. *J Am Dent Assoc Suppl* **128**:51S–5S.

Goldstein RE. (1997) In-office bleaching: where we came from, where are we to-day? *J Am Dent Assoc Suppl* **128**:11S–15S.

Haywood VB. (1992) History, safety and effectiveness of current bleaching techniques and applications of the Nightguard Vital Bleaching technique. *Quintessence Int* **23**:471–88.

Haywood VB. (1997) Nightguard Vital Bleaching: current concepts and research. *J Am Dent Assoc Suppl* **128**:19S–25S.

Haywood VB, Heymann HO. (1989) Nightguard Vital Bleaching. *Quintessence Int* **20**:173–6.

Haywood VB, Leonard RH, Neilson CF, Brunson WD. (1994) Effectiveness, side effects and long term status of Nightguard Vital Bleaching. *J Am Dent Assoc* **125**:1219–26.

Heithersay GS, Dahlstrom SW, Marrin PD. (1994) Incidence of invasive cervical resorption in bleached root filled teeth. *Austral Dent J* **39**:82–7.

IARC. (1985) Hydrogen peroxide. *Evaluation of the carcinogenic risk of chemicals to humans* **36**: 285–314.

Ito A, Wanatabe H, Naito M, Naito Y. (1981) Induction of duodenal tumors in mice by oral administration of hydrogen peroxide. *Gann* **72**:174–5.

Ito A, Wanatabe H, Naito M, Naito Y, Kawashima K. (1984) Correlation between induction of duodenal tumor by hydrogen peroxide and catalase activity in mice. *Gann* **75**:17–21.

JADA (1994) Guidelines for the acceptance of peroxide containing oral hygiene. *J Am Dent Assoc* **125**:1140–2.

JADA (1997). Reports from an International Symposium on Non-Restorative Treatment of Discoloured Teeth. *J Am Dent Assoc Suppl* **128**:1S–64S.

Kawachi T, Yahagi T, Kada T, et al. (1980) Co-operative programme on short-term assays for carcinogenicity in Japan. In: Montesano R, Bartsh H, Tomatis L, editors. *Molecular and cellular aspects of carcinogen screening tests*. IARC publication 27, pp. 323–30.

Kelleher MGD, Roe FJC. (1999) The safety-in-use of 10% carbamide peroxide (Opalescence) for bleaching teeth under the supervision of a dentist. *Br Dent J* **187**(4):190–3.

Lewinstein I, Hirschfield C, et al. (1994) The effect of hydrogen peroxide and sodium perborate on the microhardness with human enamel and dentine. *J Endodont* **20**:61–3.

Li Y. (1996) Biological properties of peroxide-containing tooth whiteners. *Food Chem Toxicol* **34**:887–904.

Li Y. (1998) Tooth bleaching using peroxide-containing agents: current status of safety issues. *Compend Contin Educ Dent* **19**(8):783–94.

Li Y. (2000) Peroxide-containing tooth whiteners: an update on safety. *Compend Cont Educ Dent* **21** (Suppl 28):S4–S9.

Nathanson D, Parra C. (1987) Bleaching vital teeth: a review of clinical study. *Compend Contin Educ Dent* **8**:490–7.

Ottoboni MA. (1989) *The dose makes the poison*. Vincent: Berkeley, CA. pp. 1–222.

Roe FJC. (1998) A brief history of the use of laboratory animals for the prediction of carcinogenic risk for man with a note on needs for the future. *Exp Toxic Pathol* **50**:271–6.

Schulte JR, Morrisette DB, et al. (1994) The effects of bleaching application time on the dental pulp. *J Am Dent Assoc* **125**:1330–5.

Shannon H, Spencer P, Gross K, Tira D. (1993) Characterisatiion of enamel exposed to 10% carbamide peroxide bleaching agents. *Quintessence Int* **24**:39–44.

Sterrett J, Price RB, Bankey T. (1995) Effects of home bleaching on the tissues of the oral cavity. *J Can Dent Assoc* **61**:412–20.

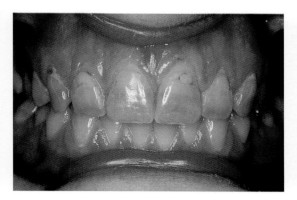

Figure 13.1
Intrinsic staining.

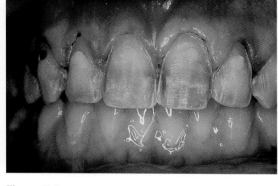

Figure 13.2
Teeth prepared for porcelain veneers.

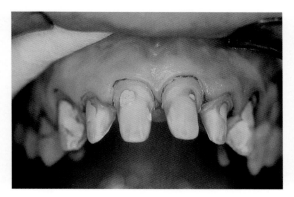

Figure 13.3
Teeth prepared for conventional crowns.

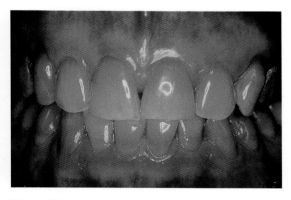

Figure 13.4
Tetracycline stained teeth prior to bleaching.

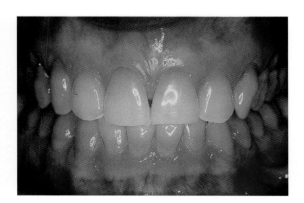

Figure 13.5
Tetracycline stained teeth after two months' Nightguard
Vital Bleaching.

14 MARKETING

INTRODUCTION

All members of the practice team can be involved in marketing bleaching programmes and bleaching services to their existing patients and prospective new patients. More patients ask questions about tooth whitening than any other dental procedure. The most commonly asked question is: 'do you think my teeth could be whiter?' or 'I don't suppose my teeth could be whiter?'

Marketing bleaching services is an excellent opportunity for practice growth and new services. The growth in patient demand for these services will stimulate further new patients for bleaching and further aesthetic treatment. This will in turn lead to increased practice revenue and profits. There are several ways of introducing the dentist-prescribed home bleaching programmes into the dental practice.

NEW PATIENTS

All new patients can be asked at their initial evaluations if they are happy with the colour of their teeth (see Chapter 4 on treatment planning). This question can be introduced on to the new patient questionnaire. Most patients, when asked, would prefer their teeth to be a lighter colour.

EXISTING PATIENTS

Explanatory leaflets about the bleaching procedures can be displayed in the dental practice. Such tools can be information sheets giving questions and answers or 'What to expect' leaflets and visual aids such as before and after photographs, models of bleaching trays and kits, brochures and posters. Information sheets on bleaching can be sent to all patients in the form of a newsletter or together with recall letters or accounts. All patients coming to the practice for their recall or continuing care programmes or routine prophylaxis visits can be advised about the new bleaching services in the practice.

DISCUSSING THE BENEFITS OF BLEACHING TREATMENT WITH PATIENTS

All members of the practice team can discuss the benefits of tooth bleaching with patients. They should be ready to articulate them should patients ask.

BENEFITS OF TOOTH BLEACHING FOR PATIENTS

- Improved appearance of the teeth
- Improved self-esteem in having an attractive smile
- The lighter colour may help patients to look younger
- The whiter smile helps patient's to smile more
- The whiter smile gives the teeth a healthy appearance and thus a healthy appearance to the rest of the face
- The whiter teeth reflect to the rest of the face and to the eyes which appear more

Table 14.1 Benefits of bleaching treatments

General
- Patient feel better about their smile
- Patients are more interested in taking care of the rest of the teeth and their bodies (Haywood 1998)
- Patients smile more to reveal the new smile, which encourages them to have a better outlook on life
- Patients often opt to have further aesthetic dental procedures

Teeth
- Teeth become lighter
- Teeth become brighter and whiter

Restorations
- Superficial cleansing of the restorations
- Reduction of the dark line around leaking composite restorations

Gingivae
- General improvement in overall gingival condition
- Improvement in oral hygiene
- Reduction in gingival bleeding
- Reduction in plaque build-up
- Some researchers have found a reduction in probing depths and bleeding, probing indices

sparkling. Beauty consultants say the colour of the teeth should match or be lighter than the colour of the whites of the eyes (Haywood 1999)
- It may result in a more healthy dentition because the patient continues excellent home care of the mouth

BENEFITS OF TOOTH BLEACHING FOR DENTISTS

- Dentists enjoy providing bleaching treatments for their patients
- This enjoyment is translated to enthusiasm
- Bleaching teeth builds relationships with patients, because the treatment is not painful or invasive
- Patients become 'friends' rather than 'nervous foes'
- Patients enjoy having the bleaching treatment and often elect to have further aesthetic dentistry
- Patients accept needed dentistry following bleaching treatment

- This results in more recommendations from patients' friends and family
- Increased practice revenue and thus better profits

BENEFITS OF TOOTH BLEACHING FOR DENTAL STAFF

- Dental staff who have had bleaching treatment become patient educators and show examples of their smiles to patients
- Treated dental staff become sales consultants and practice builders (Miles 1999)
- Dentistry becomes more enjoyable
- Increased salaries or bonuses may result because of the increased revenue generated from the dental practice

INTERNAL MARKETING

- *Treat your staff.* It is a good idea to treat a member of your staff such as the receptionist, hygienist or dental assistant. Staff can then demonstrate the lightening effects of the home bleaching (Miller 2000). It is advisable to treat one arch only so that patients can see a colour comparison.
- *Treat yourself.* By doing so, this validates the bleaching programme within the practice and provides a seal of approval.
- *Show comparative photographs.* Before and after photos of previous treated cases in the practice portfolio can be kept in the waiting room. Patients are always interested to see these photographs and the results of bleaching for other patients.
- *Patient communication.* Those who have successfully bleached their teeth may be willing to speak to prospective patients about their bleaching treatment. Most patients are so delighted, they tell their friends and family.

(See further Miller 2000.)

EXTERNAL MARKETING

The bleaching photographs of before and after cases (with patients' appropriate consent) can

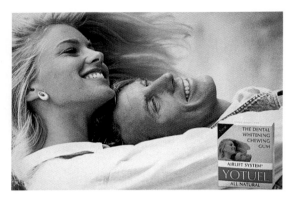

Figure 14.1

Most adverts, whatever they are advertising, feature models with attractive smiles and white teeth; having white teeth is equated with good health, youth and vitality. Patients are aware of the many adverts for white teeth in women's magazines, television and media adverts and this makes them request this service.

be sent to the local newspaper, women's magazines, or TV stations, with a press release and further information with the name and contact details of the dental practice.

MANAGING PATIENT EXPECTATIONS

It is essential to manage patient's realistic expectations of the expected results prior to commencing bleaching treatment. No promises or guarantees are given and patients are informed that every case is different (Small 1998). They should also be informed that not all teeth lighten to the same extent, particularly deeply stained dentitions (Small 1998) and multicoloured teeth. In fact, it is best to underemphasize the results that can be achieved: patients will not thus be disappointed when the shade shift is only two shades, for instance. To obtain the American Dental Association (ADA) Seal of Approval, the manufacturers of bleaching products have to demonstrate clinically that the bleaching product can demonstrate a shade change of two shades and demonstrate 6 months' clinical safety and colour maintenance (Siew 2000).

The worst that can happen is no change in the colour, and many patients are happy to try the treatment on these preconditions. Patients should be told that they should not expect a rapid shift in shade after the first bleaching treatment and a lighter shade is normally noticeable after 1 week. It is essential with any form of cosmetic or elective dentistry to assess the patient's motivation for the proposed treatment. Patients that are dysmorphophobic should not be treated. These patients have an obsessional concern about appearance and cannot accept small imperfections in their lives (Wise 1995). It is essential through the smile analysis sheets and careful planning that the patient's motivation can be assessed. Some patients have a specific goal for bleaching their teeth, such as a forthcoming wedding. Patients need to have a willingness to co-operate to achieve successful home bleaching.

Many patients have a threshold level of acceptance such that, although the discoloration is not entirely removed, they are pleased with the new lightened teeth and they are happy to discontinue treatment. It is much easier to treat these more stoical patients and to manage their expectations.

INCREASED REVENUE FROM BLEACHING TREATMENT

Providing more bleaching treatments for patients results in increased practice revenue. If just one patient per day had bleaching treatment, that would be an increase in the practice revenue: since the costs for providing this treatment are moderate, profit margins are high. An increased profit margin for the practice results in quicker repayment of loans, easier payment of both fixed and variable overheads, and more money being available for staff bonuses. There is thus a win–win situation for patients, staff, and dentist.

REFERENCES

ADA (1998) Acceptance Program Guidelines (1998) for home-use tooth whitening products.

American Dental Association, Council on Scientific Affairs, May 1998.

ADA (1994) Guidelines for the acceptance or peroxide containing oral hygiene products, American Dental Association Council on Dental Therapeutics. *J Dent Assoc* **125**(8):1140–2.

Adams M. (1999) Patient education from the hygienist's perspective. *Contemp Esthet Restor Prac Suppl.* June: 10.

Albers HF. (2000) The psychology of bleaching. *Adept Report* **6**(4):14.

Dunn J. (2000) Tooth whitening – why? (Editorial) *Comp Cont Educ Dent* **21**(Suppl 24):S2.

Haywood VB. (1999) Current status and recommendations for dentist-prescribed, at-home tooth whitening. *Contemp Esthet Restor Dent Suppl.* June, **3**:1, 2–9.

Miles LL. (1999) Whiter teeth – a total team approach. *Contemp Esthet Restor Treat Suppl.* 11.

Miller M. (editor) (2000) *Reality: the information source for esthetic dentistry,* Vol 14. Reality Publishing Company: Houston.

Siew C. (2000) ADA guidelines for the acceptance of tooth whitening products. *Comp Cont Educ Dent* **21**(Suppl 28):S44–S47.

Small B. (1998) The application and integration of at-home bleaching into private practice. *Comp Cont Educ Dent* **19**(8):799–808.

Wise MD. (1995) *Failure in the restored dentition: management.* Quintessence Publishing: London, Berlin, Chicago and Tokyo.

APPENDIX I LEGAL CONSIDERATIONS RELATING TO DENTAL BLEACHING IN EUROPE AND THE UK

Martin Kelleher

BACKGROUND

The European Community (EC) 1976 Cosmetics Directive (76/768/EEC) prohibited the use of hydrogen peroxide in cosmetics except in products and to the extent described in that Cosmetic Directive. In April 1992 Optident became the UK distributor of a product for bleaching teeth made by Ultradent (South Jordan, UT) called Opalescence. The main active ingredient of Opalescence is 10% carbamide peroxide which releases 3.5% hydrogen peroxide.

In October 1992 the Cosmetics Directive (92/86/EC) was amended to proscribe the use of carbamide peroxide in cosmetics, except in oral hygiene products and only to the limit directed, which was 0.1% hydrogen peroxide. The amount of hydrogen peroxide (about 3.5%) released by Opalescence gel exceeded this limit. Hence in November 1993, at the insistence of the Department of Trade and Industry (DTI), Opalescence was withdrawn from the UK market by Optident.

In June 1993 the Medical Devices Directive (MDD) was set up to regulate the production and marketing of medical devices. This was to be effective from 1995. An MDD mark (the CE Mark) indicated conformity to the requirements of the Medical Devices Directive. Compliance with the Directive would be verified by a notified body.

Article 4 of the MDD prohibits EC member states creating any obstacle to the placing on the market within their territory of a device bearing such a CE marking. However, under article 1 (5)(d) the MDD does not apply to cosmetics.

In October 1994 Ultradent applied to the RWTÜV (the notified body) in Germany for approval of its quality systems for Opalescence and other products. Opalescence was given a CE Mark under the MDD and it was relaunched in January 1995 with the CE Mark. The view of the DTI was that Opalescence was a cosmetic and was excluded by article 1 (5)(d). The penalty for the supply of an illegal cosmetic was stated to be six months in prison or a fine of £5000, or both. This would be enforced under the terms of the Consumer Protection Act 1987 and the 1989 Cosmetic Products safety regulations: regulation 4 (2b) prohibits the supply of a cosmetic product which contains substances set out in Schedule 2 Part 1.

THE TRIAL

In December 1996 Optident and Ultradent sued the DTI and the Department of Health (DOH) because they alleged that the DTI and DOH had breached article 4 of the MDD by obstructing the sale of Opalescence.

In 1998 the matter came to trial in the UK High Court under Mr Justice Laws. He gave his judgements as follows:

1 If the CE Mark under the MDD had been granted to Opalescence in an EEC country

must the UK authorities respect it, even though on the facts it was a cosmetic? (Answer: Yes)

2 Was Opalescence a cosmetic? (Answer: No)
3 Was it a medical device? (Answer: Yes)
4 Had the DTI and DOH obstructed its distribution? (Answer: Yes)

In Mr Justice Laws's view the MDD applied in the regulation of Opalescence rather than the Cosmetic Directive.

THE APPEAL

In 1999 the DTI and the DOH appealed against this decision on the grounds that Mr Justice Laws should have said that Opalescence was a cosmetic and that the Cosmetic Directive applied and therefore article 1 (5)(d) applied. The Appeal Court Judges Morritt, Sedley and Lyndsay reviewed Mr Justice Laws analysis and gave their answers to the questions: (1) Is it a cosmetic, (2) Is it a medical device, (3) Should the CE Mark have been respected, even if it was a cosmetic? In considering their answers they referred to the Cosmetics Directive. They quoted aspects of this.

The fifth recital of this Directive states:*

1 This directive relates only to cosmetic products and not to pharmaceutical specialities and medicinal products.
2 It is necessary to delimit the field of cosmetics from that of pharmaceuticals. These limitations follow from the detailed definition of cosmetic products which refers to their areas of application and to the purposes of their use.
3 **Products containing substances or preparations intended to be** ingested, inhaled, injected or **implanted in the human body**, do **not** come under the field of cosmetics.

NEW DEFINITION OF A COSMETIC

The new definition of a cosmetic under the EEC Directive 93/35/EC was 'A cosmetic

*Emphasis given to phrases and words in quoted text is that of the author.

product shall mean any product or substance intended to be placed in contact with the various external parts of the human body (epidermis, hair system, nails, lips and external genital organs) or with the teeth **and** the mucous membranes of the oral cavity with the view exclusively or mainly to cleaning them, perfuming them, changing their appearance and/or correcting body odours and/or protecting them or keeping them in good condition'.

APPEAL COURT'S DECISION

Lord Justices Morritt, Sedley and Lindsay presided over the question: Is Opalescence a cosmetic product within the cosmetics directive?

1 In the original High Court case Mr Justice Laws held that the effect of the use of a cosmetic was temporary, transient, superficial and reversible while the effect of Opalescence was not transient, not temporary nor reversible. The argument that a cosmetic has certain characteristics, i.e. it is temporary, superficial or reversible was accepted by Mr Justice Laws. The Appeal Court judges disgreed: they felt that the effect on a hair strand of bleaching was not temporary nor that of a depilatory necessarily reversible, nor that of a deodorant necessarily superficial.
2 A property of the mechanism of Opalescence is that it penetrates the tooth structure at least to the dentine, so that, at least in relation to non-vital teeth, it is intended to be 'implanted' so as to be excluded by reference to the fifth recital of the Cosmetics Directive.
3 The question of the possibility of danger to the zones of the body adjacent to the areas of application of the substance was then raised but **no evidence was offered of any danger posed by Opalescence**.
4 It was contended that the nature and the purpose of Opalescence was to remedy a troublesome condition which arises in specific circumstances and is different in kind from those of a cosmetic device. Mr Justice Laws produced an analogy of disfiguring birthmarks. The appeal judges

did not accept that discoloured teeth are troublesome conditions, nor a disease, nor a physical or mental handicap, but they accepted that discoloured teeth might be a social handicap.

5   The next proposition was that Opalescence was implanted inside teeth at least in non-vital bleaching. The three Appeal Court judges said Mr Justice Laws had misunderstood the technique and that the evidence was clear that all traces of Opalescence were washed out before the filling was installed. **This is true, but it is *only* after the Opalescence has bleached the teeth, which would take a number of days to do**. During that period at least it is definitely implanted within the teeth and the Appeal Court judges were therefore wrong themselves in this instance. Significantly, the Appeal Court judges did not take any expert opinions before making this erroneous decision. More specifically the hydrogen peroxide released by the gel is implanted in the teeth because all the scientific evidence is that hydrogen peroxide penetrates throughout the tooth and into the pulp within hours. In the appeal judges' view, however, even though it is clear the effect of Opalescence is not superficial or temporary, it was still a cosmetic.

THE MEDICAL DEVICES DIRECTIVE

Medical devices are divided into four classes: I, IIa, IIb, III as provided by article 9. Opalescence falls in the class IIa. The device is considered to meet the essential requirements prescribed by article III, i.e. 'must bear the CE Mark to conform within their being placed on the market'. Manufacturers are required to affix the CE Mark and to lodge with the notified body an application for assessment of its quality system, together with a number of specified documents. The function of the notified body is to audit the quality system to determine whether it meets the requirements of the annexe. Article 18 allows the case where a CE Mark has been 'unduly affixed'. Article

8 provides for safeguards when a device bearing a CE Marking fails to meet the essential requirements or standards.

DOES THE MEDICAL DEVICES DIRECTIVE APPLY TO OPALESCENCE?

This Directive states:

1   This Directive shall apply to medical devices **and their accessories**. For the purposes of this Directive, **accessories shall be treated as medical devices in their own right**. Both medical devices and their accessories are termed medical devices. For the purposes of this Directive the following definition shall apply:

(a) Medical Device means any instrument, apparatus, **appliance**, **material** or other article either used alone or in combination intended by the manufacturer to be used for *human beings* for the purpose of diagnosis, monitoring, treatment, **alleviation of or compensation for an injury or handicap** and which does not achieve its principal intended action in, or on, the human body by pharmacalogic, immunologic or metabolic means but **which may be assisted in its function by such means**.

Under article 1 (5d) the Medical Devices Directive does not apply to cosmetics. The Crown Departments in their appeal suggested that Opalescence was not a medical device within the definition contained in article 1 (2)(a). Mr Justice Laws decided that even if contrary to his decision Opalescence was a cosmetic product covered by the Cosmetics Directive, the Medical Devices Directive still applied. His view was that although, as a matter of fact, a product might on the face of it be said to be both a cosmetic and a medical device within the definitions given in the Directives, that it was equally clear that it, as a matter of law, a product could not be subject to both regimes at the same time. It followed that some mechanism had to be found to decide to which directive the product ought to be assigned as these are community wide regimes and they apply equally throughout the all member states of the EEC. If it doesn't apply equally throughout the EEC, it would mean that the Medical Device Directive applied in some countries and the Cosmetic Directive in others and that is why it could not be interpreted individually by member states. Indeed, to do so, runs totally contrary to the whole idea of CE Marking and of the freedom of movement of goods within the EEC.

The CE Marking is applied by the manufacturer. In the case of Class I devices, there is no conformity assessment, merely a declaration of conformity made by the manufacturer.

In the case of Class IIA devices (which was the Class into which Opalescence fell) an audit of the manufacturer's quality system was necessary to determine whether it met the requirement of the Annex V. The notified body assumes that the Medical Devices Directive is applicable but is not charged with determining that it is.

Further legal challenges in 2000 to the appropriateness of the CE Marking as a medical device resulted in the confirmation in Germany that this is appropriate.

CONCLUSION AND FUTURE PROSPECTS

The conclusion of the Appeal Court was that Opalescence is a cosmetic product covered by the Cosmetic Directive and is not subject to the provision of the Medical Devices Directive.

The significant argument in law is as to whether a National (e.g. British) Court can in effect second guess the correctness or otherwise of the application of a CE Mark, which has Europe-wide applications. This is part of the basis of taking it to the House of Lords, which has now been accepted for appeal.

Mr Justice Laws considered that Opalescence was a medical device within the definition because it was intended by the manufacturer to alleviate a disease or handicap. The appeal judges felt that the purpose of Opalescence is bleaching dark teeth, whatever the cause, more than the alleviation of a condition which gave rise to the dark teeth. Common sense would suggest that it is the dark teeth which is the handicap and Opalescence is effective in bleaching those.

The matter could be referred to the Court of Justice under article 234 EEC Treaty. The Appeal Judges did not consider that it be appropriate to refer this matter to the European Court of Justice.

In the mean time dentists should note that the mouthguard (tray) that is used for Nightguard Vital Bleaching is a medical device under the Medical Devices Directive: it is a certified customized device made for an individual patient from an impression of that patient's mouth; legally, that can only be done by a dentist. Even if the gel were to be considered as a cosmetic, it would still be an accessory under the Medical Devices Directive and therefore treated as a medical device in its own right provided it is used within the mouthguard.

The Chief Dental Officer in the UK clarified in 2000 that dental bleaching techniques are legal and that the dispute is in relation to the regulation of products that are used for this.

10% carbamide peroxide has now been reintroduced into the UK in an unbranded form. A legal challenge in Germany to remove the CE Marking from Opalescence was thrown out by a higher court in Germany, as noted above. Realistically, a CE Marking can only be removed by the original granting authority. The German court refused to remove the CE Marking and confirmed its appropriateness as being regulated under the Medical Devices Directive. Other EC countries (such as Sweden) have confirmed that only the country that granted the CE mark can withdraw it.

APPENDIX II   PATIENT INFORMATION AND CONSENT FORMS

WHAT TO EXPECT DURING YOUR BLEACHING TREATMENT

Your dentist has given you a bleaching kit to take home with you, together with your bleaching trays. It is essential that you follow the instructions given by your dentist and by the manufacturers in wearing the trays and applying the bleaching agent.

How long should I wear the trays for?

This depends on the amount of lightening that you desire and the original shade of the teeth. If your teeth are quite dark or very yellow/grey/tetracycline-stained, it will take longer to bleach the teeth. Tetracycline-stained teeth can take 6 months or up to 1 year to bleach. Some teeth can whiten after 1 month. If you are not experiencing any sensitivity, you may wear the trays for at least 1–2 hours and even sleep with trays in your mouth. It is very important to remove all the excess material around the gums or the palate prior to sleeping with the trays.

If you cannot wear the trays for a few days because of your hectic schedule, it does not matter; bleach your teeth according to your own schedule. Some people put the trays in after dinner and wear them for the first hour while watching TV or doing the dishes. Then, if everything is fine, they replenish the trays and sleep with them in the mouth.

What do I do if I have any sensitivity?

Sensitivity of teeth is the most common side-effect of home bleaching. In fact, many patients suffer from sensitive teeth any way; this occurs usually around the necks of the teeth where the gums have receded. If you are experiencing any sensitivity, you should stop bleaching your teeth for a few days. You can resume after about 3–4 days. If the teeth become ultra-sensitive you can place a sensitive toothpaste into the bleaching trays for an hour a day, which will usually stop the sensitivity. Alternatively, you can rub the sensitizing toothpaste into the gum margins with your finger 5 times per day for a few days.

If you are at all concerned, please call your dentist.

What happens if the teeth do not bleach evenly?

If the teeth have white spots on them before bleaching, these spots will appear whiter during the first few days; however, the contrast between the spots and the rest of the tooth will be less and eventually the spots will not be noticeable. Sometimes, the dentist can do a special procedure called microabrasion for you, where by the white spots can be more permanently removed. Ask your dentist about the procedure if you are concerned about this.

You may notice new white spots occurring on the teeth while you are undertaking the bleaching treatment, immediately after a bleaching session or in the morning if you have been wearing the trays for the whole night. These white spots were already present on the teeth before bleaching. As the teeth become lighter, they become more visible. Do not worry: as the whole tooth itself becomes lighter these spots will fade.

Some teeth may appear banded with lighter/whiter areas. Again, these bandings are originally present on the tooth. When the tooth is dark, these bandings are not obvious. As the tooth becomes lighter, the lighter parts of the tooth will lighten first, followed by the darker banded area. After a week or so these will not be noticeable any more.

How will my teeth feel?

Normally the teeth feel very clean after the bleaching procedure. The bleaching materials also have an indirect effect on the gums in helping them to heal or improving health. (This is how the technique was invented: it was first used to heal gum irritation during orthodontic treatment.)

What about my smile?

Your smile will appear brighter as a bonus. It is very rare, but sometimes the teeth do not lighten at all. If this happens and you are wearing the bleaching trays as recommended, you may need to try a different bleaching product or a slightly higher concentration of the bleaching material. The dentist can do a few power-bleaching sessions for you while you relax in the chair. Discuss this with your dentist.

If you have white fillings in the front teeth

that match the existing shade of your teeth before you bleach your teeth, they may not match the teeth afterwards. This is because your teeth can lighten, but the fillings do not. When the desired colour has been achieved, the dentist can replace these fillings with a lighter shade of filling material to match the new shade of your teeth. Normally the dentist will wait a week before changing the fillings.

How long does the bleaching last? Will I have to bleach my teeth again?

Normally the new white colour of your teeth keeps quite well. However, the effect is dependent on what has caused the teeth to discolour in the first place. If you drink lots of coffee, red wine or cola drinks, the effect may darken slightly. Some patients do a top-up treatment after 3–4 years; some patients do not need to.

The dentist will ask you to return your trays after the desired shade of lightening has been achieved. This is to ensure that you do not over-bleach your teeth.

Does bleaching harm the teeth or gums?

Safety studies have shown that bleaching teeth using the dentist-prescribed home bleaching technique is perfectly safe on the teeth, cheeks, gum and tissue of the mouth. Bleaching the teeth with the dentist-prescribed kits is equivalent to drinking one soda drink. The bleaching material has a neutral pH.

There are problems with the bleaching kits that are purchased over the counter. Although they are inexpensive, they normally contain an acid rinse that can damage the teeth or thin down the enamel of the teeth, which can be extremely harmful. (There has been one case where a patient purchased the kit over the counter and bleached the teeth. The teeth went darker and the patient continued over-using the treatment. Unfortunately the acid rinse had worn the enamel away and the darker shade was exposed dentine.)

It is not, however, advisable to bleach your teeth if you smoke. It is best to stop smoking for at least 3 weeks before commencing the bleaching procedure. Smoking causes the teeth to darken anyway and the effects will be diminished.

The technique of bleaching teeth is not for everybody. There are some situations where bleaching teeth is contraindicated (such as where the front teeth are already crowned, or there are very large fillings on the front teeth, or the teeth are already excessively worn and there is tooth surface loss). The ideal situation is where there is not much wrong with the teeth except for the colour, which has become more yellow with age.

CONSENT FORM

We are planning to whiten your teeth using carbamide peroxide solution. Please read the following instructions carefully.

1   The active ingredient is carbamide peroxide in a glycerine base. If you know of any allergy or are aware of an adverse reaction to this ingredient, please do not proceed with this treatment.
2   As with any treatment there are benefits and risks. The benefit is that teeth can be whitened fairly quickly in a simple manner. The risk involves the continued use of the peroxide solution for an extended period of time. Research indicates that using peroxide to bleach teeth is safe. There is new research indicating the safety for use on the soft tissues (gingiva, cheek, tongue, throat). The long-term effects are as yet unknown. Although the extent of the risk is unknown, acceptance of treatment means acceptance or risk.
3   The amount of whitening varies with the individual. Most patients achieve a change within 2–5 weeks. Try not to drink tea, coffee, or red wine or eat berries or curries after treatment for at least 1 month. Please use the toothpaste supplied with the kit to clean your teeth during treatment.
4   It is advisable not to smoke during the course of bleaching treatment, for at least 5–8 weeks.
5   Sensitivity may result after a few days. This is usually slight and temporary. If this should occur, refrain from using the bleaching treatment for 3–4 days or apply desensitizing toothpaste or the proprietary desensitizing agent/fluoride gel to the tray and then wear overnight.
6   Do not use the bleaching treatment if you are pregnant. There have been no adverse reactions, but long-term clinical effects are unknown.
7   Wear the tray overnight (or according to the manufacturer's instructions).
8   After the desired amount of tooth whitening has been achieved, you will be requested to return the bleaching trays to your dentist. It may be necessary to do a top-up treatment in 18–24 months, depending on the amount of staining.

I have read the above information and agree to return for examination in _____ days after treatment begins and at any recommended time afterwards. I have read and received a copy of this information sheet.

I consent to treatment and assume the risks described above.

I consent to photographs being taken. I understand that they may be used for documentation and for illustration of my treatment.

Signed: _____ (Patient)

Date: _____

INDEX

Page numbers in *italic* refer to figures.

abrasion 6, 42, 229
access cavities *85*, 160, *168*, *170–1*, 174–5
acetone-based adhesives 40, 225
acid etching *155*, 162
acid rinse in OTC kits 33, 260
acne treatment and staining 4
activating/energizing source 133, 161
active sensitivity treatment 97–8
adverse effects *see* side effects
advertisements 251–2
aesthetic dentistry 24, 61, 209
    further demand 95, 250, 251
aesthetics 62, 64, 225–6
ageing discoloration 6, *20*, *55*, *56*
    power bleaching, in-office *216–17*
alcohol-based adhesives 40
alginate impressions 91, *105*, 119–20
alginator machines 119
allergies 41, 62, 90, *102*
amalgam restorations
    effects of bleaching materials 41, *59*, *187–8*
    and staining 5, *18–19*
amelogenesis imperfecta 2, *11*
American Dental Association 28, 247
    Council on Scientific Affairs 144
    Council on Therapeutics (1994) 42
    Seal of Approval 247
analgesics in power bleaching 136
antibacterial effect of CPS 41
antibiotic staining 1, 2–3, *23*
    see also minocycline; tetracycline
aprismatic layer, loss of 37
aspirations *see* patients' expectations
assessment of shade *see* shade assessment
assisted bleach technique 136, *151*, *185–6*
attrition 6, *21*

banding of teeth 65, 95
barrier preparation 160, *170*, 173–4, *181*
benefits of bleaching 133, 250–1
beverage staining 7, 8, 233, 234
    before and after bleaching *22* , *109*, *112*, *114*
    power bleaching, in-office *148–9*, *216–17*
    reducing occurrence 90

bleaching 24–30, *114*, *146*, 193, 260
    daytime/overnight 93
    uneven 259–60
    in vitro experiments *49*, *52–3*
bleaching logs, patients' 92, 93, *102*
bleaching materials 31–60, 92, 133
    effects of 37–8, 40–1
bleaching potential 36
bleaching time, length of 39
bleaching trays 25, *51*, 91, *198*, 247, 258
    with dentures *128*
    design options 116–19, *192*
    equipment and method 119–21, 229
    fabrication and use 118, 119, *123–31*, *199*
        incorrect *108*, *129*
    and inside/outside bleaching 174
    intolerance to 134
    materials 118, 119, 120–1, *129*
    in power bleaching 136
    properties, ideal 116
    with reservoirs 116–18, *124–6*, *130*
    return of 94–5, 260
    seating *82*, 92–3, *106*, *199*
    wearing times 36, 93, 259
bonding 224
    post-bleach 37, 40, 139, 162, 225
brightness 38
Brite Smile 33
bruxing habit 95, 119
burns *see* tissue damage

calcium loss with CPS 37
cancer risk 244–5
carbamide peroxide 38, 41, 133, 206
    in bleaching gel 31
    safety issues 244–5, 246–7
carbamide peroxide solution (CPS) 25, 34, 41–2,
        247
    adverse effects 245–6, 247
    vs. hydrogen peroxide 34–5
    movement through teeth 35, *51*
Carbopol (carboxypolymethylene) 32
caries *see* dental caries
case reports
    bleaching and composite restorations 229–34
    dual-activated/in office bleaching 139

casting 120, 121
   see also alginate impressions
catalase and H_2O_2 162, 175
CE (Communite European) Safety Mark 29, 255–6, 257,
   258
cement barriers 160, *170, 181, 183–4*
cements, luting 41
cervical resorption 25, 38, 174, 175, 176
'chameleon effect' 208
chemical burns *see* tissue damage
chemical composition of enamel 37
chemical discoloration 7
chewing gum with CPS 41
chlorhexidine 7, *23, 78*, 229
chlorine 24
chromogens 7, 8
classification
   of H_2O_2 dental products 28
   of tetracycline staining 3, *12–14*
   of tooth discoloration 1–2, 8, *11*
clinical evaluations 35–6, 44
clinical examination of teeth 90–1, *152*
   for microabrasion technique 195
   see also under examinations
closed chamber technique 176
closed mouth techniques 91
Coastal Dental Study Group 28
coffee staining *see* beverage staining
colorimeters 137
colour 1–2, *11*
   change
      amalgams 41
      monitoring 28, 95
      rate 36, 38
      stabilization 43, 176
   classification 1–2
   components of 68
   map 226, 230, *236*
   regression 24, 39, 135, 139, 207
   see also shade
colour interference 67, 225
combination walking bleach technique 25, 26
combining bleaching techniques 173–92, *183*, 228
   at-home and in-office 132
   with composite resin restorations 224–43
   with microabrasion 173, 177
   power and home bleaching 27, 177
   with restorative dentistry 205–23
communication *see* discussion
compliance 62, 177
   in combined treatment 228
   in power bleaching 132, 134
   reviews, bleaching 175
   and tetracycline stain treatment 95–6
components of smile 62, 64, *75*
composite curing light 139, *154, 155, 157*
   maintenance of 228

composite restorations *12, 77, 236, 238*
   and bleaching 40, 224–43, *241, 242, 243*
   new, in lighter shade 65, 91
   and staining *20*
   unsuitable for bleaching *57*
compressive bleaching technique 136–7, *146*
consent forms 66, 92, 161, 261
conservative dentistry 205, 224, 231
Consumer Protection Act 255
contact points 227
contours/recontouring 207, 228, 230, 233
costs
   of combined techniques 177, 178, 207
   composite restorations 224, 226
   factors affecting fees 68–9
   fee planning 69
   home bleaching 88
   in-office techniques 132, 134
   of lasers 141
   of microabrasion 195
   quoting fees per arch 66, 69
   re-treatment 95, 135
   see also payment; revenue
counselling 38
cracks, surface 89, 91, 208, 233
crowns, teeth prepared for *249*

darkening of teeth 134, 144
deaths from H_2O_2 ingestion 244
degradation of peroxides 31, *54*, 133
dental caries 5, *17, 204*
dental health evaluation 61
dental history of new patient 62
dental procedures and discoloration 5–6, *17*
dental work and CPS 41
dentifrice 33
dentine 1, 97, *111*
   defects 2, 5, *11*
   deposition 6, *80*, 226
   effects of bleaching materials 37–8
dentine, artificial 230, 231, *240*
dentinogenesis imperfecta 2, *11*
Department of Health 28, 255, 256
Department of Trade and Industry 28, 255, 256
dessication of teeth 33, 133
diagnostic wax-up 65, 207
diastema closure *84*, 226–7, 232, 233, *236, 237*
direct resin veneer and reshaping 225–6
discoloration 2, 8, *11–23*
   aetiology 1, 9, 62
   ageing 6, *20, 55, 56, 216–17*
   artificial, in vitro *49, 52–3*
   bleaching agent selection 92
   causes and colours 4, 143
   chemical 7
   dental procedures 5–6, *17*
   enamel changes 6

erosion and 6, *21*
illness and 3
metals 7
minocycline 3–4, *150*
multiple causes 96, 178, *185*, *192*, *222–3*
oral hygiene and 7, *22*, *23*
pulp necrosis 4–5
rebound 134, 176
reparative dentine 6
salivary changes 6
smoking *21*, *109*
tannins and 7
trauma and 3, *84*
see also staining
discoloration questionnaire 90
discomfort/pain, post-treatment 136, 141
discussion with patients 61–2, 93, 251
    of benefits of bleaching 250–1
    of treatment planning 66, *82*, 159, 161
disease and pre-eruptive staining 1
Drufomat-TE 120
dual-activated bleaching system 133, 139
dual-activated in-office technique 137–9
dysmineralizations *see* mineralizations, abnormal
dysmorphophobic patients 252

EC Cosmetics Directives 255, 256
electrode, radiosurgery 133
enamel 1, 34, *58*, *59*
    changes 6
    defects, developmental 2, 197
    effects of bleaching materials 37
    effects of microabrasion 195
    thickness 1, 65, 196
'enamel glaze' effect 195
enamel resistance and microabrasion 197
endodontic materials 5, *18*, *19*
endodontic treatments 4, 137, 161–2
energizing/activating source 133, 161
enzymes in toothpastes 43
erosion *57*, *77*
    by acid rinses 33
    with CPS 37
    and discoloration 6, *21*
    with OTC bleaching kits 34, *50*, *56*
ethanol 225, 229
ethyl vinyl acetate (Eva) 120
eugenol staining 5
European Community *see* EC
examinations, intraoral 65, *73*, *78*, 90–1, 224
    see also clinical examination of teeth
existing restorations 65, *153*, *214–15*
expectations *see* patients' expectations
extrinsic staining 1, 2, 4, 8, 62

finances/fees *see* costs; payment; revenue
flavourings in bleaching gel 33

fluoride application 37, 196–7
    and bond strength 40
    for sensitivity 98, *111*
fluorosis 2, *12*, 39, *114*
    combined bleaching techniques 177–8
    and early bleaching 26, 27
    and laser-assisted bleaching 141
Food and Drug Administration (FDA) 28, 141
food staining 7, *23*, 90

gagging 119, 134
gels, bleaching 31–3, 133
gingival health/disease 65, *114*, 119, 208
gingival irritation 97, 98, *108*, 118
gingival margin immaturity *84*
gingival scaffold 64, *76*, *77*, *147*
gingival ulceration 96
glass ionomers *166*
    cement barriers *170*, *181*, *183–4*
    and CPS 41
Gly-Oxide 25, 27, 42
glycerine vehicle 33, 41
Gnathastone 120
golden proportions *75*, *78*, 226–7
    gauge 64, *78*

H_2O_2 *see* hydrogen peroxide
haemorrhage, intrapulpal 4, *16*
haemosiderin staining 176
halogen curing light 29
hardness of teeth 246
heat
    and Hi-Lite bleach 139
    and non-vital bleaching 162
    and resorption 245–6
    sources 133–4, 140
Hi-Lite bleach 137, 138, 139, 143, 144
history of bleaching 24–30
home bleaching 39, 66, 88–114, 232, 233
    advanced cases/problems 91, 95–9
    advantages/disadvantages 88–9
    after microabrasion *200*
    agents for 36
    alternatives to 89
    and diastemma closure *110*
    history of 25, 26, 28–9
    indications/contraindications 89, 260
    inside-outside technique 174
    instruction and consent form 259–61
    and microabrasion technique 197
    of multiple problem teeth *114*
    of naturally yellow teeth *113*, *199*
    patient response to 38–9
    and power bleaching 27, 177
    protocol 90–5
    with restoration *109*, *241*, *242*, *243*
home bleaching trays *see* bleaching trays

hybrid composites 226, 228
hydrochloric acid 26, 27, 194–5
hydrogen peroxide 31, 32, 34
    vs. CPS 34–5
    high concentrations 132, 133, 245–6
    history of bleaching 24, 25, 26, 27
    pulp penetration 38
    safety issues *147*, 244, 245
    toothpastes 43
hydrogen peroxide strip system 33–4
Hydroxylite 32
hypercalcification, dentine 5, *16*
hypocalcification, enamel 2, *12*, *236*
hypoplasias 2, *12*, *16*, 197, *204*

illness and pre-eruptive discoloration 3
impressions, alginate 91, *105*, 119–20
in-office techniques 132–58
    dual-activated 137–9
indicator dye 132, 137, 139, *154*, *157*
information as marketing 250
information, patient 258, 259–61
informed consent forms 66, 92, 161, 261
inside-outside bleaching technique 25, 27, *85–7*,
        173–6
    combination methods *181–8*, *187–8*
    and pulp necrosis 4
    and restorative dentistry *222–3*
    tooth coss-sections *180*
instructions 92, 228, 259–61
intermediate restorative material 41, *59*
internal bleaching 25, 38, *103*
intracoronal bleaching 25, 159–72, *166*, *170–1*
    after cleft palate repair *221*
    effects 162, *165*
    indications/contraindications 159, *172*
    preparation *167*, *168*, *239*
    and pulp necrosis 4
intrinsic staining 1, 2, 4, *249*
ion exchange binding mechanism 8
irritation
    gingival 97, 98, *108*, 118
    soft tissue 97, 136

Kaffir D stone 120
Klusmier, Dr W 25, 26, 28

Labarraque's solution 24, 26
laser activated bleaching 29, 141
laser bleaching technique 27, 140–2, 144
laser types 141
laxative effect of CPS 41
leaking restorations 5–6, 40
legal considerations 255
light activated bleaching 29, *191*
light and Hi-Lite bleach 138–9
light and tetracycline staining 3

light curing of composite 228
lightening, degree of 66
lightness 38
lights
    bleaching lamps 29
    composite curing 139, *154*, *155*, *157*, 228
    halogen curing 29
    plasma arc 27, 29, 135
    xenon power arc 29
lip framework 64, *76–7*
longevity of CPS results 247

macroabrasion 207–8
Maillard reaction 8, *17*
maintenance 95, 144, 176, 206, 228–9
marginal defects, repair of 206
marketing 250–4
matrix bleaching 88
mechanisms of action
    bleaching induced damage 162
    bleaching materials 34–5
    power bleaching 135
    tetracycline stain bleaching 96
medical devices, bleaches as 29
Medical Devices Directive 255, 257–8
medical history of new patients 62
medication and pre-eruptive staining 1
medications, current 62
megabrasion 207–8
mercury release 41
metal staining 7
metallic/non-metalic stains 8
metamerism 67
methacrylate staining with CPS 40, 41
Micro Clean Kit 194
microabrasion technique *16*, 27, 193–204, *198*, *220*
    adjunctive treatment 197
    in combination 173, 177, 197, *200*
    hydrochloric acid 194, 196
    indications/contraindications 194, *204*
microfill composites 226, 228
Microstone 120
mineralizations, abnormal *198*
    and microabrasion 193, *201–2*, *203*
minocycline discoloration 3–4, *150*
model casting and trimming 120
morphology changes 205
motivation, patient 173, 209, 252
mouthguard 88, 258
mouthwashes *23*, 25, *78*
multiple discolorations 96, 178, *185*, *192*
mutagenicity 244–5

Nathoo stain classification 8, *11*
Natural Elegance 43
Nightguard Vital Bleaching 25, 27, 28, *51*, 88
    clinical evaluations 36

as medical device 258
  safety issues 244, 245–6
Nite White 35
non-scalloped trays 118, *126*, *131*
non-vital bleaching 162–3, 230
  history of 24, 25, 26, 27
  intracoronal 159–72
  options 162, 176
  tissue protection in 159, 161, 162
non-vital teeth 90, 173
Nu-Smile 33

obturation, endodontic 162
odontoblast damage 140
odontogenesis *see* pre-eruption
Opalescence 29, 32, *55*, 229, 232
  clinical evaluations 35, 36
  legal case surrounding 255–8
  and Medical Devices Directive 257–8
  in vitro experiments *53*, *54*
Opalescence Quick 31
Opalescence Xtra *152*
Opalustre 194, *201–2*
oral health/disease 61, 208
oral hygiene 7, *22*, 23
oral prophylaxis *23*, 92, *153*
orthodontic consultation 228
orthodontic treatment *78–9*
  with bleaching *201*, 208–9, *219–20*
over-the-counter (OTC) bleaching kits 27, 33
  safety concerns over 28, *50*, *56*
overbleached teeth 68, 225
overnight bleaching 93, 247
oxidising agents in early bleaching 24
oxygen release with Carbopol 32

pain/discomfort, post-treatment 136, 141
pain fibres 97
parafunctional changes and staining 6, *21*
passive sensitivity treatment 97, 98
patient evaluation/selection 38, 137–8, 196
patient information 258, 259–61
patient review 93–5, 162, 174, 175, 176
patients' expectations 61, 66, 137, 196, 252
patients, new 61–2, 250
patients' responses 38–9, 138
payment for extended bleaching 96
pellicle, surface *22*, 42–3
  chemical removal of 43
periodontal disease 208
periodontal treatment with bleaching *189*, 208,
  218
peroxides
  ADA guidelines on 247
  in toothpastes 43
  see also carbamide peroxide; hydrogen peroxide;
    pyrozone

pH
  of acid rinses 33
  and composite restorations 229
  of OTC bleaches 37
  of sodium perborate preparations 160
  and urea 32
phosphoric acid etching 197
photographing teeth 67
photographs, before and after 91, 93, 251–2
pigment dispersants in bleaching gel 33
pigments oxidised by H_2O_2 34
pins and posts causing staining 6
pitting of enamel 37
placement of reservoir 118
planning *see* treatment planning
plaque discoloration 7, *22*
plasma arc light 27, 29, 135
'polishing cream' 33
polychromatic nature of teeth 1
polyphenols and staining 7
Polyx 32
porcelain restorations 41, 206
porcelain veneers *50*, *56*, 206–7
post-treatment follow-up 28
potassium nitrate 98
power bleaching 27, 29, 132–58, *153*, *191*
  advantages/disadvantages 134–5, *147*
  in combination 173
  equipment/materials 133–4, *154*
  indications 134
  prior to home bleaching 92, *150*, *190*
  procedure 135–6, *148–9*
  side effects 41–2, 135, *147*, *151*
  using heat 140
pre-eruption stains 1, 2–3
Prema kit 194, *198*
preservatives in bleaching gel 33
press-down machine 120
Prevident 500 Plus 98
procedures
  bleaching and composite restorations 229–30, 232,
    233–4
  dual-activated technique 138–9
  inside-outside technique 173–5
  laser bleaching technique 141–2
  microabrasion technique 195–7
  power bleaching, in-office 135–6
prophylaxis, oral *23*, 92, *153*
prophylaxis toothpastes 43
proportions, golden 226–7
protective wear 134, 138, *148*, *153*, *190*, 196
Proxigel 25
pulp
  chamber 25
  damage to 140
  effects of bleaching materials 38
  necrosis 4–5, 143

pulp *contd*
  penetration 37
  remnants 5, *182*
  tester, electric *80*
  transient sensitivity of 35
pumice 43
pyrozone (ether peroxide) 24, 25, 26

questionnaires 62, *71*, 90
  for new patients 61, *72*, 250
Quick-Start 31, 136

radiographic analysis *81*, *103*, *165*
  pre-treatment 65, *80*, *239*
re-bleaching/re-whitening 39, 95, 260
rebound discoloration 134, 176
recalling of patients 94–5
record sheet, bleaching 92, *101*
regression, colour 24, 39, 135, 139, 207
rehydration 134
Rembrandt Lighten *52–3*
remineralization 37, 197, 206
reservoirs, bleaching tray 116–18, *199*
reshaping and direct resin veneer 225–6
residual oxygen and bond strength 40
resin, block-out 120, *123*, *128*, *129*
resin tags 40, 225
resorption 38, *103*, 245–6
  cervical 25, 38, 174, 175, 176
restorations
  assessment of 159
  damage to 162
  defective 206, 207
  existing 65, *77*, *78*, 260
  proportions 227
  replacement *103*, 138
  shade matching post-bleach 206
restorative dentistry *57*, 206
  bleaching, integrated with 205–23
  effects of bleaching materials 40–1
  extensive/complex 208, *212–13*
  inside-outside technique and *222–3*
  tooth replacement 210–13, *214–15*
retractors, lip and cheek 136, *148*, 230
revenue implications of bleaching 251, 252
reviews, bleaching 93–5, 162, 174, 175, 176
root resorption, external 38, 162
rubber dam 31, *153*, *155*, *156*

safer non-vital bleaching 162–3
safety 244–9, 260
  carbamide peroxide 244–5, 246–7
  guidelines for tooth bleaching agents 28
  hydrogen peroxide *147*, 244, 245
  and laser-assisted bleaching 144
  Nightguard Vital Bleaching 244, 245–6
  OTC kits 28, *50*, *56*

of peroxide-containing toothpastes 43
  and power bleaching 134
saliva 32, 39, 195
salivary changes and discoloration 6
scalloped trays 118, *123–31*, *199*
schedule, bleaching 94
sealant, surface penetrating 228
seating of bleaching tray 92–3
selection of shade *see* shade selection
sensitivity 90, 97–8, 142, 259
  bleach dose and frequecy 36, 38
    CPS 246
    hydrogen peroxide 43
  and dessication 133
  and home bleaching 89
  in power bleaching 29, 135, 140
  and tetracycline stain treatment 96
  and tray type 97, 119
sensitivity treatment 97–8, *111*
sequence of treatment 177, 205
shade *11*, 64
  assessment 67–8, *81–2*, *86*, 91
    for inside-outside technique 174
    pre-restoration 224–5
    restorations 159, 161
  relapse 39
  selection 67–8, *107*, 208
    in multiple discoloration *222–3*
    of restorations after bleaching 230–1
  stabilization 43, 176, 205
  value 68
  see also colour
shade guides, proprietary 67, *104*, 137, 206
shade matching/maintenance 206
shade tabs in photographs 67
shelf-life of H_2O_2 133, 135
shortened trays 119, *126*
side effects 28, 66, 93, 96–7
  bleaching agents 35, *147*
  glycerine vehicle 33
  intracoronal bleaching 162
  power bleaching 41–2, 135, *147*, *151*
  tetracycline stain treatment 96
silver restorative materials 5
single discolored tooth *84*, 143–4, *158*, *183*
smile analysis/evaluation 62, 64, *75–7*, 207
  and tetracycline staining 142
smile analysis sheets 62, *74*, 252
smile components 62, 64, *75*
smoking *56*, 233, 234, 260
  and CPS 42
  discoloration of teeth 7, 8, *21*, *109*
  treatment planning and 62, 90
Snapstone 120
sodium bicarbonate 43
sodium dioxide 24
sodium lauryl sulphate 43

sodium perborate 25, 26, 160
Sof-Tray material 119, 120
soft tissue damage 31, 247
soft tissue irritation 97, 136
    minimised with scalloped trays 118
soft tissue protection 31, 135, 138
solvents for sealer dissolution 160
spacers 229
    see also reservoirs
staining
    of composite restorations 229
    endodontic materials and 5, *18*, *19*
    extrinsic 2, 4, 8, 62
    functional changes and 6
    intrinsic 1, 2, 4, *249*
    leaking restorations 5–6
    parafunctional changes and 6, *21*
    see also specific staining agents
stains
    after odontogenesis 3–9
    classification 8, *11*
    during odontogenesis 2–3
    response to bleaching 39
stannous fluoride 2, 8
subjectivity of aesthetics 61
success rates 39, 66–7, 88
superoxyl 24, 26
surfactant in bleaching gel 33
swimmers' calculus 7

tannins and posteruptive discoloration 7
taste sensation, altered 97
tea staining *see* beverage staining
temperature activated bleaching 29
temperature and intracoronal bleaching 161
temporomandibular joint dysfunction *130*, 232
    and tray thickness 119
tetracycline staining *23*, 142–3, *155*, *249*
    bleaching 27, 39, 95–6, *111*, *156*, 173
        planning of treatment 69
    classification 3, *12–14*
    and combination bleaching *183*
    on extracted teeth *15*
    home bleaching *14*, *106*, *107*, *110*
    and intracoronal bleaching 161, 246–7
    and laser-assisted bleaching 141
    power bleaching 142–3
    pre-bleaching assessment 65
    in pre-eruptive teeth 2–3
thermo/photo bleaching procedure 161
thermocatalytic technique 25, 26, *171*
thickening agents in bleaching gel 32
thickness, enamel 1, 65, 196
3D Master Shade System 68
timing of inside-outside technique 174
tissue damage 134, *147*, 162, 247

tissue irritation 97, 136
    minimised with scalloped trays 118
tissue protection 31
    dual-activated technique 138
    laser bleaching technique 141
    in microabrasion 196
    in non-vital bleaching 159, 161, 162
    in power bleaching 133, 135, 142, *147*
titanium dioxide 33, 43
titrating bleaching treatment *190*
tobacco/nicotine staining 7, 8
tooth, areas of *11*
toothpastes, whitening 42–4
'touch-up' bleaching of composites 229
toxicity 244–5
transillumination 137, *152*
translucency of enamel 1, *11*
    decrease with bleaching 38
    measurement 91
    pre-bleaching assessment 65
translucent restorations 208
trauma and discoloration 3, *84*
tray-forming machine, vacuum 121, *124*
trays, bleaching *see* bleaching trays
treatment 66
    further 95
    planning 61–87, *82*, *84*, 91
        complex 173, 178
        discussion of 66, *82*, 93, 159, 161
        microabrasion technique 196
        restorative dentistry 205
        smoking and 62, 90
    of sensitivity 98–9
    times/timing 35–6, 142, 174, 196
Triad 2000 light box 120
trolamine 32

urea 31, 32–3, 244

veneered teeth 207
veneers, direct composite 226, *243*, *249*
viscosity of Carbopol 32
Vita Shade Guide 68, 91, *104*, 229
vital bleaching technique *55*, *56*, 229
vital teeth 24, 26, 27
vitality testing 4, 65, *80*, 90, 144, 232

waiting room bleach technique 136
walking bleach procedure 25, 26, 159–60, *166*, *169*
wear problem in teeth 42, *57*, *237*
White & Brite 27
whiteness 38
width-to-length ratio 227, 233, *237*
windows, trays with 119, *126*, *131*

xenon power arc light 29